Cardiac Imaging
A Core Review

Browse the other titles in our Core Review Series at your local Wolters Kluwer website or bookseller.

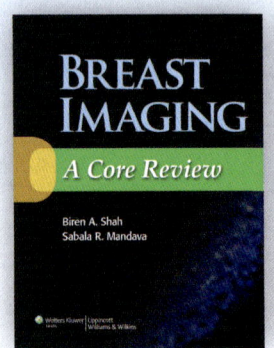 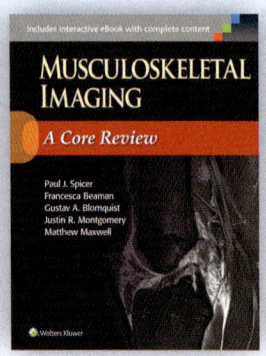 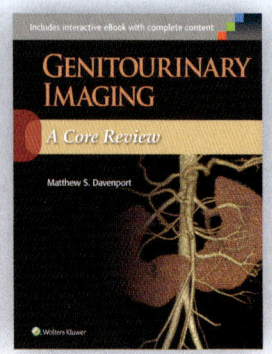 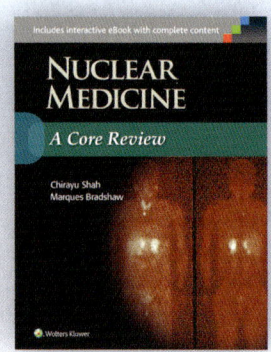 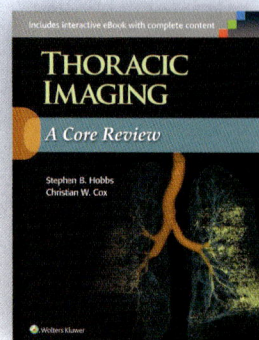

Breast Imaging: A Core Review
Biren A. Shah • Sabala R. Mandava
ISBN: 978-1-4511-7639-1

Musculoskeletal Imaging: A Core Review
Paul J. Spicer • Francesca Beaman
Gustav A. Blomquist
Justin R. Montgomery
Matthew Maxwell
ISBN: 978-1-4511-9267-4

Genitourinary Imaging: A Core Review
Matthew S. Davenport
ISBN: 978-1-4511-9407-4

Nuclear Medicine: A Core Review
Chirayu Shah • Marques Bradshaw
ISBN: 978-1-4963-0062-1

Thoracic Imaging: A Core Review
Stephen Hobbs • Christian Cox
ISBN: 978-1-4698-9883-4

Gastrointestinal Imaging: A Core Review
Wendy Hsu • Felicia Cummings
ISBN: 978-1-4963-0718-7
Publishing in 2016

Radiology Physics and Safety: A Core Review
Kenneth Lewis • Tianling Gu
Jerome Jones
ISBN: 978-1-4963-1884-8
Publishing in 2016

Vascular Interventional Radiology: A Core Review
Kevin Stadtlander • Daniel Siragusa
ISBN: 978-1-4963-0721-7
Publishing in 2017

Ultrasound: A Core Review
Ruchi Shrestha • Ka-Kei Ngan
ISBN: 978-1-4963-0981-5
Publishing in 2017

Pediatric Imaging: A Core Review
Steven Blumer • Gerald Behr
David Biko
ISBN: 978-1-4963-0980-8
Publishing in 2017

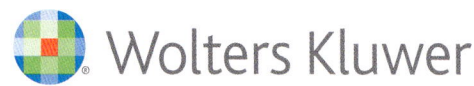

Cardiac Imaging
A Core Review

EDITORS

Joe Y. Hsu, MD
Director of Cardiac CT/MR
Kaiser Permanente Los Angeles Medical Center
Los Angeles, California

Amar Shah, MD
Assistant Professor
New York Medical College
Valhalla, New York

Jean Jeudy, MD
Associate Professor
University of Maryland School of Medicine
Cardiothoracic Imaging
Department of Diagnostic Radiology and Nuclear Medicine
University of Maryland Medical Center
Baltimore, Maryland

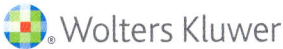

Wolters Kluwer

Philadelphia · Baltimore · New York · London
Buenos Aires · Hong Kong · Sydney · Tokyo

Acquisitions Editor: Ryan Shaw
Product Development Editor: Lauren Pecarich
Production Project Manager: Priscilla Crater
Senior Manufacturing Coordinator: Beth Welsh
Design Coordinator: Elaine Kasmer
Prepress Vendor: SPi Global

Copyright © 2016 by Wolters Kluwer

All rights reserved. This book is protected by copyright. No part of this book may be reproduced or transmitted in any form or by any means, including as photocopies or scanned-in or other electronic copies, or utilized by any information storage and retrieval system without written permission from the copyright owner, except for brief quotations embodied in critical articles and reviews. Materials appearing in this book prepared by individuals as part of their official duties as U.S. government employees are not covered by the above-mentioned copyright. To request permission, please contact Wolters Kluwer at Two Commerce Square, 2001 Market Street, Philadelphia, PA 19103, via email at permissions@lww.com, or via our website at lww.com (products and services).

10 9 8 7 6 5 4 3 2 1

Printed in China

Library of Congress Cataloging-in-Publication Data
Cardiac imaging (Hsu)
  Cardiac imaging : a core review / editors, Joe Y. Hsu, Amar Shah, Jean Jeudy.
    p. ; cm. — (Core review series)
  Includes index.
  ISBN 978-1-4963-0061-4 (pbk)
  I. Hsu, Joe Y., editor. II. Shah, Amar, editor. III. Jeudy, Jean, editor. IV. Title. V. Series: Core review series.
  [DNLM: 1. Cardiac Imaging Techniques—methods—Problems and Exercises. 2. Cardiovascular Diseases—Problems and Exercises. 3. Diagnostic Techniques, Cardiovascular—Problems and Exercises. WG 18.2]
  RC683.5.R33
  616.1'207540076—dc23
                                                                              2015028031

This work is provided "as is," and the publisher disclaims any and all warranties, express or implied, including any warranties as to accuracy, comprehensiveness, or currency of the content of this work.

This work is no substitute for individual patient assessment based upon healthcare professionals' examination of each patient and consideration of, among other things, age, weight, gender, current or prior medical conditions, medication history, laboratory data and other factors unique to the patient. The publisher does not provide medical advice or guidance and this work is merely a reference tool. Healthcare professionals, and not the publisher, are solely responsible for the use of this work including all medical judgments and for any resulting diagnosis and treatments.

Given continuous, rapid advances in medical science and health information, independent professional verification of medical diagnoses, indications, appropriate pharmaceutical selections and dosages, and treatment options should be made and healthcare professionals should consult a variety of sources. When prescribing medication, healthcare professionals are advised to consult the product information sheet (the manufacturer's package insert) accompanying each drug to verify, among other things, conditions of use, warnings and side effects and identify any changes in dosage schedule or contraindications, particularly if the medication to be administered is new, infrequently used or has a narrow therapeutic range. To the maximum extent permitted under applicable law, no responsibility is assumed by the publisher for any injury and/or damage to persons or property, as a matter of products liability, negligence law or otherwise, or from any reference to or use by any person of this work.

LWW.com

To my wife Jennifer—You are the source of my inspiration! Thanks for your unwavering support.

To my children James, Katherine, and Kira—Your smile and laughter give me the reason to keep trying.

To my teachers—"If I have seen further it is by standing on the shoulders of giants."

To my residents—Thanks for challenging me to be better.

—Joe Y. Hsu

To my wife, I can not thank you enough for all that you say and do.

To the late Pragna Shah, thank you for everything you have done.

To my mentors and residents, thank you for everything you have done and continue to do to help me learn.

—Amar Shah

Thank you to so many…

To my beautiful wife and daughters for their love and support (and I love you just as deeply).

To my mentors for their inspiration; and to all my residents and fellows who have allowed me to inspire them.

—Jean Jeudy

CONTRIBUTORS

John P. Fantauzzi, MD
Assistant Professor
Department of Radiology
Albany Medical College/Albany Medical Center Hospital
Albany, New York

Ami Gokli, MD
Staten Island University Hospital
Staten Island, New York

Nikhil Goyal, MD
Section Chief, Cardiac Imaging
Department of Radiology
Staten Island University Hospital
Staten Island, New York

SERIES FOREWORD

Cardiac Imaging: A Core Review is the fifth book added to the *Core Review Series*. This book covers the most important aspects of cardiac imaging in a manner that I am confident will serve as a useful guide for residents to assess their knowledge and review the material in a question-style format that is similar to the ABR Core examination.

Dr. Joe Hsu, Dr. Amar Shah, and Dr. Jean Jeudy have succeeded in producing a book that exemplifies the philosophy and goals of the *Core Review Series*. They have done an excellent job in covering key topics and providing quality images on a subject matter that many residents find most challenging. The multiple-choice questions have been divided logically into chapters so as to make it easy for learners to work on particular topics as needed. Each question has a corresponding answer with an explanation of not only why a particular option is correct but also why the other options are incorrect. There are also references provided for each question for those who want to delve more deeply into a specific subject. This format is also useful for radiologists preparing for the Maintenance of Certification (MOC).

The intent of the *Core Review Series* is to provide the resident, fellow, or practicing physician a review of the important conceptual, factual, and practical aspects of a subject by providing approximately 300 multiple-choice questions, in a format similar to the ABR Core examination. The *Core Review Series* is not intended to be exhaustive but to provide material likely to be tested on the ABR Core examination, and that would be required in clinical practice.

As the Series Editor of the *Core Review Series*, I have had the pleasure to work with many outstanding individuals across the country who contributed to the series. This series represents countless hours of work and involvement by many, and it would not have come together without their participation.

Dr. Joe Hsu, Dr. Amar Shah, Dr. Jean Jeudy, and their contributors are to be congratulated on doing an outstanding job. As like the other books in the *Core Review Series*, I believe *Cardiac Imaging: A Core Review* will serve as an excellent resource for residents during their board preparation and a valuable reference for fellows and practicing radiologists.

Biren A. Shah, MD, FACR
Series Editor

PREFACE

The new American Board of Radiology (ABR) core examination is an all-encompassing core exam, which challenges residents to prove their comprehensive knowledge across the entire specialty. The transition to this new format introduces image-rich, computer-based presentations requiring knowledge of anatomy, pathophysiology, and principles of radiological physics. As opposed to the "fact-based" focus of the previous written examination, there is now a greater emphasis on higher level comprehension of subject matter including synthesis of information, differential diagnosis, and management decisions.

Despite this historic change, the availability of quality review material is still lacking. Our goal with this book is to provide a refined source of material that reflects the level of comprehensive information that residents will encounter on the core examination. The questions provided in this book are grouped into key subtopics in cardiac imaging. Many cases are image based, and a subset offers higher-order questions where the user must commit to an answer before advancing to the following associated question.

The curation of exam questions is an arduous process. Study material must be reviewed for clarity and accuracy. References must be relevant and reflect current clinical understanding and practices. In organizing our content, we have strived to provide the best in quality on the topic. The psychometric integrity of the questions in this book reflects the same standards of the ABR, ensuring residents will have quality questions to study from.

We hope that this book serves not only as a key resource for the initial qualifying exam but also as a practical guide preparing for the ABR's Certifying exam and Maintenance of Certification (MOC) exam.

Thank you to the many individuals who without their contributions and support, this book would not have been written. Additionally, we extend tremendous thanks to the staff at Lippincott Williams & Wilkins for providing this opportunity and beneficial help along the way. Finally, we are deeply grateful to our families, who have encouraged us through long hours of work and supported us each step along the way.

Joe Y. Hsu, MD
Amar Shah, MD
Jean Jeudy, MD

ACKNOWLEDGMENTS

The authors would like to thank Dr. Biren Shah for his patience and guidance throughout this whole process. We would also like to thank the staff at Lippincott Williams & Wilkins for their commitment and discipline in making this book possible. Finally, we would like to thank the staff at SPi Global for their editorial support.

CONTENTS

Contributors vii
Series Foreword ix
Preface xi
Acknowledgments xiii

1 Basics of Imaging: Radiography, CT, and MR 1

2 Normal Anatomy, Including Variants, Encountered on Radiography, CT, and MR 12

3 Physiologic Aspects of Cardiac Imaging 32

4 Ischemic Heart Disease 50

5 Cardiomyopathy 67

6 Cardiac Masses 97

7 Valvular Disease 120

8 Pericardial Disease 137

9 Congenital Heart Disease 153

10	**Acquired Disease of the Thoracic Aorta and Great Vessels**	**181**
11	**Devices and Postoperative Appearance**	**200**

Index   217

1 Basics of Imaging: Radiography, CT, and MR

QUESTIONS

1. What is the purpose of double-inversion recovery in black blood imaging?
   A. To improve blood pool signal
   B. To suppress fat
   C. To suppress blood flow
   D. To improve temporal resolution

2. With conventional filtered-back projection (FBP), what is the relationship of tube current to noise?
   A. Directly proportional
   B. Inversely proportional
   C. No direct relationship
   D. Exponentially proportional

3. A patient is coming back for a follow-up CT. You looked at a prior CT, and it was very noisy. What parameter can you change on the follow-up CT to reduce the noise by a factor of 2 (assuming filtered-back projection was used)?
   A. Increase the effective mAs by a factor of 2.
   B. Increase the effective mAs by a factor of 4.
   C. Decrease the kVp by 40%.
   D. Decrease the kVp by 20%.

4. Assuming a rotation time of 0.3 seconds and mA of 700, what is the effective tube current-time product if the pitch is 0.2?
   A. 2,100 mA
   B. 1,050 mA
   C. 210 mA
   D. 42 mA

5. In filter-back projection, changing the type of reconstruction algorithm/kernel can affect the spatial resolution and what else?
   A. Radiation dose
   B. Noise of image
   C. Temporal resolution

6. How is dose length product (DLP) related to scan length?
   A. It is not related.
   B. It is directly proportional.
   C. It is inversely proportional.

7. How does one calculate an estimated effective dose in millisieverts?
   A. Multiply the dose length product by a conversion factor.
   B. Divide the dose length product by a conversion factor.
   C. Multiply the CT volume dose index by a conversion factor.
   D. Divide the CT volume dose index by a conversion factor.

8. In a patient with contraindication to beta-blockers, which medication can be given to slow the heart rate?
   A. Atenolol
   B. Nitroglycerin
   C. Verapamil
   D. Sildenafil

9. The image below is from a phase-contrast image in a patient with suspected pulmonic stenosis. Which of the following statements is most accurate about the image?

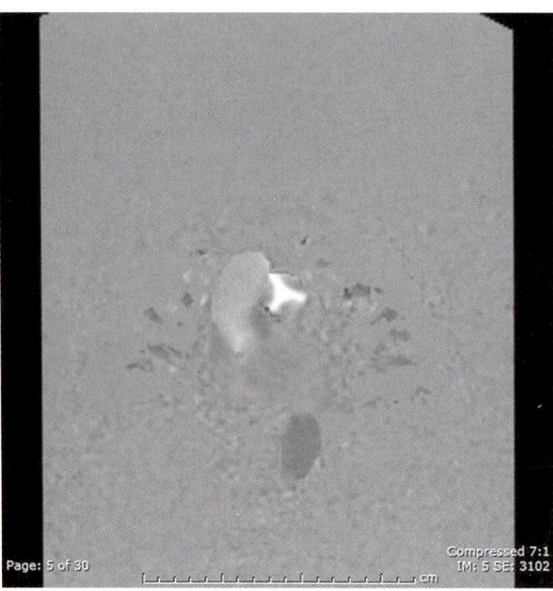

   A. The velocity-encoding gradient was set too low.
   B. The image shows no net phase shift of the blood.
   C. Bipolar gradients were applied to obtain the image.
   D. There is stenosis of flow across the valve.

10. Your department needs a new CT scanner in the emergency department and wants to offer cardiac CTA. A vendor says the single-source scanner has a temporal resolution of 200 msec when using a single-segment reconstruction. If this statement is true, what must the rotation speed of the scanner be?
    A. 200 msec
    B. 300 msec
    C. 400 msec
    D. 500 msec

11 A 55-year-old male with a history of atypical chest pain undergoes a retrospective cardiac CTA at your institution on a 64-slice scanner. As you inject contrast, the heart rate increases to 85 beats per minute during the entire scan acquisition. Your technologist reconstructs the data, and you are still able to interpret the exam. What strategy did your technologist employ?
   A. Use a sharp kernel/filter.
   B. Multi-segment reconstruction.
   C. Increased the pitch during the exam.
   D. Use tube modulation.

12 Your technologist completes a short-axis balanced steady-state free precession cardiac MRI (cMRI) sequence to calculate cardiac function. While scanning the apex of the heart, the technologist notices a mass in the liver with bright signal and asks you if this sequence can confidently characterize the lesion. Your response is which of the following?
   A. Yes, since the sequence is only T2 weighted, the mass is a cyst.
   B. Yes, it is a cyst since the sequence is not susceptible to calcification or metallic artifact.
   C. No, the mass contains calcification, which accounts for its bright signal.
   D. No, although the sequence has relative T2 weighting, it has both T2 and T1 properties.

13 A postprocessing technique that chooses the maximum voxel value in a defined thickness and uses it as the displayed value is called
   A. Curved multiplanar reformatted image
   B. Maximum-intensity projection image
   C. Shaded surface display image
   D. Volume-rendered image

14 A patient undergoes a cardiac CTA. The patient has no coronary artery disease in the vessels; however, while postprocessing the data, your 3D tech makes a pseudolesion in the left anterior descending coronary artery. Which post processing technique did your 3D tech most likely used?
   A. Curved planar reformat
   B. Maximum-intensity projection
   C. Minimal-intensity projection
   D. Volume-rendered

15 A patient arrives for a cardiac MRI to evaluate the mitral valve and aortic valve. Your sequence has a TR of 5 msec and the views per segment is 20. What is the temporal resolution of your scan?
   A. 4 msec
   B. 15 msec
   C. 25 msec
   D. 100 msec

16 A patient who sustained a large LAD myocardial infarction undergoes a cardiac MRI to evaluate for late gadolinium enhancement (LGE) and scar assessment. After contrast is administered, the inversion time is chosen. The 10-minute delayed enhanced image shows the infarcted tissue to be increased in signal relative to the normal myocardium. Which best accounts for the above scenario?
   A. The inversion time is too long.
   B. The inversion time is correct.
   C. The inversion time is too short.

17 Nephrogenic systemic fibrosis (NSF) is a systemic disease that has been associated with gadolinium deposition. What is a clinical feature of the disease?

   A. Facial scarring
   B. Pulmonary fibrosis
   C. Retroperitoneal fibrosis
   D. Skin thickening of the extremities

18 A change in contrast flow rate from 6 mL/s to 4 mL/s would result in which of the following?

   A. Initial increase and then decrease in arterial enhancement
   B. Increase in iodine molecules given per time
   C. No change in arterial enhancement
   D. Reduced iodine flux

19 Which of the below shows the ideal contrast bolus geometry?

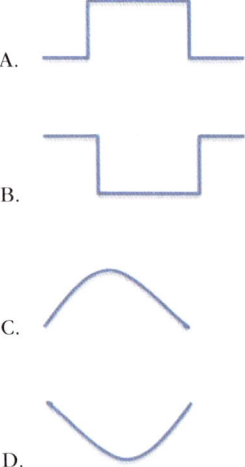

   A.

   B.

   C.

   D.

20 What is the most likely cause of transient interruption of the contrast bolus from an injection in the right antecubital fossa?

   A. Increased flow from the IVC
   B. Increased flow from the SVC
   C. Increased flow from the brachiocephalic vein
   D. Increased flow from the coronary sinus

21 What is the impact on the specific absorption rate (SAR) by a patient undergoing a scan on a 3T scanner compared to a 1.5T scanner assuming flip angle and TR are held constant?

   A. Higher SAR
   B. Lower SAR
   C. No impact on SAR
   D. Mixed impact on SAR

22 Which of the following patterns of pharmacokinetics is characteristic of gadolinium when administered to a patient with normal myocardium?

   A. Intravascular injection—extracellular space
   B. Intravascular injection—extracellular space-intracellular space
   C. Intravascular injection—intracellular space-extracellular space
   D. Intravascular injection—intracellular space

23 Why does gadolinium have paramagnetic properties when placed in a magnetic field?
    A. Excess protons in the nucleus
    B. Unpaired electrons in the outer shell
    C. Uneven number of neutrons
    D. Emission of positrons

24 A patient is undergoing screening by an MRI technologist for cardiac MRI. In which zone does this take place?
    A. Zone 1
    B. Zone 2
    C. Zone 3
    D. Zone 4

25 With balanced steady-state free precession sequences, what is the relationship of longitudinal magnetization (LM) to the transverse magnetization (TM)?
    A. LM = TM
    B. LM > TM
    C. TM < LM

26 How does parallel imaging reduce scan time?
    A. Increase phase-encoding steps
    B. Use of geometry of phased array coils
    C. Modify the field of view

27 A 45-year-old male with a BMI of 27 undergoes a cardiac CTA (CCTA) in the emergency department. What instructions do you give your technologist to reduce radiation exposure?
    A. Scan from the thoracic inlet to diaphragm.
    B. Use a kVp of 100 rather than 120.
    C. Use retrospective gating.
    D. Do calcium scoring.

28 You perform a cardiac CTA (CCTA) using retrospective gating to evaluate cardiac function. In order to minimize dose, you use tube modulation. What best describes the effect of tube modulation?
    A. Changes mAs based on BMI
    B. Changes mAs depending on cardiac cycle
    C. Maintains uniform mAs
    D. Increases mAs with arrhythmia

29 While at the scanner, your technologist increases the number of phase-encoding steps. The increase in phase-encoding steps causes which of the following?
    A. Increase in acquisition time
    B. Imaging a larger field of view
    C. Lower spatial resolution
    D. Smaller voxel size

30 A patient with a history of acute renal insufficiency is referred for a cardiac MRI with and without contrast. You can perform the exam with contrast if the

A. Albumin is normal.
B. GFR exceeds 60 mL/min.
C. Patient is on dialysis.
D. Patient signs a consent.

31 A patient is undergoing a cardiac MRI with a device that is MR conditional. Your new MR technologist states the patient can undergo the exam

A. With a physician in the room
B. With certain scan parameters
C. Without restriction

ANSWERS AND EXPLANATIONS

1. **Answer C.** Double-inversion recovery sequence in black blood cardiac imaging is designed to suppress the signal from blood flow.

   Reference: Ginat DT, Fong MW, Tuttle DJ, et al. Cardiac imaging: part 1, MR pulse sequences, imaging planes, and basic anatomy. *AJR Am J Roentgenol* 2011;197(4):808–815. doi: 10.2214/AJR.10.7231.

2. **Answer B.** With filtered-back projection, tube current is inversely proportional to noise. That is, increasing the mA by factor of 4 will yield half the noise (1/square root of 4). Tube current determines the number of photons generated and noise.

   Reference: Litmanovich DE, Tack DM, Shahrzad M, et al. Dose reduction in cardiothoracic CT: review of currently available methods. *Radiographics* 2014;34(6):1469–1489. doi: 10.1148/rg.346140084.

3. **Answer B.** With filtered-back projection, tube current is inversely proportional to noise. That is, increasing the mA by factor of 4 will yield half the noise (1/square root of 4). Relationship of kVp to noise is complex, but in general, decreasing the kVp will increase the noise if other factors are held constant.

   Reference: Litmanovich DE, Tack DM, Shahrzad M, et al. Dose reduction in cardiothoracic CT: review of currently available methods. *Radiographics* 2014;34(6):1469–1489. doi: 10.1148/rg.346140084.

4. **Answer B.** Effective tube current-time product is obtained by multiplying the rotation time by the mA and then dividing by the pitch. So in this case 0.3 × 700 = 210 mA, which is then divided by 0.2, giving 1,050 mA.

   Reference: Litmanovich DE, Tack DM, Shahrzad M, et al. Dose reduction in cardiothoracic CT: review of currently available methods. *Radiographics* 2014;34(6):1469–1489. doi: 10.1148/rg.346140084.

5. **Answer B.** Reconstruction algorithm/kernel does not affect radiation dose since it is applied after the study is already obtained. It can affect spatial resolution and noise depending on which algorithm/kernel is used.

   Reference: Litmanovich DE, Tack DM, Shahrzad M, et al. Dose reduction in cardiothoracic CT: review of currently available methods. *Radiographics* 2014;34(6):1469–1489. doi: 10.1148/rg.346140084.

6. **Answer B.** DLP is obtained by multiplying the CTDIvol by the scan length; therefore, it is directly proportional.

   Reference: Litmanovich DE, Tack DM, Shahrzad M, et al. Dose reduction in cardiothoracic CT: review of currently available methods. *Radiographics* 2014;34(6):1469–1489. doi: 10.1148/rg.346140084.

7. **Answer A.** Effective dose gives a general population risk rather than patient-specific risk. It is obtained by multiplying the DLP by a conversion factor (f). The conversion factor is obtained by Monte Carlo simulation, and the best estimates (f) factor should be size specific.

   Reference: Litmanovich DE, Tack DM, Shahrzad M, et al. Dose reduction in cardiothoracic CT: review of currently available methods. *Radiographics* 2014;34(6):1469–1489. doi: 10.1148/rg.346140084.

8. **Answer C.** In patients with contraindication to beta-blocker (such as second-degree heart block, severe asthma, decompensated heart failure), a calcium channel blocker can be used. Verapamil is a calcium blocker agent. Atenolol is a beta-blocker so it should not be used if there is contraindication to beta-blocker. Nitroglycerin is used for vasodilatation of the coronaries and will not slow the heart rate. Sildenafil (Viagra) should not be used concurrently with nitroglycerin as it could cause severe hypotension.

   Reference: Taylor CM, Blum A, Abbara S. Patient preparation and scanning techniques. *Radiol Clin North Am* 2010;48(4):675–686. doi: 10.1016/j.rcl.2010.04.011.

9   **Answer C.**   Phase-contrast images are used to measure blood flow and velocity. In cardiac imaging, they are most commonly used to evaluate the peak velocity in cases of valve stenosis and the regurgitant fraction in cases of valve insufficiency. A bipolar gradient is applied, and results in stationary objects experiencing no net phase shift while moving objects will experience a phase shift proportional to their velocity, which yields signal. If the velocity-encoding gradient is set too high or low, aliasing will occur (which is not on the image below).

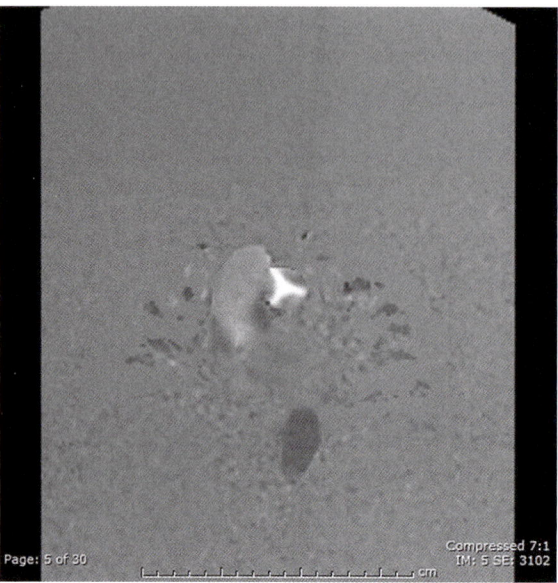

Reference: Lotz J, et al. Cardiovascular flow measurement with phase-contrast MR imaging: basic facts and implementation. *Radiographics* 2002;22(3):651–671.

10 **Answer C.**   With a single-source CT scanner, the image can be generated once 180 degrees of data have been acquired. The temporal resolution is calculated by dividing the rotation speed of the scanner by 2 (Temporal resolution = Rotation speed/2). In our example, 200 msec = Rotation speed/2; 400 msec = Rotation speed.

Reference: Lin E, Alessio A. What are the basic concepts of temporal, contrast, and spatial resolution in cardiac CT. *Cardiovasc Comput Tomogr* 2009;3(6):403–408.

11 **Answer B.**   Patients with an elevated heart rate who undergo retrospective cardiac CTA can have the data analyzed using multisegment reconstruction techniques. When using multisegment reconstruction, the image will be created using data from multiple heart beats. This will produce an image that potentially has better temporal resolution than single segment reconstruction. Multisegment reconstruction requires the study be acquired with a low pitch. The use of multiple heart beats makes this techniques susceptible to motion artifact and heart rate variability.

Reference: Mahesh M, Cody DD. Physics of cardiac imaging with multiple-row detector CT. *Radiographics* 2007;27(5):1495–1509.

12 **Answer D.**   The balanced steady-state free precession sequence is a gradient-echo sequence that is susceptible to metallic artifact and has weighted T2/T1 signal. While the sequence is relatively T2 weighted, it will also have T1 properties.

References: Chavan GB, Babyn PS, Jankharia BG, et al. Steady-state MR imaging sequences: physics, classification, and clinical applications. *Radiographics* 2008;28(4)1147–1160.

Bieri O, Scheffler K. Fundamentals of balanced steady state free precession MRI. *J Magn Reson Imaging* 2013;38:2–11. doi: 10.1002/jmri.24163.

13 Answer B. The maximum-intensity projection image uses the maximum voxel value to create a displayed value. The technique is useful to evaluate vessels; however, if the vessel is densely calcified or if there is metallic material, this technique may obscure the vessel lumen.

Reference: Calhoun PS, Kuszyk BS, Heath DG, et al. Three-dimensional volume rendering of spiral CT data: theory and method. *Radiographics* 1999;19(3):745-764.

14 Answer A. The abnormality most likely occurred on the curved planar-reformatted image. This technique places the long axis of the vessel (i.e., coronary artery) on a single image, allowing it to be visualized along its entire course. It allows stenosis to be readily visualized; however, it is susceptible to pseudolesions from an inability to show the vessel along its true long axis. This can result from unsuccessful vessel extraction, or motion artifact.

Reference: Dalrymple NC, Prasad SR, Freckleton MW, et al. Introduction to the language of three-dimensional imaging with multidetector CT. *Radiographics* 2005;25(5):1409-1428.

15 Answer D. Temporal Resolution = TR × Views per segment
Temporal resolution is determined by how quickly the image is obtained (like shutter speed in a camera). Better temporal resolution is required to visualize fast moving structures such as valve leaflets.

References: Lee VS. *Cardiovascular MRI: Physical principles to practical protocols.* Lippincott Williams & Wilkins, 2006:291.

Slavin GS, Bluemke DA. Spatial and temporal resolution in cardiovascular MR imaging: review and recommendations. *Radiology* 2005;234(2):330-338. doi:10.1148/radiol.2342031990.

16 Answer C. Delayed enhanced images are used to evaluate for myocardial scar formation. If the inversion time is chosen correctly, normal myocardium will be dark (its signal is nulled) and abnormal myocardium will be bright. If the inversion time is too short, the infarcted tissue can be dark and the myocardium bright. If the inversion time is too long, both the myocardium and infarcted tissue will be bright.

Reference: Kim RJ, Shah DJ, Judd RM. How we perform delayed enhanced images. *J Cardiovasc Magn Reson* 2003;5(3):505-514.

17 Answer D. NSF is characterized by thickening and hardening of the skin, which is symmetric and involves the upper and lower extremities. The skin can be nodular and the disease process can involve the trunk; however, the face is usually spared.

Reference: Nainani N, Panesar M. Nephrogenic systemic fibrosis. *Am J Nephrol* 2009;29:1-9 doi:10.1159/000149628.

18 Answer D. The iodine flux is the number of iodine molecules administered per unit time and is related to the flow rate and the iodine concentration of the contrast agent. A higher flow rate will result in more molecules of iodine given per unit time and a greater amount of enhancement. Conversely, a decrease in flow rate will result in fewer molecules of iodine given per unit time and a reduced amount of enhancement.

Reference: Roberto P. *Multidetector-row CT angiography.* Springer Science & Business Media, 2006:44.

19 Answer A. Contrast bolus geometry is defined as the pattern of enhancement measured in a region of interest when looking at Hounsfield units versus time. In CTA, the ideal geometry is immediate and maximal enhancement that persists over time (steady state) of the study and does not change. However, this does not occur in the real world, typically one will get a rise in enhancement, short peak, and subsequent downslope.

Reference: Cademartiri F, van der Lugt A, Luccichenti G, et al. Parameters affecting bolus geometry in CTA: a review. *J Comp Assist Tomogr* 2002;26(4)598-607.

20 Answer A. Transient interruption of the contrast bolus occurs when deep inspiration increases central venous return from the IVC. This results in disruption of bolus and is most commonly witnessed during exams for pulmonary embolism. As a result, the right ventricle and pulmonary artery will experience a decrease in attenuation compared to the SVC and can render the study nondiagnostic.

Reference: Wittram C, Yoo AJ. Transient interruption of contrast on CT pulmonary angiography: proof of mechanism. *J Thoracic Imaging* 2007;22(2):125-129.

21 Answer A. The higher field strength will contribute to a higher overall SAR. SAR is a function of field strength, flip angle, and TR. A doubling of the field strength or flip angle will lead to a 4× increase in the SAR.

Reference: Bitar R, Leung G, Perng R, et al. MR pulse sequences: what every radiologist wants to know but is afraid to ask. *Radiographics* 2006;26(2):513-537.

22 Answer A. When gadolinium is injected, it will be transported via systemic circulation to the myocardium. Upon reaching the myocardium, gadolinium will permeate the extracellular space; however, in healthy myocardium, there is no intracellular uptake. Infarcted myocardium will not be able to prevent gadolinium from crossing the cell membranes, and as a result gadolinium will permeate and remain in the intracellular space.

Reference: Edelman RR. Contrast-enhanced MR Imaging of the heart: overview of the literature. *Radiology* 2004;232(3):653-668.

23 Answer B. Gadolinium has paramagnetic properties due to unpaired outer shell electrons. When in a magnetic field, gadolinium becomes temporarily magnetized. The interaction between the outer shell of electrons and adjacent hydrogen nuclei leads to the T1-shortening properties of gadolinium.

Reference: Biglands JD, Radjenovic A, Ridgway JP. Cardiovascular magnetic resonance physics for clinicians: part II. *J Cardiovasc Magn Reson* 2012;14:66 doi:10.1186/1532-429X-14-66.

24 Answer B. The patient is screened in zone 2. In zone 1, there is no risk and the general public can enter the space. In zone 2, screening takes place. In zone 3, the magnetic field is sufficiently strong and can be hazardous to unscreened patients and personnel (console area). In zone 4, the magnetic field is strongest and all ferromagnetic objects must be excluded.

Reference: Kanal E, Barkovich AJ, Bell C, et al. ACR guidance document on MR safe practices: 2013. *Magn Reson Imaging* 2013;37:501-530.

25 Answer A. On balanced steady state free precession sequence, a steady state is achieved by having the TR lower than the tissue T2 relaxation time. Since the TR is less than T2, there is not enough time for TM to decay before the next RF excitation pulse, resulting in the TM going back into the LM with the next excitation. At the same time, a portion of LM is flipped into the transverse plain.

Reference: Chavan GB, Babyn PS, Jankharia BG, et al. Steady-state MR imaging sequences: physics, classification, and clinical applications. *Radiographics* 2008;28(4):1147-1160.

26 Answer B. Parallel imaging techniques reduce scan time by decreasing the number of phase-encoding steps. Parallel imaging uses multielement receiver coil arrays with a geometric distribution to achieve this. The number of phase-encoding steps can be reduced by a defined factor, and the missing k-space information is filled in by interpolating the data.

Reference: Biglands JD, Radjenovic A, Ridgway JP. Cardiovascular magnetic resonance physics for clinicians: Part II. *J Cardiovasc Magn Reson* 2012;14:66. doi:10.1186/1532-429X-14-66.

27 Answer B. The patient can be scanned with a lower kVp based on the patient's body mass index. The scan length should be decreased (carina to diaphragm) and a lower mAs or auto mAs tool should be used to reduce dose. Retrospective gating will give more radiation than prospective ECG triggering. Doing a calcium score will add radiation from a noncontrast study.

Reference: Budoff M. Maximizing dose reductions with cardiac CT. *Int J Cardiovasc Imaging* 2009;25(Suppl 2):279–287.

28 Answer B. Patients who undergo retrospective gating will be imaged through systole and diastole. Tube modulation minimizes dose during systole but provides enough dose to calculate function and maximizes dose during diastole to evaluate the coronary arteries.

Reference: Mayo JR, Leipsic JA. Radiation does in cardiac CT. *AJR Am J Roentgenol* 2009;192:646–653.

29 Answer A. Image acquisition time = TR (Repetition time × Number of phase-encoding steps). A greater number of phase-encoding steps will increase the acquisition time and improve the spatial resolution. The greater spatial resolution will require a greater number of repetitions and results in a longer acquisition time.

Reference: Biglands JD. Cardiovascular magnetic resonance physics for clinicians: part I. *J Cardiovasc Magn Reson* 2010;12:71 doi:10.1186/1532-429X-12-71.

30 Answer B. Patients with acute renal injury or chronic renal insufficiency should have a GFR checked prior to undergoing a cardiac MRI. A GFR >30 mL/min has been recommended to be used as a minimum threshold. If the GFR is lower than this value, gadolinium contrast should not be administered due to the system risk of nephrogenic systemic fibrosis.

Reference: http://www.fda.gov/Drugs/DrugSafety/ucm223966.htm

31 Answer B. Devices are grouped into three categories: (1) MR safe; (2) MR conditional; and (3) MR unsafe. A MR safe device poses no threat in any environment. A MR conditional device has no known hazards under specific conditions of use. A MR unsafe device poses hazards in all environments.

Reference: American Society for Testing and Materials (ASTM) International, Designation: F2503-05. *Standard practice for marking medical devices and other items for safety in the magnetic resonance environment*. West Conshohocken, PA: ASTM International, 2005.

2 Normal Anatomy, Including Variants, Encountered on Radiography, CT, and MR

QUESTIONS

1a What is the dominance of this patient?

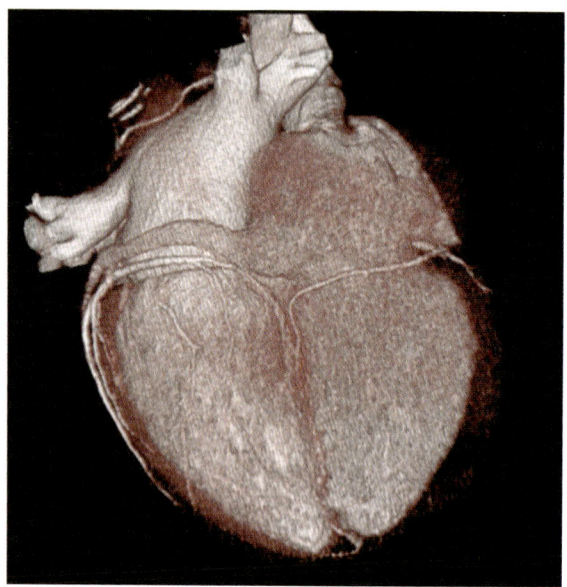

A. Left
B. Right
C. Codominant
D. Nondominant

1b How often is this type of anatomy present?
A. 10% to 20%
B. 40% to 50%
C. 80% to 90%

2 What is the normal relationship of tricuspid and mitral valves?
A. They are located on the same level.
B. Tricuspid valve is more apically located than the mitral valve.
C. Mitral valve is more apically located than the tricuspid valve.

3 What is the normal relationship of the left pulmonary artery to the bronchi
   A. Hyparterial
   B. Eparterial
   C. Isoarterial

4 Which cardiac valve is the most posteriorly located?
   A. Aortic
   B. Mitral
   C. Pulmonic
   D. Tricuspid

5 Which cardiac valve is the most superiority located?
   A. Aortic
   B. Mitral
   C. Pulmonic
   D. Tricuspid

6 What is the valve at the ostium of the coronary sinus?
   A. Eustachian
   B. Thebesian
   C. Vieussens
   D. Marshall

7 This structure located in the right atrium is most likely which of the following?

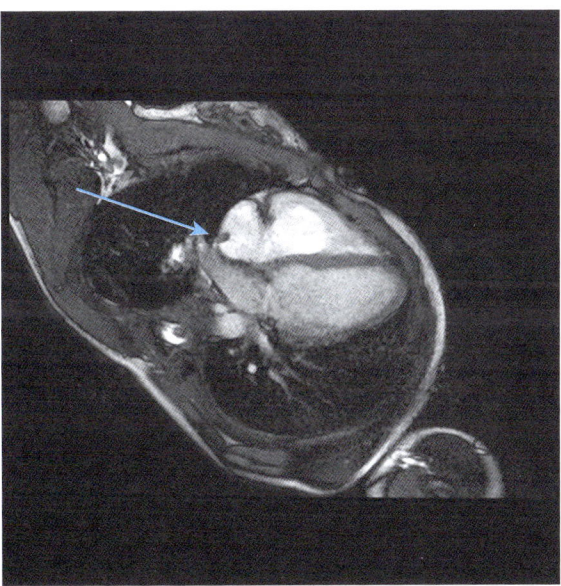

   A. Crista terminalis
   B. Thrombus
   C. Myxoma
   D. Central line

8 Which pulmonary vein is seen draining into the left atrium?

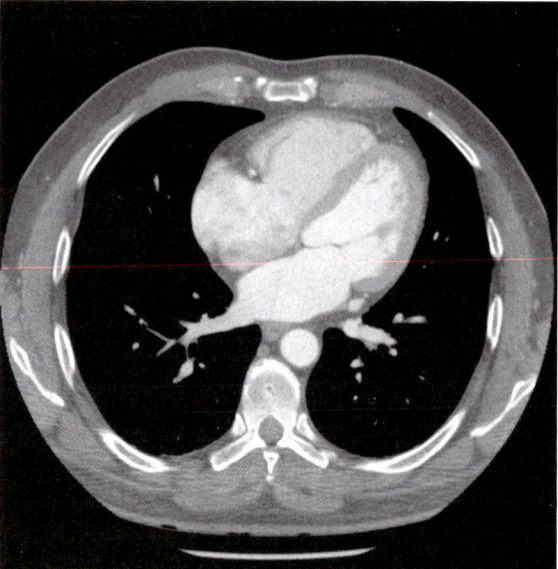

A. Right superior pulmonary vein
B. Right inferior pulmonary vein
C. Scimitar vein

9 Which of the valves has been treated in the below radiograph?

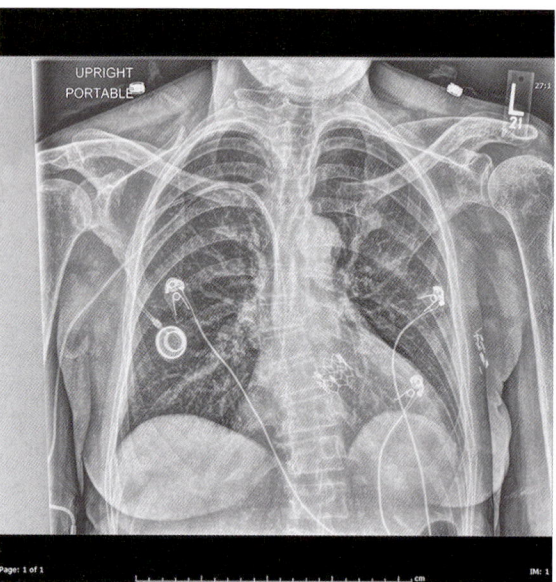

A. Aortic valve
B. Mitral valve
C. Pulmonic valve
D. Tricuspid valve

10 The anatomic structure that contains the abnormality is the

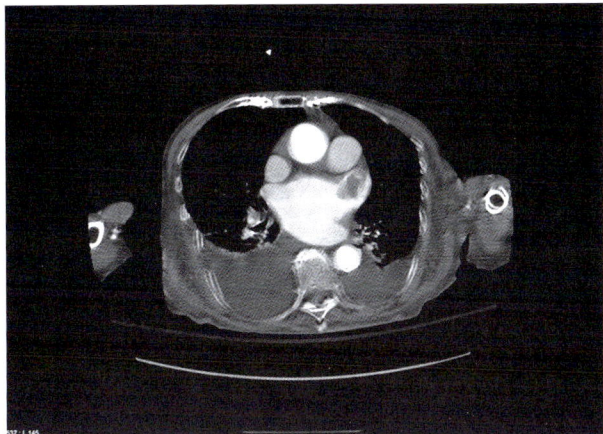

   A. Aorta
   B. Left atrial appendage
   C. Pulmonary vein
   D. Right atrium

11 The arrow points to what structure?

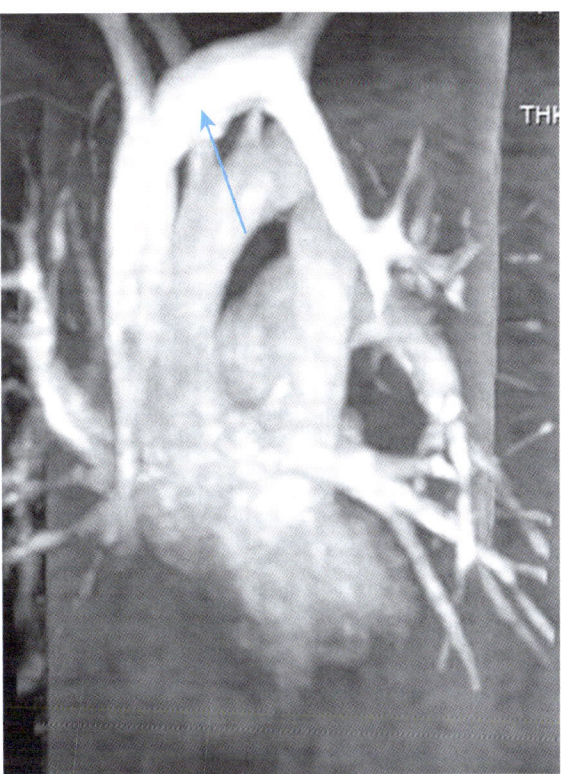

   A. Aorta
   B. Brachiocephalic vein
   C. Left upper lobe pulmonary vein
   D. Superior vena cava

12 The image shows an oblique coronal image of the aorta. The aortic root is defined as:
    A. Between the annulus and sinotubular junction
    B. Between the brachiocephalic artery and aortic isthmus
    C. Between the sinotubular junction and aortic isthmus
    D. Between the aortic isthmus and diaphragmatic hiatus

13 The vessel arising from the right coronary artery supplies which structure?

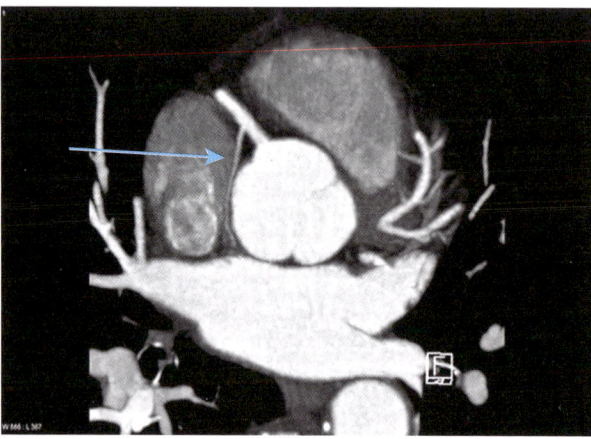

    A. Anterior wall of the right ventricle
    B. Infundibulum
    C. Left atrium
    D. Sinoatrial node

14 This short-axis balanced steady-state free precession is at the level of the midcavity of the papillary muscle. Which coronary artery typically supplies the structure the arrow is pointing to?

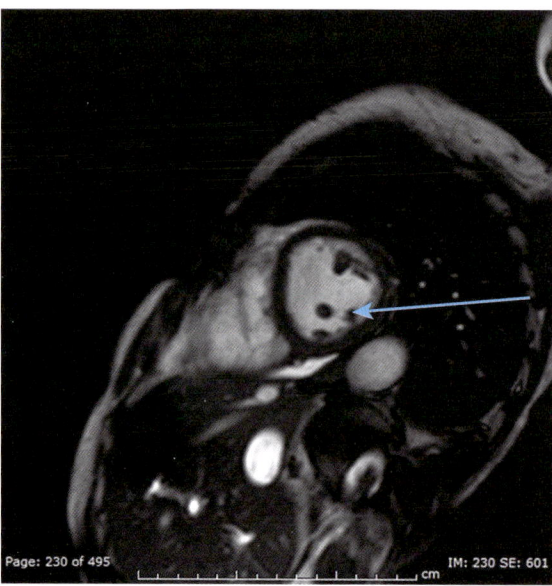

    A. Left anterior descending coronary artery
    B. Left circumflex coronary artery
    C. Left main coronary artery
    D. Right coronary artery

15 What is the best description for this cardiac plane?

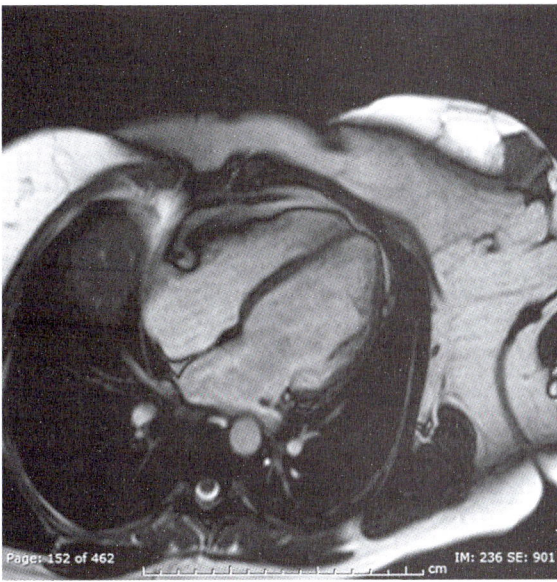

A. Four-chamber plane
B. Three-chamber plane
C. Two-chamber plane
D. Short-axis plane

16 The arrow points to which anatomic structure?

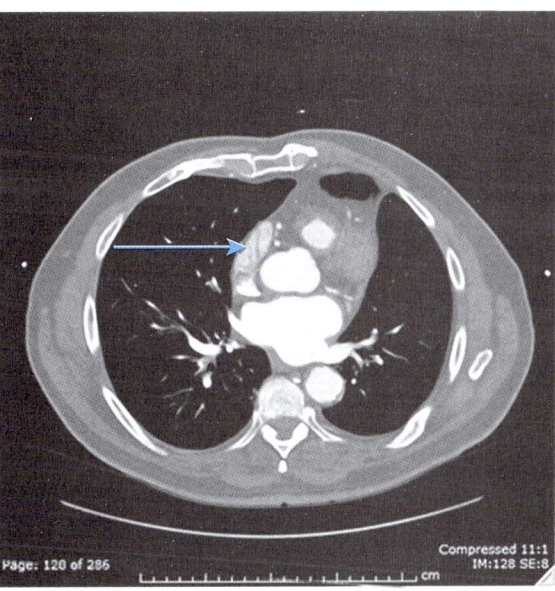

A. Chiari network
B. Eustachian valve
C. Right atrial appendage
D. Superior vena cava

17 The arrow in the four-chamber balanced steady-state free precession sequence shows what findings?

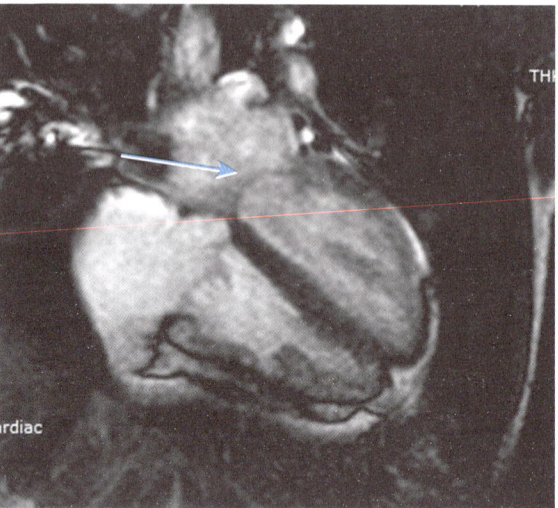

A. Normal mitral valve
B. Mitral valve prolapse
C. Normal tricuspid valve
D. Tricuspid valve prolapse

18 The arrow in the two-chamber balanced steady-state free precession image shows which leaflet of the mitral valve?

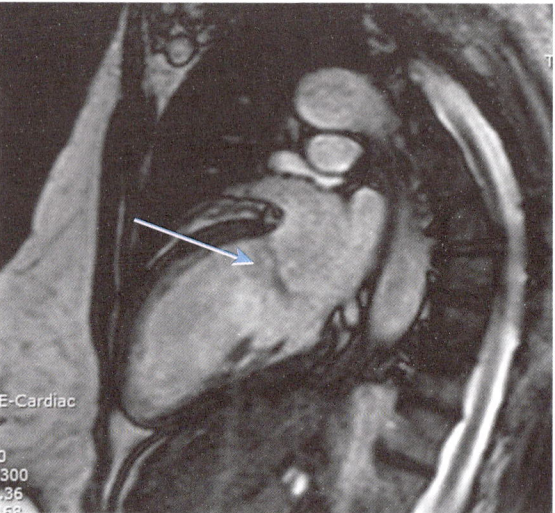

A. Anterior leaflet of the mitral valve
B. Posterior leaflet of the mitral valve
C. Aortic leaflet of the mitral valve
D. Septal leaflet of the mitral valve

19 This image from a balanced steady-state free precession sequence shows a bicuspid aortic valve. What structure is indicated by the arrow?

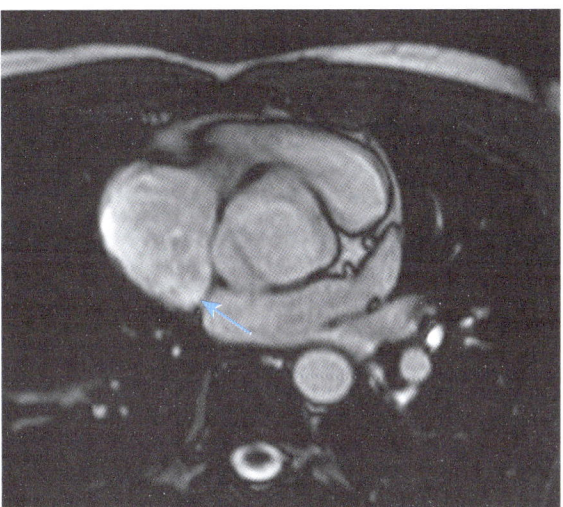

A. Interatrial septum
B. Noncoronary cusp
C. Mitral attachment
D. Crista terminalis

20 The arrow shows an abnormality in what structure?

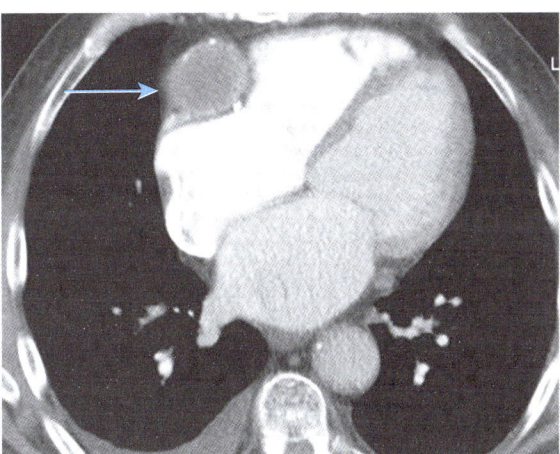

A. Atrioventricular groove
B. Right atrium
C. Superior vena cava
D. Tricuspid valve

21 The image shows an abnormality in what part of the heart?

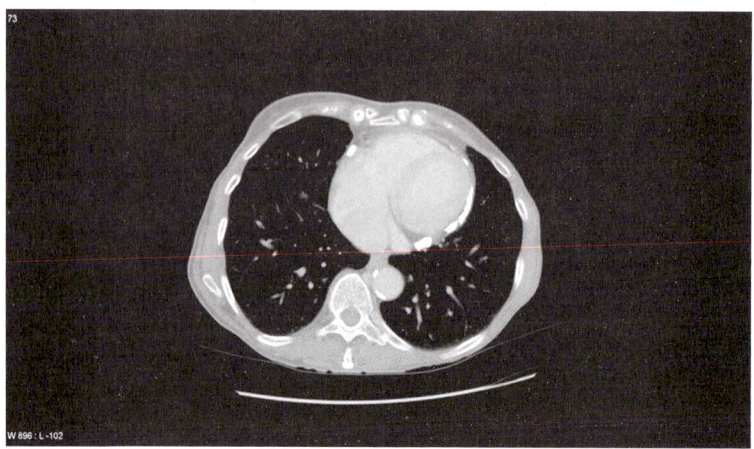

A. Coronary artery
B. Myocardium
C. Pericardium
D. Endocardium

22 The arrow points to what normal anatomic structure?

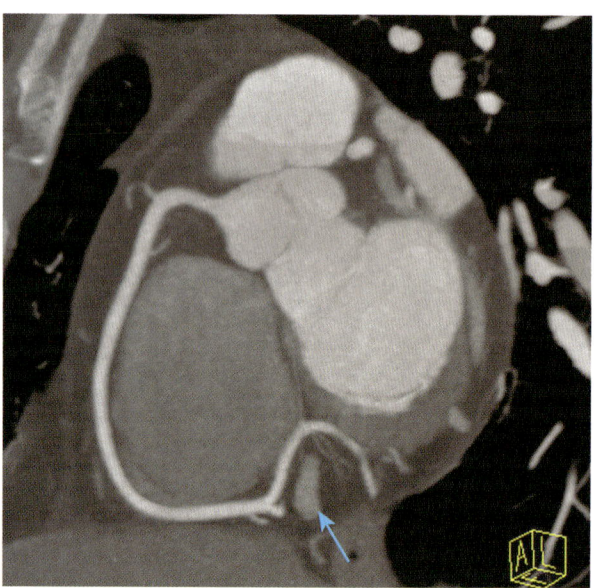

A. Great cardiac vein
B. Middle cardiac vein
C. Posterolateral vein
D. Vein of Marshall

23 The arrow points to what structure?

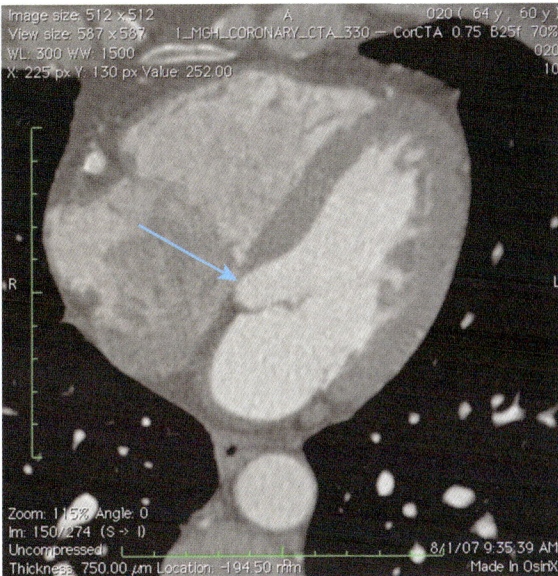

A. Fossa ovalis
B. Membranous septum
C. Mitral valve
D. Chordae tendineae

24 The arrow shows which coronary artery?

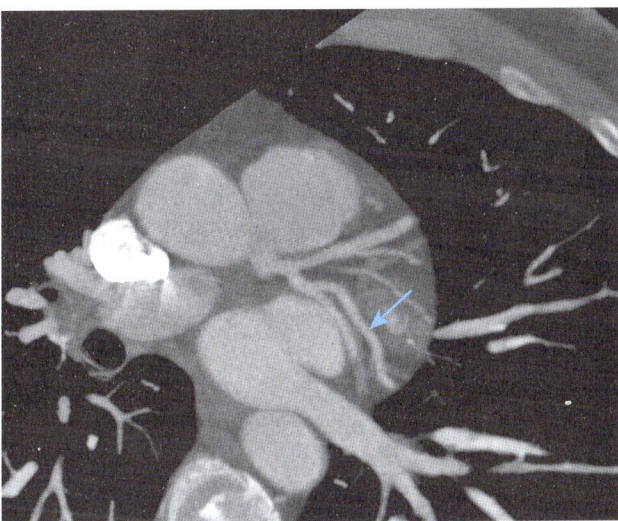

A. Circumflex
B. Diagonal
C. Left anterior descending
D. Obtuse marginal

25 The angiographic image below shows which coronary artery?

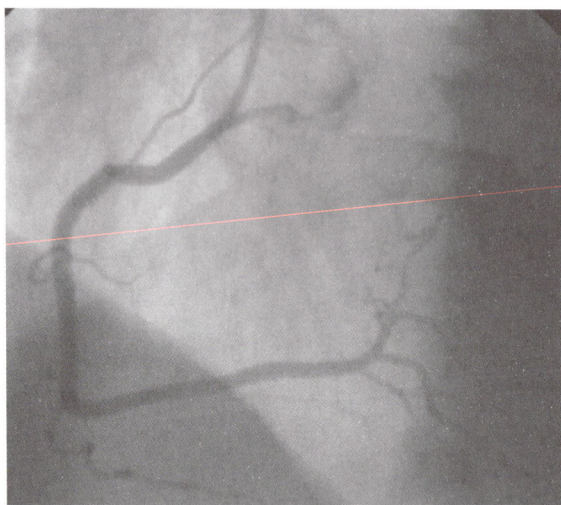

A. Right coronary artery
B. Left anterior descending
C. Left circumflex
D. Ramus intermedius

26 What structure is shown in the image?

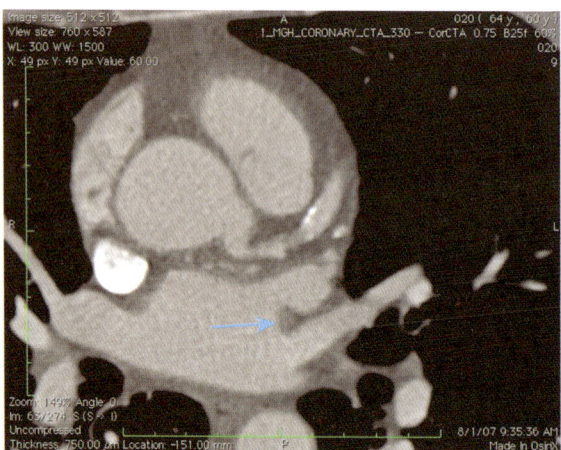

A. Inferior pulmonary vein
B. Left atrial appendage
C. Ligament of Marshall
D. Fossa ovalis

27 The angiogram from an RAO caudal position shows an arrow on which coronary artery?

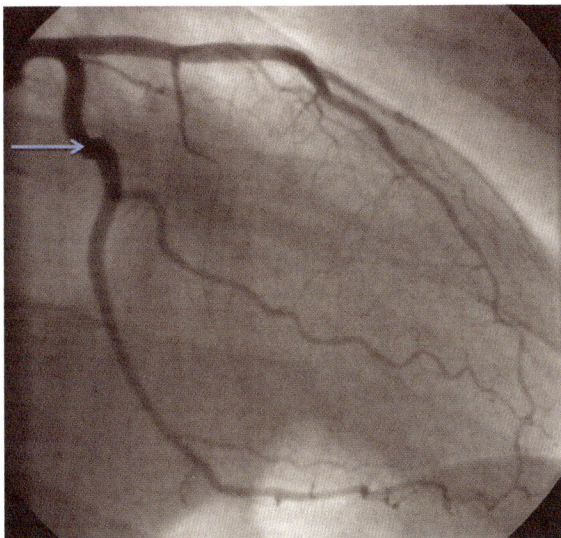

A. Right coronary artery
B. Left anterior descending
C. Left circumflex
D. Ramus intermedius

28 The arrow points to what anatomic structure?

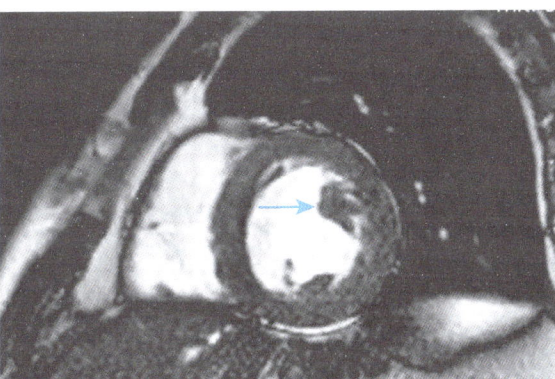

A. Anterolateral papillary muscle
B. Chordae tendineae
C. Lateral wall
D. Moderator band

ANSWERS AND EXPLANATIONS

1a Answer C. Volume-rendered image shows both RCA and LCX supplying the PDA. This is consistent with a codominant anatomy.

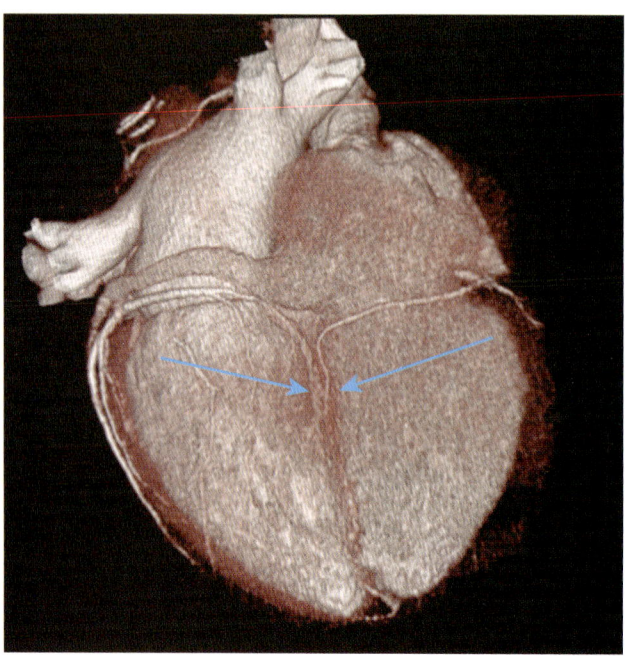

1b Answer A. Codominant anatomy occurs in roughly 10% to 20% of patients.

References: O'Brien JP, Srichai MB, Hecht EM, et al. Anatomy of the heart at multidetector CT: what the radiologist needs to know. *Radiographics* 2007;27(6):1569–1582. Review.

Pannu HK, Flohr TG, Corl FM, et al. Current concepts in multi-detector row CT evaluation of the coronary arteries: principles, techniques, and anatomy. *Radiographics* 2003;23:S111–S25. Review.

2 Answer B. The tricuspid valve is more apically located than the mitral valve. This can be helpful in identifying the valves/ventricles in patients with ventricular inversion. The AV valves (tricuspid and mitral) will go with their respective morphologic ventricles (tricuspid with morphologic RV, mitral with morphologic LV).

References: O'Brien JP, Srichai MB, Hecht EM, et al. Anatomy of the heart at multidetector CT: what the radiologist needs to know. *Radiographics* 2007;27(6):1569–1582. Review.

Schallert EK, Danton GH, Kardon R, et al. Describing congenital heart disease by using three-part segmental notation. *Radiographics* 2013;33(2):E33–E46. doi: 10.1148/rg.332125086.

3 Answer A. Normal relationship of the left pulmonary artery to the left mainstem and left lobar bronchi is hyparterial (the bronchi is inferior to the bronchi). The normal relationship of the right pulmonary artery to the right main stem bronchus is eparterial (artery is superior to the bronchus). This can be used when evaluating patients with situs anomalies to determine the right and left side.

References: Lapierre C, Déry J, et al. Segmental approach to imaging of congenital heart disease. *Radiographics* 2010;30(2):397–411. doi: 10.1148/rg.302095112. Review.

Schallert EK, Danton GH, Kardon R, et al. Describing congenital heart disease by using three-part segmental notation. *Radiographics* 2013;33(2):E33-E46. doi: 10.1148/rg.332125086.

4 **Answer B.** The most posteriorly located valve is the mitral valve. The pulmonic valve is located anterior and superior to the aortic valve. The mitral valve is located posterior to the aortic valve. The tricuspid valve is the most lateral right-sided valve (typically right of the spine).

References: Lapierre C, Déry J, Guérin R, et al. Segmental approach to imaging of congenital heart disease. *Radiographics* 2010;30(2):397-411. doi: 10.1148/rg.302095112. Review.

Schallert EK, Danton GH, Kardon R, et al. Describing congenital heart disease by using three-part segmental notation. *Radiographics* 2013;33(2):E33-E46. doi: 10.1148/rg.332125086.

5 **Answer C.** The most superiorly located valve is the pulmonary valve. One mnemonic for remembering the pulmonary valve position is "my Pal Sal." The pulmonic valve (PAL) is superior and anterior and to the left (SAL) relative to the aortic valve in normal anatomy.

References: Lapierre C, Déry J, Guérin R, et al. Segmental approach to imaging of congenital heart disease. *Radiographics* 2010;30(2):397-411. doi: 10.1148/rg.302095112. Review.

Schallert EK, Danton GH, Kardon R, et al. Describing congenital heart disease by using three-part segmental notation. *Radiographics* 2013;33(2):E33-E46. doi: 10.1148/rg.332125086.

6 **Answer B.** The valve at the ostium of the coronary sinus is the Thebesian valve. The eustachian valve is at the inferior vena cava. The Vieussens valve is at the junction of the coronary sinus and the great cardiac vein. The ligament of Marshall is the developmental remnant of the left superior vena cava.

Reference: Shah SS, Teague SD, Lu JC, et al. Imaging of the coronary sinus: normal anatomy and congenital abnormalities. *Radiographics* 2012;32(4):991-1008. doi: 10.1148/rg.324105220.

7 **Answer A.** This posterior right atrial structure is the crista terminalis, which is a muscular ridge separating the muscular and smooth portion of the right atrium. It can often be mistaken for a right atrial mass/thrombus but is a normal structure. While thrombus can be associated with the crista terminalis, it would typically be larger and associated with history of central line placement. Right atrial myxoma can occur in the posterior right atrial wall but are typically larger and along the interatrial septum.

Reference: Malik SB, Kwan D, Shah AB, et al. The right atrium: gateway to the heart—anatomic and pathologic imaging findings. *Radiographics* 2015;35(1):14-31. doi: 10.1148/rg.351130010.

8 **Answer B.** The vein seen draining into the left atrium is the right inferior pulmonary vein. This can be determined due to the fact that inferior pulmonary veins drain the lower lobe, which is posteriorly located. Therefore, any vein that is approaching from the posterior lung will be draining the lower lobe and thus inferiorly located. Any vein draining anteriorly would be the superior pulmonary veins. The scimitar vein typically will drain into the right atrium/IVC.

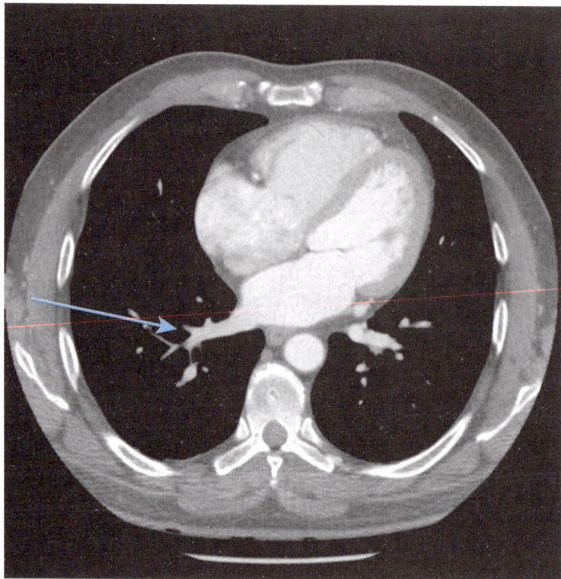

Reference: Porres DV, Morenza OP, Pallisa E, et al. Learning from the pulmonary veins. *Radiographics* 2013;33(4):999–1022. doi: 10.1148/rg.334125043. Review.

9 Answer A. The patient has undergone transaortic valve replacement (TAVR) secondary to aortic stenosis. The procedure is performed in patients who are high risk for surgery who cannot undergo an open aortic repair. The percutaneous valve is seated in the left ventricular outflow tract and ascending aorta.

References: Leipsic J, Wood D, Manders D, et al. The evolving role of MDCT in transcatheter aortic valve replacement: a radiologists' perspective. *AJR Am J Roentgenol* 2009;193:3, W214–W219.

Mehlman DJ. A guide to the radiographic identification of prosthetic heart valves: an addendum. *Circulation* 1984;69(1):102–105.

10 Answer B. The left atrium is enlarged and within the left atrial appendage is a thrombus. Thrombus can develop in the left atrial appendage in patients with recurrent atrial fibrillation and can undergo systemic embolization.

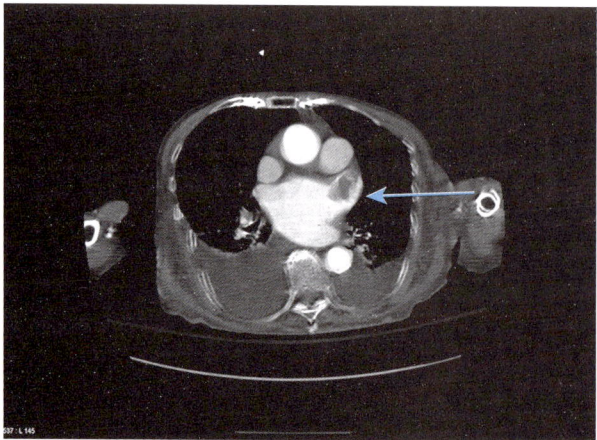

Reference: Garcia MJ. Detection of left atrial appendage thrombus by cardiac computed tomography. A word of caution. *J Am Coll Cardiol* 2009;2(1):77–79. doi: 10.1016/j.jcmg.2008.10.003.

11 Answer B. Patient has left upper lobe anomalous pulmonary venous return (arrow on the right). The anomalous vein drains into the left brachiocephalic vein and subsequently to the SVC and right atrium. The pattern of drainage creates a left-to-right shunt.

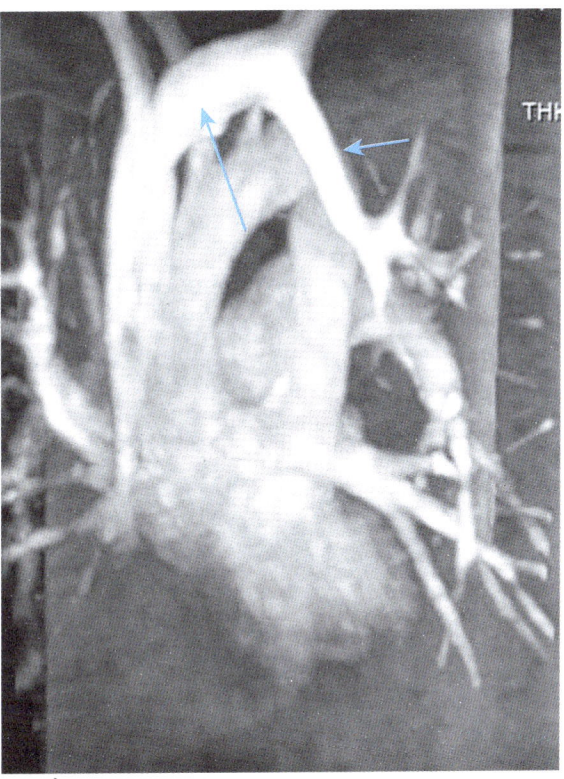

Reference: Dillman JR, Yarram SG, Hernandez RJ. Imaging of pulmonary venous developmental anomalies. *AJR Am J Roentgenol* 2009;192(5):1272–1285.

12 Answer A. The aortic root is defined as the segment between the aortic annulus (basal ring of the annulus and the sinotubular junction. It includes the basal ring of the annulus (aortic cusp insertion), the aortic valve cusps, and the sinuses of valsalva.

Reference: Charitos EI, Seivers HH. Anatomy of the aortic root: implications for valve-sparing surgery. *Ann Cardiothorac Surg* 2012;2(1):53–56.

13 Answer D. The sinoatrial nodal artery most commonly arises from the RCA and courses toward the interatrial septum. The artery can also arise from the left circumflex coronary artery.

Reference: Kini S, Bis, KG, Weaver L. Normal and variant coronary arterial and venous anatomy on high resolution CT angiography. *AJR Am J Roentgenol* 2007;188(6):1665–1674.

14 Answer D. There are two papillary muscles in the left ventricle, the anterolateral and posteromedial papillary muscles. The anterolateral papillary muscle has a shared blood supply from the left anterior descending and left circumflex coronary artery. The posteromedial papillary muscle is supplied by the right coronary artery (in right dominant patients) and is more prone to rupture following myocardial infarction given its single vascular supply.

References: Czarnecki A, Thakrar A, Fang T, et al. Acute severe mitral regurgitation: consideration of papillary muscle architecture. *Cardiovasc Ultrasound* 2008;6:5.

Fradley MG, Picard MH. Rupture of the posteromedial papillary muscle leading to partial flail of the anterior mitral leaflet. *Circulation* 2011;123(9):1044–1045.

15 **Answer A.** This is a four-chamber plane, which shows the right atrium, right ventricle, left atrium, and left ventricle. The plane allows for evaluation of the mitral and tricuspid valves and to evaluate the right ventricular free wall, interventricular septum, and lateral wall of the left ventricle.

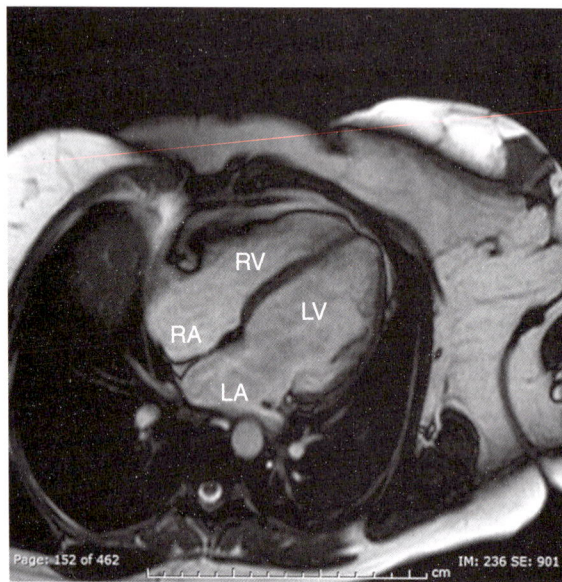

Reference: Nasif MS, Oliveira AC Jr, Carvalho AC, et al. Cardiac magnetic resonance and its anatomical planes: How do I do it? *Arq Bras Cardiol* 2010;95(6):756-763.

16 **Answer C.** The structure represents the right atrial appendage. The right atrial appendage extends anteriorly from the right atrium and contains multiple pectinate muscles. It is adjacent to the ascending aorta to the right of the midline and will maintain a broad conical shape. The right atrial appendage can be associated as a nidus of arrhythmia and can serve as a target for pacing.

Reference: Manolis AS, Varriale P, Baptist SJ. Necropsy study of right atrial appendage: morphology and measurements. *Clin Cardiol* 1988;11:788-792.

17 **Answer B.** The image shows prolapse of the mitral valve, which extends beyond 2 mm posterior the plane of the mitral valve. The mitral valve divides the left atrium from the left ventricle.

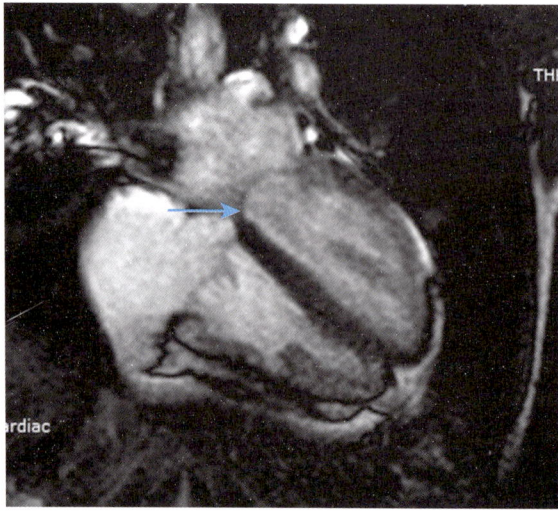

Reference: Ring L, Rana SB. Anatomy of the mitral valve: understanding the mitral valve complex in mitral regurgitation. *Eur Heart J Cardiovasc Imaging* 2010;11(10):i3–i9. doi: 10.1093/ejechocard/jeq153.

18   **Answer A.**   The mitral valve is a bileaflet structure (anterior and posterior leaflet), which has a "D"-like shape. The anterior leaflet is smaller than the posterior leaflet and is typically thin measuring less than 2 mm in thickness. The mitral valve leaflets are connected to the papillary muscle by thin fibrous bands known as the chordae tendineae. There is no aortic or septal leaflets of the mitral valve.

Reference: Ring L, Rana SB. Anatomy of the mitral valve: understanding the mitral valve complex in mitral regurgitation. *Eur Heart J Cardiovasc Imaging* 2010;11(10):i3–i9. doi: 10.1093/ejechocard/jeq153.

19   **Answer A.**   The arrow is pointing to the interatrial septum. The interatrial septum is directed toward the noncoronary cusp. In the below image, the left coronary cusp and right coronary cusp are fused.

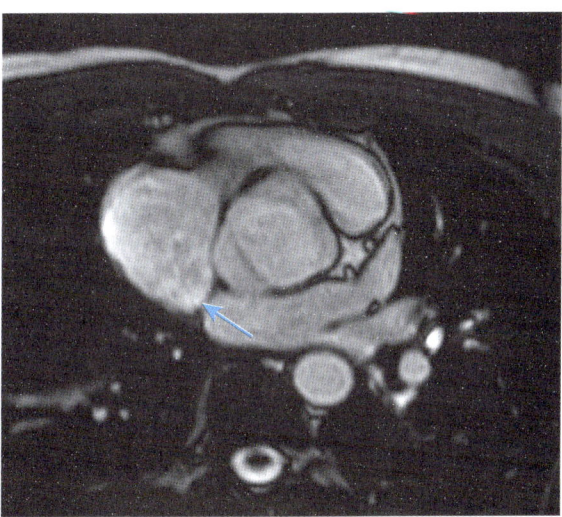

Reference: Ziad FI, John MM, Douglas PZ. *Clinical arrhythmology and electrophysiology: A companion to Braunwald's heart disease series*. Saunders W.B.:582.

20   **Answer A.**   The image shows a coronary artery bypass graft aneurysm in the right atrioventricular groove. The aneurysm causes mild mass effect on the right atrium and right ventricle.

Reference: Halpern EJ. *Clinical cardiac CT: anatomy and function*. Thieme, 2011.

21   **Answer C.**   The patient has calcifications of the pericardium. Pericardial calcifications are most commonly secondary to prior infection. Other causes include hemorrhage, uremia, neoplasm, or autoimmune syndrome.

Reference: Czum JM, Silas AM, Althoen MC. Evaluation of the pericardium with CT and MR. *ISRN Cardiol* 2014;2014:174908. doi: 10.1155/2014/174908

22   **Answer B.**   The arrow points to the middle cardiac vein. The middle cardiac vein can also be referred to as the posterior interventricular vein and courses with the posterior descending artery in the posterior interventricular groove. The coronary sinus drains into the right atrium.

Reference: Habib A, Lachman N, Christensen KN, et al. The anatomy of the coronary sinus venous system for the cardiac electrophysiologist. *Europace* 2009;11(Suppl 5):v15–v21. doi: 10.1093/europace/eup270.

23   **Answer B.**   The interventricular septum contains two components, a membranous segment and a muscular segment. The majority of the septum is the muscular segment, which separates the right and left ventricle from each other.

The most superior and posterior segment of the septum is the membranous portion, which is at the base of the heart between the inlet and outlet components of the muscular septum and inferior to the right and noncoronary cusps of the aortic valve.

Reference: Minette MS, Sahn DJ. Ventricular septal defects. *Circulation* 200614;114(20):2190–2197.

24 Answer D. The image shows the left main coronary artery with a normal bifurcation into the left anterior descending (LAD) and left circumflex coronary artery (LCx). The first obtuse margin division is shown to arise from the LCx. The obtuse marginal divisions typically supply the inferolateral wall.

Reference: Kini SKG, Bis KG, Weaver L. Normal and variant coronary arterial and venous anatomy on high-resolution CT angiography. *Am J Roentgenol* 2007;188(6):1665–1674.

25 Answer A. The coronary artery is the right coronary artery and gives rise to the PDA and PLV divisions (blue and red arrows) and the conus branch (yellow arrow). The view above is a "c" view of the right coronary artery, which can be obtained from CTA datasets through using multiplanar reformatting to mimic the angiographic left anterior oblique (LAO) view.

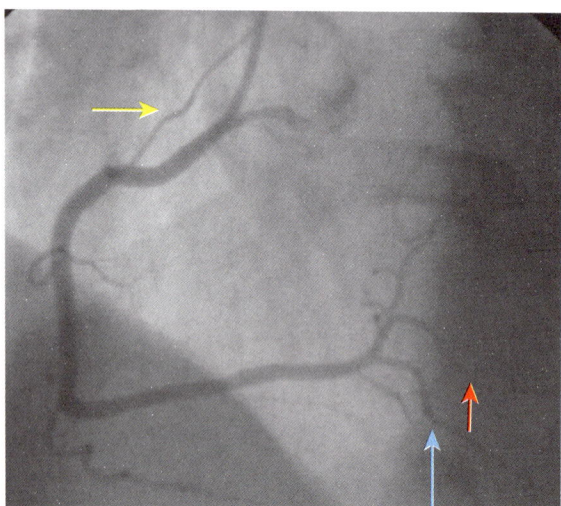

Reference: Kern M. Angiographic projections made simple: an easy guide to understanding oblique views. Cath Lab Digest 2011;19(8).

26 Answer C. This structure represents the ligament of Marshall. The ligament of Marshall is a normal structure which is positioned between the left atrial appendage ostium and the left superior pulmonary vein. It is the embryonic residua of the left-sided SVC and if enlarged can mimic a mass or thrombus.

Reference: Ho SY, Cabrera JA, Sanchez-Quintana D. Advances in arrhythmia and electrophysiology: left atrial anatomy revisited. *Circ Arrhythm Electrophysiol* 2012;5:220–228. doi: 10.1161/CIRCEP.111.962720

27 Answer C. This RAO caudal position shows the left main bifurcating into the left circumflex and left anterior descending coronary artery. The blue arrow shows the left circumflex coronary artery, while the green arrow shows the LAD. The obtuse marginal and diagonal divisions are highlighted in yellow and red, respectively.

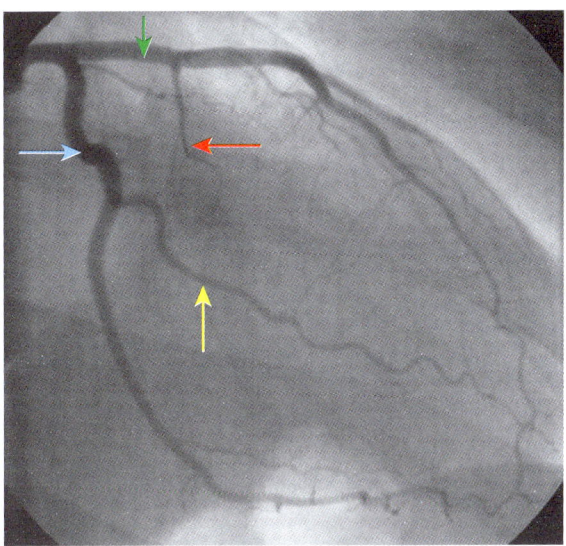

28 Answer A. The left ventricle has two papillary muscles, the anterolateral and posteromedial papillary muscles. The arrow points to the anterolateral papillary muscle. The mitral valve attaches to the papillary muscle via the thin fibrous chordae tendineae.

Reference: Moore KL, Dalley AF, Agur AM. *Clinically oriented anatomy*, 3rd ed. Baltimore, MD: Lippincott Williams & Wilkins, 2007.

3 Physiologic Aspects of Cardiac Imaging

QUESTIONS

1a A 50-year-old male underwent a gated cardiac CTA (CCTA) acquisition using a 64-slice CT scanner. The gray box shows the only phase of the cardiac cycle during which images were obtained. What characterizes this phase of the cardiac cycle?

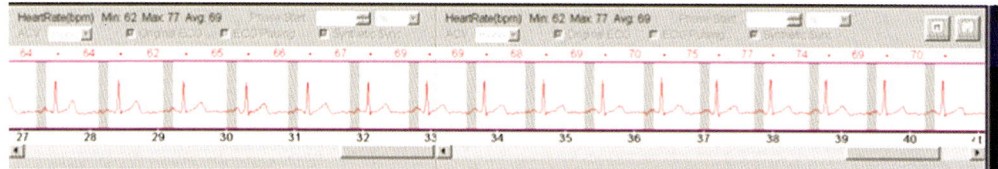

A. Atrial relaxation
B. Open mitral valve
C. Closed tricuspid valve
D. Ventricular contraction

1b A 50-year-old male underwent a gated cardiac CTA (CCTA) acquisition using a 64-slice CT scanner. The gray box shows the only phase of the cardiac cycle during which images were obtained. Why would the images be obtained using such an approach?

A. Allows ejection fraction to be calculated
B. Improves temporal resolution
C. Lower impact of elevated heart rate
D. Reduces radiation dose

1c Patients undergoing a cardiac CTA (CCTA) can receive a lower radiation dose through which of the following strategies?

A. Decreasing the pitch
B. Employing retrospective gating
C. Increasing mAs
D. Reducing kVp

2a The abnormality on the image is associated with which of the following?

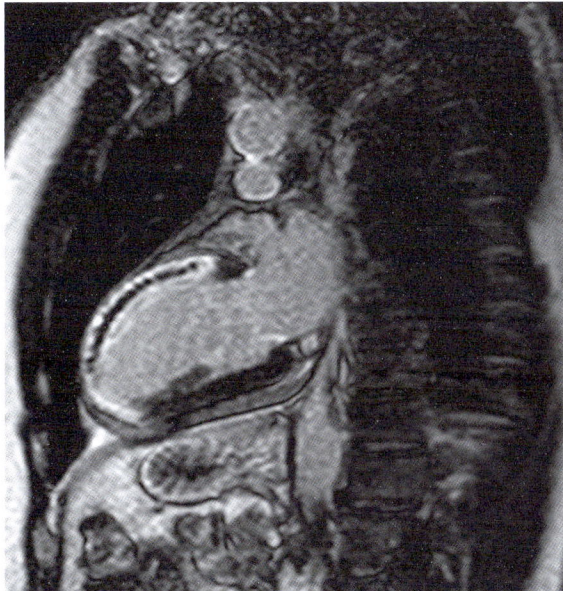

A. An ejection fraction >55%
B. Elongated mitral valve leaflet
C. Left ventricular wall thickening
D. Wall motion abnormalities

2b A severely decreased left ventricular systolic ejection fraction measures less than which value?

A. 55%
B. 50%
C. 45%
D. 40%
E. 35%

3a Which of the following findings would be expected?

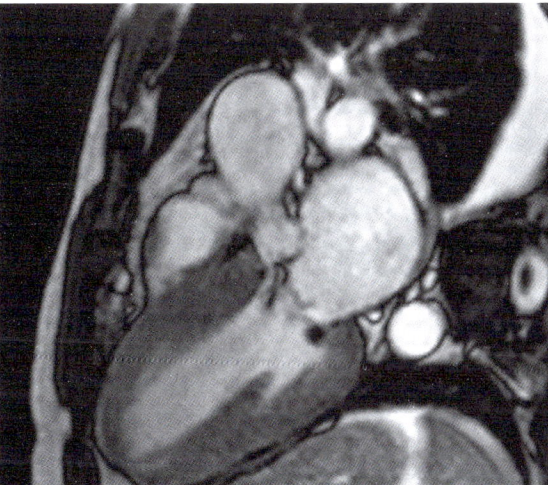

A. Decreased left ventricular filling pressure
B. Dilated ascending aorta
C. Narrowing of the left ventricular outflow tract
D. Thickening of the aortic valve leaflets

3b Which of the following physiologic changes occurs in the left heart in hypertrophic obstructive cardiomyopathy (HOCM)?

A. Decreased myocardial mass
B. Elevated left atrial pressure
C. Increased left ventricular compliance
D. Decreased atrial kick

3c Which of the following left ventricular changes in hypertrophic obstructive cardiomyopathy (HOCM) is most associated with the highest risk of sudden cardiac death?

A. Diastolic dysfunction
B. Mitral leaflet elongation
C. Mitral regurgitation
D. Septal thickening

4 Which of the following describes isovolumetric contraction of the ventricles?

A. Corresponds to the trough of the QRS complex.
B. The mitral and tricuspid valves are open.
C. Ventricular pressure increases.
D. Ventricular volume decreases.

5 Which of the following is characteristic of atrial systole?

A. By the T wave on an electrocardiogram
B. Contributes 20% to 30% of ventricular volume
C. Decreasing atrial pressure
D. Overlaps with early ventricular systole
E. Increases afterload

6 Which of the following conditions increases the ventricular preload?

A. Decreased atrial contraction
B. Decreased ventricular compliance
C. Deep inspiration
D. Elevated heart rate
E. Ligating an arterial-venous fistula
F. Reduced atrial pressure

7 Aliasing on phase contrast cardiac MRI occurs if the angular phase shift is

A. >120 degrees and the velocity within that pixel is then misregistered
B. >150 degrees and the velocity within that pixel is then misregistered
C. >180 degrees and the velocity within that pixel is then misregistered
D. >210 degrees and the velocity within that pixel is then misregistered

8 In preparation for a cardiac CTA, a patient was administered 100 mg of metoprolol via an oral tablet. Which of the following describes the mechanism of metoprolol?

A. Increases the heart rate
B. Stimulates the beta-1 receptors
C. Exerts positive inotropic effects
D. It is a cardioselective beta blocker

9a Which of the following criteria would indicate treatment for the condition shown in the image?

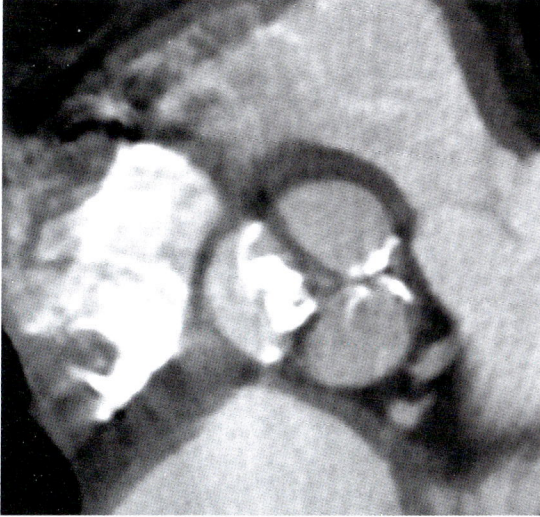

A. A valve area of 1.3 cm²
B. A valve calcium score of 2,000
C. A velocity gradient of 45 mm Hg
D. A velocity jet of 3 m/sec
E. A bicuspid valve

9b The above patient has aortic stenosis and underwent a cardiac MRI. The velocity across the valve was calculated to measure 150 cm/sec. Given the velocity, what is the estimated pressure gradient?

A. 5.5 mm Hg
B. 6 mm Hg
C. 8 mm Hg
D. 9 mm Hg

10a The below image was obtained in diastole. Which of the following describes the underlying process?

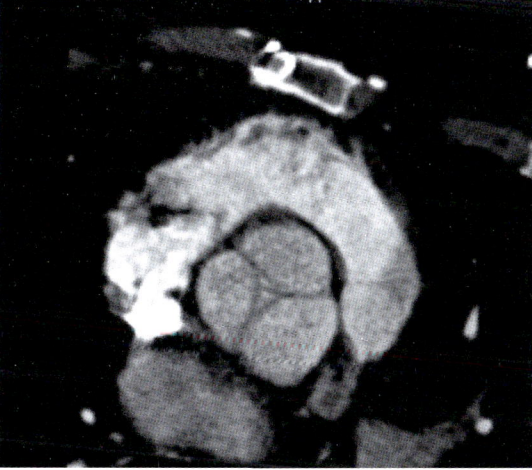

A. Aortic stenosis
B. Bicuspid aortic valve
C. Increased end-diastolic volume
D. Pulmonic insufficiency
E. Pulmonic stenosis

10b Aortic insufficiency can be quantified using phase contrast MRI. Which of the below indicates severe aortic insufficiency?

    A. A bicuspid aortic valve
    B. A dilated left ventricle measuring 6.5 cm
    C. A regurgitant volume of 65 mL
    D. An aortic valve area of 0.9 cm^2

11a The following artifact is caused by

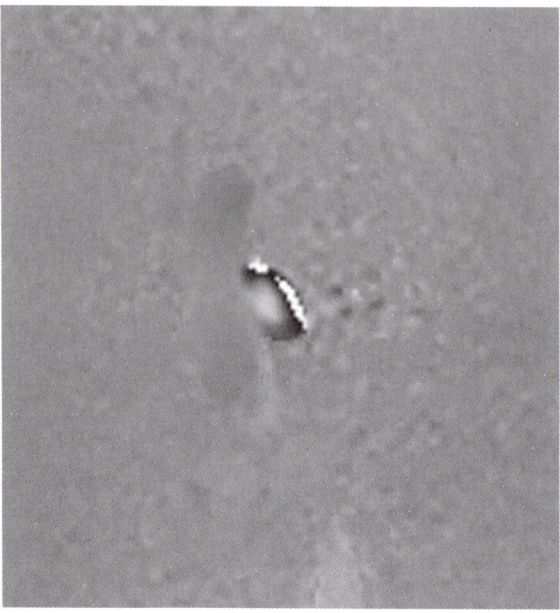

    A. An incorrect inversion time
    B. An incorrect velocity map
    C. Incomplete fat saturation
    D. Too high temporal resolution
    E. Too low spatial resolution

11b A phase contrast cardiac MRI (CMRI) sequence produces two sets of images. What set of images are produced by the phase contrast acquisition?

    A. Magnitude image and phase velocity map
    B. Magnitude image and volume map
    C. Magnitude image and velocity gradient map
    D. Magnitude image and pressure gradient map

12 A patient is given intravenous beta blockers in preparation for a cardiac CTA. What is the impact of this agent on the Frank Starling Curve?

    A. Shifts the Frank-Starling curve upward and to the right
    B. Shifts the Frank-Starling curve downward and to the right
    C. Shifts the Frank-Starling curve upward and to the left
    D. Shifts the Frank-Starling curve downward and to the left

13a A patient underwent a coronary venogram and it showed abnormal connection between the coronary sinus and which structure?

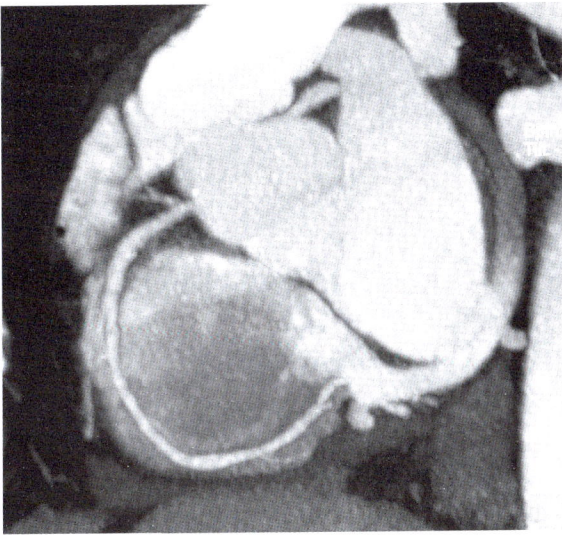

A. Left atrium
B. Left circumflex coronary artery
C. Right atrium

13b The patient underwent a cardiac MRI to determine the left to right shunt. The calculated Qp/Qs was 1.2. What is the next step?

A. No further treatment
B. Percutaneous cardiac intervention
C. Surgical treatment
D. Stress echocardiogram

14 A patient underwent a cardiac CCTA secondary to an abnormal nuclear medicine stress test. The stress test showed a perfusion defect involving which vascular territory (territories)?

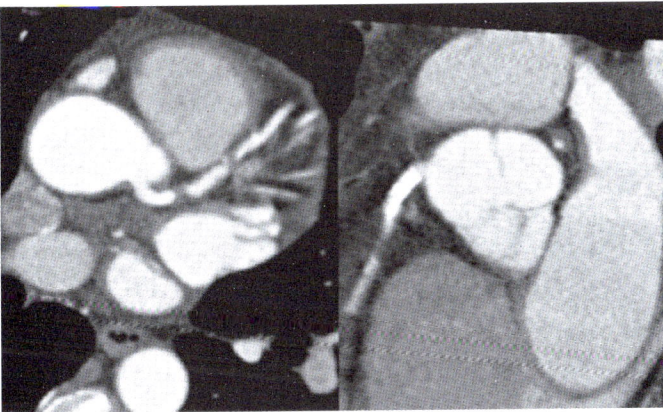

A. Left anterior descending coronary artery
B. Left circumflex coronary artery
C. Left anterior descending coronary artery and left circumflex coronary artery
D. Left circumflex and right coronary arteries
E. Left circumflex coronary artery, left anterior descending coronary, artery and right coronary artery

15a The patient underwent a cardiac CCTA secondary to an abnormal nuclear medicine stress test. The stress test showed a perfusion defect involving which vascular territory (territories)?

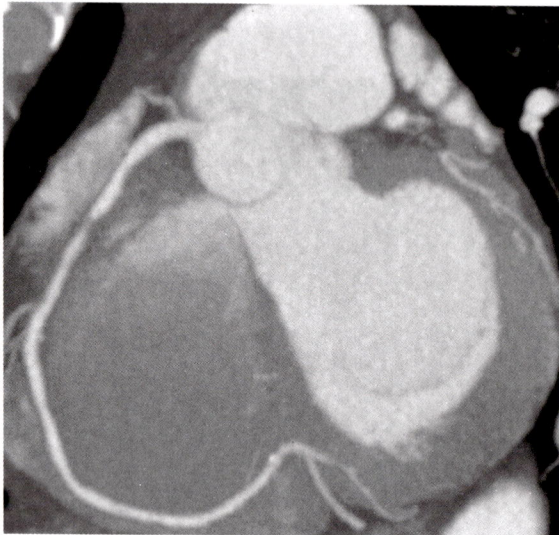

A. Left anterior descending coronary artery
B. Left circumflex coronary artery
C. Left anterior descending coronary artery and left circumflex coronary artery
D. Right coronary artery
E. Left circumflex coronary artery, left anterior descending coronary artery, and right coronary artery

15b What amount of narrowing in cardiac CTA indicates flow-limiting stenosis in a non-ostial segment of the coronary artery?

A. 40%
B. 50%
C. 60%
D. 70%

16 Sublingual nitroglycerin (SL-NTG) is administered during a cardiac CTA (CCTA). The patient experiences headaches after it is administered and asks to speak to a physician to explain why they were given the medication. What explanation do you give to the patient regarding the benefits of SL-NTG use?

A. Decreases motion of the coronary arteries
B. Improves visualization of the coronary arteries
C. Improves ventricular function
D. Reduces radiation exposure

17 A patient with history of atypical chest pain, severe asthma, and type 2 diabetes arrives for a cardiac CTA with a resting heart rate of 50 beats/min. The patient took sildenafil within the last 24 hours. A fellow asks if sublingual nitroglycerin (SL-NTG) can be administered to the patient. Your response is

A. No, due to hypotension
B. No, it is can induce arrhythmia
C. No, it increases the preload
D. No, due to respiratory arrest

18 Which anatomic configuration accounts for the finding below?

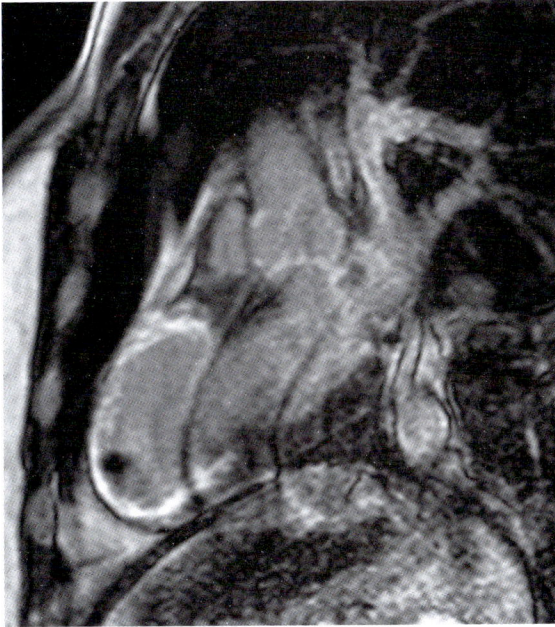

A. Anomalous left circumflex coronary artery
B. False ventricular aneurysm
C. Right dominant coronary artery
D. Wrap around left anterior descending coronary artery

19a A patient underwent an MRI following an abnormal echocardiogram. What is the diagnosis?

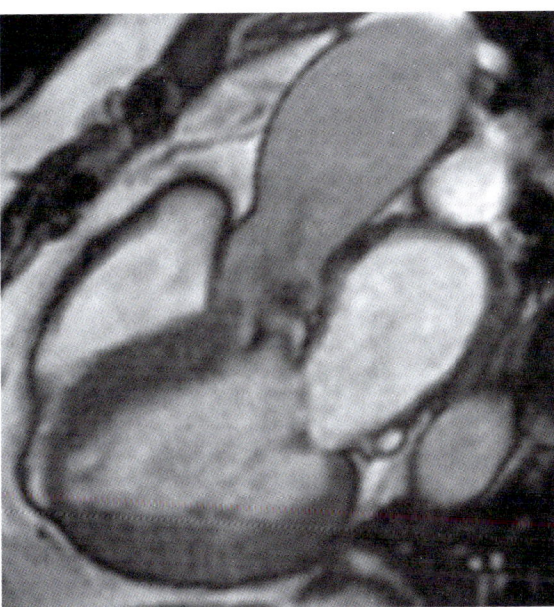

A. Hypertrophic cardiomyopathy
B. Left ventricular noncompaction
C. Mitral valve prolapse
D. Subaortic membrane

19b How does a subaortic membrane impact cardiac hemodynamics?
   A. Homogenous flow across the left ventricular outflow tract
   B. Increases afterload
   C. Increases left ventricular ejection fraction
   D. No impact on mitral regurgitation
   E. Reduces inotropy

20 You complete a cardiac MRI (CMRI) and need to report the ejection fraction. The end systolic volume is 40 mL. The end diastolic volume is 100 mL. The stroke volume is 60 mL. The myocardial mass is 65 g. The automated computer system reports an error and you must manually calculate the ejection fraction. What is the ejection fraction?
   A. 40%
   B. 55%
   C. 60%
   D. 65%
   E. 70%

21 Atrial fibrillation is the most common cardiac arrhythmia. Patients with atrial fibrillation have ectopic electrical-stimulating foci that overwhelm the function of what normal cardiac structure?
   A. Atrioventricular node
   B. Bundle of His
   C. Purkinje fibers
   D. Sinoatrial node

22 A patient is referred for a cardiac MRI (CMRI) to determine the left ventricular myocardial mass. How is myocardial mass calculated?
   A. (Epicardial myocardial volume – endocardial myocardial volume) × specific density of myocardium
   B. (Endomyocardial volume – epicardial myocardial volume) × specific density of myocardium
   C. (Epicardial myocardial volume) × specific density of myocardium
   D. (Endocardial myocardial volume) × specific density of myocardium

23 Which of the following best describes diastolic dysfunction?
   A. Cardiac MRI is advantageous compared to echocardiography in establishing the diagnosis.
   B. Left ventricular filling rate decreases early in the disease process.
   C. Left atrial size is normal.
   D. Systolic ejection fraction is reduced.

24 A 55-year-old male undergoes a cardiac MRI (CMRI) and the left ventricular size is measured. What is the minimum value at which the cavity is considered to be dilated?
   A. 5.0 cm
   B. 5.5 cm
   C. 6.0 cm
   D. 6.5 cm

25a A patient underwent a gated cardiac CTA (CCTA) which showed a mass. Based on the image, what is the effect of the mass??

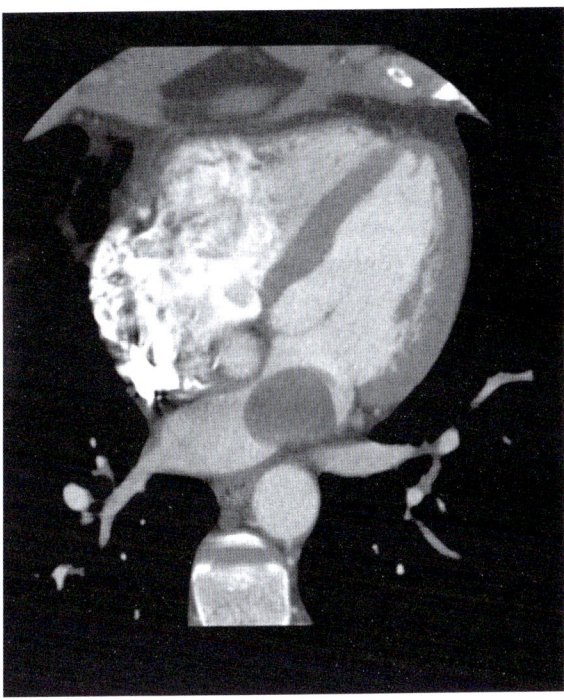

A. Obstructed left ventricular outflow tract
B. Obstructed pulmonary vein
C. Obstructed SVC
D. Obstructed tricuspid valve

25b The mass obstructed the pulmonary vein inflow and lead to pulmonary edema. Which of the following values indicates a normal pulmonary venous wedge pressure?

A. 10 mm Hg
B. 20 mm Hg
C. 30 mm Hg
D. 40 mm Hg

26 A 55-year-old male undergoes a cardiac MRI (CMRI) to quantify his aortic insufficiency. Which of the following be expected?

A. Preserved stroke volume
B. Increased preload
C. Decreased cavity size
D. Preserved afterload
E. No change in isovolumetric relaxation

27 A 28-year-old competitive cyclist arrives for a cardiac MRI (CMRI). Which morphologic changes in the heart are expected?

A. Decrease in cavity size and wall thickness
B. Increase in cavity size and wall thickness
C. Increase in cavity size and decrease in wall thickness
D. No change in cavity size and wall thickness

ANSWERS AND EXPLANATIONS

1a Answer B.   The image shows the EKG tracing from a cardiac CTA acquisition. The gray box corresponds to late ventricular diastole, just prior to ventricular contraction. During late diastole, the mitral and tricuspid valves are open. During the late phase of diastole, the atrial has a minimal contraction allowing to fill the ventricles. The ventricles contract during systole, which corresponds to the QRS complex.

Reference: Klabunde R. *Cardiovascular physiology concepts*. Lippincott Williams & Wilkins, 2011: 62–63. ISBN-10: 1451113846.

1b Answer D.   The patient was imaged using prospective triggering in order to reduce the radiation dose. During prospective triggering only a short segment of the cardiac cycle, usually diastole, is imaged resulting in no imaging in the remainder of the cardiac cycle and as a result no radiation being given. This method contrasts to retrospective gating during which the entire cardiac cycle is imaged resulting in a higher radiation dose since both systole and diastole are imaged.

References: Hirai N, et al. Prospective versus retrospective ECG-gated 64-detector coronary CT angiography: assessment of image quality, stenosis, and radiation dose. *Radiology* 2008;248(2): 424–430. doi: 10.1148/radiol.2482071804.

Menke J, et al. Head-to-head comparison of prospectively triggered vs retrospectively gated coronary computed tomography angiography: meta-analysis of diagnostic accuracy, image quality, and radiation dose. *Am Heart J* 2013;165(2):154–163. doi: 10.1016/j.ahj.2012.10.026.

1c Answer D.   Radiation dose can be reduced by decreasing the mAs, decreasing the kVp, using prospective triggering, and reducing the scan length. Reducing the pitch will increase the amount of radiation to the imaged area.

References: Labounty TM, et al. Coronary CT angiography of patients with a normal body mass index using 80 kVp versus 100 kVp: a prospective, multicenter, multivendor randomized trial. *AJR Am J Roentgenol* 2011;197(5):W860–W867. doi: 10.2214/AJR.11.6787.

Leipsic J, et al. A prospective randomized controlled trial to assess the diagnostic performance of reduced tube voltage for coronary CT angiography. *AJR Am J Roentgenol* 2011;196(4):801–806. doi: 10.2214/AJR.10.5786.

2a Answer D.   The image shows delayed enhancement along the left anterior descending coronary artery territory from an acute myocardial infarction with microvascular obstruction and no myocardial thinning indicating an acute infarction. Myocardial infarction and delayed enhancement are associated with wall motion abnormalities and decreased ventricular function.

References: Boagert J, et al. Remote myocardial dysfunction after acute anterior myocardial infarction: impact of left ventricular shape on regional function: a magnetic resonance myocardial tagging study. *J Am Coll Cardiol* 2000;35(6):1525–1534. doi: 10.1016/S0735-1097(00)00601-X.

Marra MP, Lima JAC, Iliceto S. MRI in acute myocardial infarction. *Eur Heart J* 2011;32(3): 284–293. doi: http://dx.doi.org/10.1093/eurheartj/ehq409. First published online: 26 November 2010. doi: 10.1016/S0735-1097(00)00601-X.

2b Answer E.   A severly decreased ejection measures less than 35%. Patients with a severly decreased ejection fractions are at higher risk for arrhythmia and may require device placements (AICD's).

3a Answer C.   The three-chamber image shows narrowing along the left ventricular outflow tract. There is also dephasing artifact along the left ventricular outflow tract indicating turbulent flow and velocity elevation in this patient with a diagnosis of hypertrophic cardiomyopathy.

References: Bogaert J, Olivotto I. MR Imaging in Hypertrophic Cardiomyopathy: from Magnet to Bedside. *Radiology* 2014;273(2):329-348. doi: 10.1148/radiol.14131626.

Chun EJ, et al. Hypertrophic cardiomyopathy: assessment with MR imaging and multidetector CT. *Radiographics* 2010;30(5):1309-1328. doi: 10.1148/rg.305095074.

3b **Answer B.** Patients with hypertrophic cardiomyopathy have an increased myocardial mass, an elongated mitral valve leaflet, and decreased left ventricular compliance. The increased mass makes it difficult for blood to fill the left ventricle during diastole and leads to diastolic dysfunction. Patients with diastolic dysfunction have increased left atrial pressure and an increased left atrial kick in an attempt to further fill the left ventricle.

References: Bogaert J, Olivotto I. MR Imaging in Hypertrophic Cardiomyopathy: from Magnet to Bedside. *Radiology* 2014;273(2):329-348. doi: 10.1148/radiol.14131626.

Chun EJ, et al. Hypertrophic cardiomyopathy: assessment with MR imaging and multidetector CT. *Radiographics* 2010;30(5):309-1328. doi: 10.1148/rg.305095074.

3c **Answer D.** Patients with HOCM are at risk for sudden cardiac death. The features most associated with cardiac death include prior cardiac arrest, recurrent syncope, family history of cardiac death, left ventricular hypertrophy (wall thickness > 30 mm), and increased pressure along the left ventricular outflow tract gradient (30 mm Hg).

References: Bogaert J, Olivotto I. MR Imaging in Hypertrophic Cardiomyopathy: from Magnet to Bedside. *Radiology* 2014;273(2):329-348. doi: 10.1148/radiol.14131626.

Chun EJ, et al. Hypertrophic cardiomyopathy: assessment with MR imaging and multidetector CT. *Radiographics* 2010;30(5):1309-1328. doi: 10.1148/rg.305095074.

Frenneaux MP. Assessing the risk of sudden cardiac death in a patient with hypertrophic cardiomyopathy. *Heart* 2004;90(5):570-575. doi: 10.1136/hrt.2003.020529.

4 **Answer C.** During isovolumetric contraction of the ventricles, the pressure within the ventricle rises; however, the volume within the ventricle does not change. During isovolumetric contraction, the tricuspid and mitral valves are closed. The pressure in the ventricles, however, is not yet greater than the systemic pressure, and as a result, the aortic and pulmonic valves are closed.

References: http://www.cvphysiology.com/Heart%20Disease/HD002b.htm

http://www.austincc.edu/emeyerth/isovolum.htm

5 **Answer B.** Atrial systole occurs when the small amount of muscle within the atria contract correlating to the "P" wave on an EKG. During atrial systole, atrial contraction, in combination with decreased ventricular pressure, contributes to up to 20% to 30% of blood flowing into the ventricles. Atrial systole, therefore, contributes to ventricular volume, which increases the preload, not the afterload.

Reference: http://www.cvphysiology.com/Heart%20Disease/HD002a.htm

6 **Answer C.** Preload is altered by the volume of blood within the ventricle. Factors that increase central venous return will increase blood in the ventricle and thereby increase the preload. A noncompliant ventricle will cause less blood to be in the ventricle. An elevated heart rate will afford less time and less blood to fill the ventricle. Ligating a fistula will decrease venous return, thereby decreasing blood volume and preload. Reduced atrial pressure and decreased atrial contraction will result in less blood filling the ventricles and a reduced preload.

References: Suzanne C, O'Connell S, Bare BG, et al. *Brunner & Suddarth's textbook of medical-surgical nursing, Volume 1*, 2010:824.

http://cvphysiology.com/Cardiac%20Function/CF007.htm

7 Answer C. During a phase contrast acquisition, the Venc should be set at a value greater than the maximum expected velocity. Once the sequence is started, protons in the blood will experience a phase shift proportional to their velocity, while non moving objects have no phase shift in response to the pulses. If the velocity of blood is higher than the Venc, the phase shift will be >180 degrees and aliasing will occur. As long as the Venc is larger than the fastest velocity of blood, no aliasing will occur.

References: Ferreira PF, et al. Cardiovascular magnetic resonance artefacts. *J Cardiovas Magn Reson* 2013;15:41. doi: 10.1186/1532-429X-15-41.

Lee VS. *Cardiovascular MR: Physical principles to practical protocols*. Lippincott Williams & Wilkins, 2006;206.

8 Answer D. Metoprolol is a type of beta blocker that can be administered orally or intravenously to patients undergoing cardiac CTA. Metoprolol acts by selectively blocking the beta-1 receptor. As a result, the heart rate and blood pressure will decrease and it will have a net negative ionotropic effect on the heart.

References: Marx JA. "Cardiovascular drugs". *Rosen's emergency medicine: concepts and clinical practice*, 8th ed. Philadelphia, PA: Elsevier/Saunders, 2014. Chapter 152. ISBN 1455706051.

http://www.nlm.nih.gov/medlineplus/druginfo/meds/a682864.html

9a Answer C. The image shows a tricuspid aortic valve at end ventricular systole in a patient with severe aortic stenosis. The valve leaflets are thickened and calcified with only a small open valve area. Severe aortic stenosis is diagnosed with a valve area measuring <1.0 cm^2 (by valve planimetry). Other values characteristic of aortic stenosis can be quantified by cardiac MRI and include a velocity gradient >40 mm Hg or a velocity jet >4.0 m/sec.

References: Feuchtner G. Imaging of cardiac valves by computed tomography. *Scientifica* 2013;2013:13. Article ID 270579. doi: 10.1155/2013/270579.

John AS. Magnetic resonance to assess the aortic valve area in aortic stenosis: how does it compare to current diagnostic standards? *J Am Coll Cardiol* 2003;42(3):519–526. doi: 10.1016/S0735-1097(03)00707-1.

9b Answer D. The pressure gradient can be calculated using the modified Bernoulli equation (pressure gradient (mm Hg) = $4v_{max}^2$) where the maximum velocity (v_{max}) is reported in meters per second

Using the above equation and values: 150 cm/sec = 1.5 m/sec
Pressure gradient = $4(1.5 \text{ m/sec})^2$
Pressure gradient = 9 mm Hg

References: Feuchtner G. Imaging of cardiac valves by computed tomography. *Scientifica* 2013;2013:13. Article ID 270579. doi: 10.1155/2013/270579.

John AS. Magnetic resonance to assess the aortic valve area in aortic stenosis: how does it compare to current diagnostic standards? *J Am Coll Cardiol* 2003;42(3):519–526. doi: 10.1016/S0735-1097(03)00707-1.

10a Answer C. The image shows an aortic valve in diastole. At this moment, the aortic valve should be fully closed (complete coaptation); however, centrally, the valve is open. Incomplete coaptation of the valve is a sign of aortic insufficiency. Aortic insufficiency will result in an increased end diastolic volume and ventricular dilation secondary to backflow of blood from the aorta into the ventricle. The severity of aortic insufficiency can be quantified by cardiac MRI using a phase contrast sequence.

References: Cawley PJ, et al. Valvular heart disease: changing concepts in disease management cardiovascular magnetic resonance imaging for valvular heart disease technique and validation. *Circulation* 2009;119:468–478. doi: 10.1161/CIRCULATIONAHA.107.742486.

Feuchtner G. Imaging of cardiac valves by computed tomography. *Scientifica* 2013;2013:13. Article ID 270579. doi: 10.1155/2013/270579

10b Answer C. Aortic insufficiency can be graded from mild to severe. Severe aortic insufficiency can be diagnosed by a regurgitant volume >60 mL/beat or a regurgitant fraction >50%. Other features associated with aortic insufficiency include holodiastolic flow reversal in the descending aorta, incomplete leaflet coaptation, increased end-diastolic volume, and ventricular dilation.

References: Cawley PJ, et al. Valvular heart disease: changing concepts in disease management cardiovascular magnetic resonance imaging for valvular heart disease technique and validation. *Circulation* 2009;119:468-478. doi: 10.1161/CIRCULATIONAHA.107.742486.

Maurer G. Aortic regurgitation. *Heart* 2006;92(7):994-1000. doi: 10.1136/hrt.2004.042614.

11a Answer B. The image is from a phase contrast cardiac MRI acquisition. The sequence produces two data sets (magnitude image and phase velocity maps). When acquiring the data set, the user sets the Venc (velocity range measured by the sequence). The Venc should be set at a value greater than the maximum expected velocity. If the actual velocity is greater than the Venc, aliasing will occur. This can be solved by repeating the sequence with a higher Venc.

References: Ferreira PF, et al. Cardiovascular magnetic resonance artefacts. *J Cardiovas Magn Reson* 2013;15:41. doi: 10.1186/1532-429X-15-41.

Lee VS. *Cardiovascular MR: Physical principles to practical protocols*. Lippincott Williams & Wilkins, 2006:206.

11b Answer A. The phase contrast cardiac MRI acquisition produces two data sets (magnitude image and phase velocity maps). The images are viewed and the vessel of interest is evaluated with contour lines placed over the area of interest.

References: Ferreira PF, et al. Cardiovascular magnetic resonance artefacts. *J Cardiovas Magn Reson* 2013;15:41. doi: 10.1186/1532-429X-15-41.

Lee VS. *Cardiovascular MR: Physical Principles to practical protocols*. Lippincott Williams & Wilkins, 2006:206.

12 Answer B. Beta blockers are negative inotropic agents. As a result, once beta blockers are administered, they will decrease myocardial contractility. The Frank-Starling curve is a graphical tool that shows how cardiac output changes in response to changes in heart rate or stroke volume. The administration of beta blockers will reduce contractility and heart rate resulting in a shift of the curve down and to the right. A positive inotrope would shift the curve up and to the left.

References: Marx JA. *"Cardiovascular drugs". Rosen's emergency medicine: Concepts and clinical practice*, 8th ed. Philadelphia, PA: Elsevier/Saunders, 2014. Chapter 152. ISBN 1455706051.

http://www.nlm.nih.gov/medlineplus/druginfo/meds/a682864.html

http://www.cvphysiology.com/Cardiac%20Function/CF003.htm

13a Answer A. The image shows an unroofed coronary sinus with abnormal connection between the left atrium and the coronary sinus. This results in a left to right shunt with a connection between the left and right atrium via the coronary sinus defect. An unroofed coronary sinus can be associated with a left SVC.

References: Kim H, Choe YH, Park SW, et al. Partially unroofed coronary sinus: MDCT and MRI findings. *AJR Am J Roentgenol* 2010;195(5):W331-W336. doi: 10.2214/AJR.09.3689.

Ootaki Y, et al. Unroofed coronary sinus syndrome: diagnosis, classification and surgical treatment. *J Thorac Cardiovas Surg* 2003;126(5):1655-1656.

13b Answer A. The Qp/Qs is the ratio of the flow in the pulmonary circulation to the flow in the systemic circulation. It is obtained by using phase contrast sequence to measure the flow in the pulmonary artery and the aorta. A Qp/Qs value of 1.5 or greater suggests the shunt is significant and may trigger an intervention.

References: Kim H, Choe YH, Park SW, et al. Partially unroofed coronary sinus: MDCT and MRI findings. *AJR Am J Roentgenol* 2010;195(5):W331–W336. doi: 10.2214/AJR.09.3689.

Ootaki Y, et al. Unroofed coronary sinus syndrome: diagnosis, classification and surgical treatment. *J Thorac Cardiovas Surg* 2003;126(5):1655–1656.

Rajiah P, Kanne JP. Cardiac MRI: Part 1, cardiovascular shunts. *AJR Am J Roentgenol* 2011;197(4):W603–W620. doi: 10.2214/AJR.10.7257.

14 Answer C. The patient has a prior cardiac stent in the right coronary artery. The left main coronary artery contains noncalcified plaque, which narrows the lumen by 50%. Stenosis of 50% or greater in the left main coronary artery or of either coronary ostia will cause a significant reduction in flow (significant stenosis). The left main coronary artery gives rise to the left anterior descending and left circumflex coronary arteries. Given that the stenosis is proximal to these vessels, these territories will have perfusion defects.

References: Fathala A. Myocardial perfusion scintigraphy: techniques, interpretation, indications and reporting. *Ann Saudi Med* 2011;31(6):625–634. doi: 10.4103/0256-4947.87101.

Kinis S, et al. Normal and variant coronary arterial and venous anatomy on high-resolution CT angiography. *AJR Am J Roentgenol* 2007;188:1665–1674.

15a Answer D. The image shows noncalcified plaque in the proximal right coronary artery. The plaque causes more than 70% narrowing of the proximal right coronary artery indicating a significant stenosis and the territory likely to contain a perfusion defect.

References: Fathala A. Myocardial perfusion scintigraphy: techniques, interpretation, indications and reporting. *Ann Saudi Med* 2011;31(6):625–634. doi: 10.4103/0256-4947.87101.

Kinis S, et al. Normal and variant coronary arterial and venous anatomy on high-resolution CT angiography. *AJR Am J Roentgenol* 2007;188:1665–1674.

15b Answer D. A flow-limiting stenosis by CTA that does not involve the ostium or left main correlates with stenosis >70%. Plaque causing 70% on CCTA are likely to cause compromised flow when evaluated by invasive coronary angiography.

References: Kinis S, et al. Normal and variant coronary arterial and venous anatomy on high-resolution CT angiography. *AJR Am J Roentgenol* 2007;188:1665–1674.

http://www.scct.org/advocacy/coverage/PubGuidelines.pdf

16 Answer B. Sublingual nitroglycerin is given to dilate the coronary arteries thereby improving their visualization. In particular, sublingual nitroglycerin helps improve the visualization of the distal divisions of the coronary arteries. Beta blockers are given to decrease motion of the coronary arteries. No medication is routinely given to improve ventricular function or decrease radiation dose.

References: Chun EJ, et al. Effects of nitroglycerin on the diagnostic accuracy of electrocardiogram-gated coronary computed tomography angiography. *J Comput Assist Tomogr* 2008;32(1):86–92. doi: 10.1097/rct.0b013e318059befa.

Decramer I, et al. Effects of sublingual nitroglycerin on coronary lumen diameter and number of visualized septal branches on 64-MDCT angiography. *Am J Roentgenol* 2008;190:219–225.

17 Answer A. Sublingual nitroglycerin should not be administered to a patient who has taken sildenafil within 24 hours secondary to the risk of severe hypotension. Sublingual nitroglycerin dilates the coronary arteries and improves their visualization. If a patient has taken tadalafil, sublingual nitroglycerin should be administered for at least 48 hours due to the longer half-life of the drug and the risk of hypotension.

References: Cheitlin MD, Hutter AM, Brindis RG, et al. ACC/AHA Expert Consensus Document. Use of sildenafil (viagra) in patients with cardiovascular disease. *Circulation* 1999;99:168–177. doi: 10.1161/01.CIR.99.1.168.

Kloner RA, et al. Time course of the interaction between tadalafil and nitrates. *J Am Coll Cardiol* 2003;42(10):1855–1860.

18 Answer D. The image shows a two-chamber view of the left ventricle. There is delayed enhancement along the anterior wall from the base to the apex and along the inferior wall at the apex.

The remainder of the inferior wall is normal. This distribution of infarction can occur if the left anterior descending coronary artery wraps around the apex. A right coronary artery territory infarct could not cause the extensive involvement of the anterior wall. An anomalous left circumflex coronary artery infarct would involve the inferolateral wall, which is not shown on this image.

References: Hoyt J. Left anterior descending artery length and coronary atherosclerosis in apical ballooning syndrome (Takotsubo/stress induced cardiomyopathy). *Int J Cardiol* 2010;145(1): 112-115. doi: 10.1016/j.ijcard.2009.06.018. Epub 2009 Jul 1.

Kinis S, et al. Normal and variant coronary arterial and venous anatomy on high-resolution CT angiography. *AJR Am J Roentgenol* 2007;188:1665-1674.

19a Answer D. The balanced steady-state image in the three-chamber plane shows a linear low signal structure extending into the left ventricular outflow tract just below the aortic valve. This image is most indicative of a subaortic membrane. The mitral valve is normal, and the myocardium and the septum are normal. The subaortic membrane can obstruct the left ventricular outflow tract and if symptomatic can be resected. Membranes can recur after treatment and are associated with congenial heart disease (ventricular septal defect, patent ductus arteriosus and coarctation of the aorta).

References: Tarcin OT, et al. Discrete subaortic stenosis. *Tex Heart Inst J* 2003;30(4):286-292.

http://www.uptodate.com/contents/subvalvar-aortic-stenosis-subaortic-stenosis

19b Answer B. A subaortic membrane can obstruct flow across the aortic valve, and its physiologic effects can be similar. The membrane can cause turbulent flow across the left ventricular outflow tract with the decreased flow across the valve leading to a reduced ejection fraction. The obstruction can lead to increased mitral regurgitation if the process is long standing or if the obstruction is significant. There is no impact on inotropy of the heart.

References: Aboulhosn J, Child JS. Left ventricular outflow obstruction: subaortic stenosis, bicuspid aortic valve, supravalvar aortic stenosis, and coarctation of the Aorta. *Circulation* 2006;114: 2412-2422. doi: 10.1161/CIRCULATIONAHA.105.592089.

http://www.cardioaccess.com/OpImages/Diagrams/diagSM.html

20 Answer C. The ejection fraction is calculated by the following formula:

[(End Diastolic Volume − End Diastolic Volume) / End Diastolic Volume] × 100

EF = (100 − 40) / 100 × 100

EF = 60%

At end diastole, the ventricular volume will be at its maximum, while at end systole, the ventricular volume will be at its minimum. The difference between these entities is the stroke volume. A normal ejection fraction measures 55%. A diminished ejection fraction can be associated with reduced mortality and an increased of developing ventricular thrombus or arrhythmia.

Reference: Guyton AC, Hall JE. *Textbook of medical physiology*, 11th ed. Elsevier Saunders, 2006:108. ISBN 0-7216-0240-1.

21 Answer D. Atrial fibrillation is the most common sustained arrhythmia, and its incidence is increasing with the progressively aging population. Atrial fibrillation can be associated with stroke, and up to 20% to 25% of strokes are caused by atrial fibrillation. In atrial fibrillation, the atria are constantly being activated in a chaotic manner by arrhythmogenic foci at the pulmonary vein ostia, the coronary sinus, or along the atria. The electrical impulses bypass the normal electrical coordinated conduction process that begins in the SA node. This results in too many signals reaching the AV node and ventricles resulting in the ventricles beating too fast (>100 beats/min).

References: Schotten U, et al. Pathophysiological mechanisms of atrial fibrillation: a translational appraisal. *Am Physiol Soc* 2011;91(1):265-325. doi: 10.1152/physrev.00031.2009.

Waktare J. Cardiology patient page: atrial fibrillation. *Circulation* 2002;106:14-16. doi: 10.1161/01.CIR.0000022730.66617.D9.

22 **Answer A.** Cardiac MRI (CMRI) can be used to calculate myocardial mass by calculating the difference between epicardial and endocardial volumes and multiplying the value by the specific density of the myocardium (1.05 g/mL). CMR accurately quantifies myocardial mass because the entire myocardium can be visualized and high spatial resolution.

References: Bezante GP, et al. Left ventricular myocardial mass determination by contrast enhanced colour Doppler compared with magnetic resonance imaging. *Heart* 2005;91(1):38-43. doi: 10.1136/hrt.2003.023234.

Higgins CB, Sakuma H. Heart disease: functional evaluation with MR imaging. *Radiology* 1996;199:307-315.

23 **Answer B.** Diastolic dysfunction occurs when the left ventricle cannot fill with blood during ventricular diastole secondary to ventricular stiffness or impaired ventricular relaxation. As a result, the stroke volume and end diastolic volume are reduced, and patients have heart failure with a normal ejection fraction. The left atrium will progressively enlarge during the course of diastolic dysfunction.

References: European Study Group on Diastolic Heart Failure. How to diagnose diastolic heart failure. *Eur Heart J* 1998;19:990-1003.

Zile MR, Brutsaert DL. Clinical cardiology: new frontiers new concepts in diastolic dysfunction and diastolic heart failure: part I diagnosis, prognosis, and measurements of diastolic function. *Circulation* 2002;105:1387-1393. doi: 10.1161/hc1102.105289.

24 **Answer C.** A chamber measuring >5.5 cm is considered dilated. Dilated cardiomyopathy (DCM) can also manifest with heterogeneous wall thickness, wall thinning, preserved right ventricular mass, and late gadolinium enhancement. Three patterns of late gadolinium enhancement can occur and include mid wall late gadolinium enhancement, subendocardial delayed enhancement or no late gadolinium enhancement.

References: Francone M. Role of cardiac magnetic resonance in the evaluation of dilated cardiomyopathy: diagnostic contribution and prognostic significance. *ISRN Radiol* 2014;2014:16. Article ID 365404. doi: 10.1155/2014/365404.

McCrohon JA, Moon JCC, Prasad SK, et al. Differentiation of heart failure related to dilated cardiomyopathy and coronary artery disease using gadolinium-enhanced cardiovascular magnetic resonance. *Circulation* 2003;108(1):54-59.

25a **Answer B.** The image shows a myxoma adjacent to the inflow of the left inferior pulmonary vein partially blocking its inflow to the left atrium. The most common location for a cardiac myxoma is the left atrium, and while it can be attached to the interatrial septum via a broad base, it can prolapse through the mitral valve, embolize or obstruct the pulmonary veins.

References: Grebenec ML, et al. Cardiac myxoma: imaging features in 83 patients. *Radiographics* 2002;22(3):673-689.

Stevens LH, et al. Left atrial myxoma: pulmonary infarction caused by pulmonary venous occlusion. *Ann Thorac Surg* 1987;43(2):215-217.

25b Answer A. Hemodynamics are an essential part of cardiac physiology. Normal values for the heart include

RA, 1-8 mm Hg; LA, 4-12 mm Hg
RV, 15-30/1-8 mm Hg; LV, 100-140/4-12 mm Hg
PA, 15-30/4-12 mm Hg; Ao, 100-140/60-80 mm Hg

When the pulmonary capillary wedge pressure, which is usually similar to the left atrial pressure, approaches 20 mm, the patient will develop interstitial edema, and when the value is >20 mm Hg, the patient will have alveolar edema.

Reference: Grossman W (ed.). *Cardiac catheterization and angiography*, 3rd ed. Philadelphia, PA: Lea & Febiger, 1986. http://www.uptodate.com/contents/cardiac-catheterization-techniques-normal-hemodynamics

26 Answer B. Aortic insufficiency will result in an increased stroke volume, increased preload (due to the volume from the regurgitant fraction), progressive dilation of the left ventricular cavity (from the regurgitant volume), increased afterload (initially due to the increased pressure needed by the myocardium to eject the increased blood volume), and loss of an isovolumetric relaxation phase since blood is continuously entering the ventricle.

Reference: Bekeredjian R, Grayburn PA. Contemporary reviews in cardiovascular medicine valvular heart disease aortic regurgitation. *Circulation* 2005;112:125-134. doi: 10.1161/CIRCULATIONAHA.104.488825.

27 Answer B. The heart of competitive athletes can undergo a series of changes secondary to the cardiovascular activity. In most cases, the left atrium, left ventricle, and right ventricle will dilate and the myocardial mass will increase.

Reference: Maron BJ, Pelliccia A. Contemporary reviews in cardiovascular medicine the heart of trained athletes cardiac remodeling and the risks of sports, including sudden death. *Circulation* 2006;114:1633-1644. doi: 10.1161/CIRCULATIONAHA.106.613562.

4 Ischemic Heart Disease

QUESTIONS

1. In the below images the abnormality of the right coronary artery is most closely associated with which of the following in this patient with chest pain but no EKG changes?

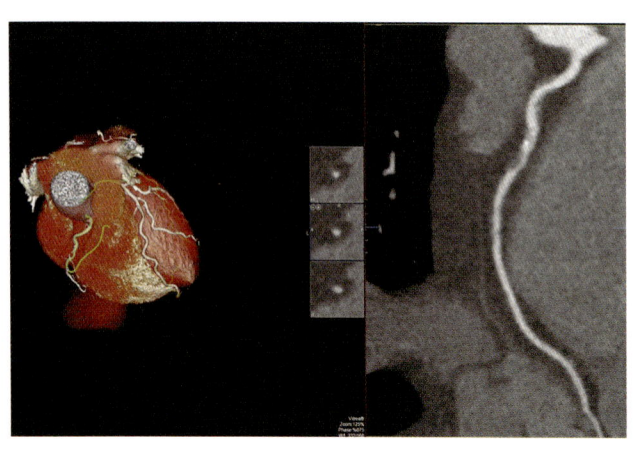
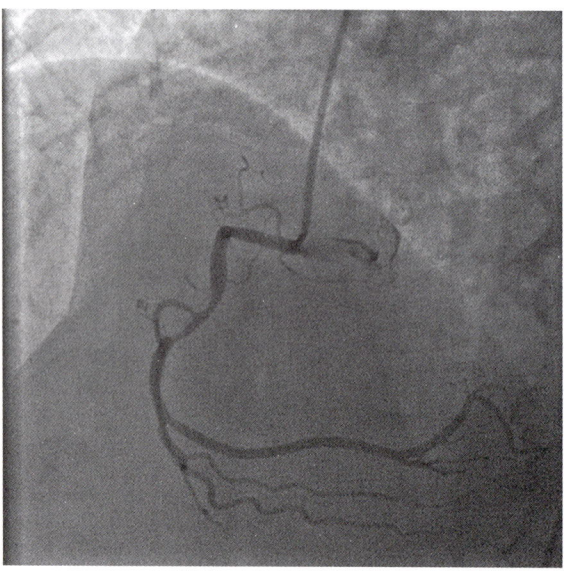

   A. Lateral wall hypokinesis
   B. Significant restriction of blood flow to the inferior wall
   C. RCA occlusion
   D. ST elevation myocardial infarction (STEMI)

2. The use of which of the following drugs precludes the use of sublingual nitroglycerin for cardiac CTA?

   A. Metformin
   B. Sildenafil
   C. Diltiazem
   D. Atorvastatin

3   What treatment could be initiated for the condition shown in this patient with chest pain with exercise?

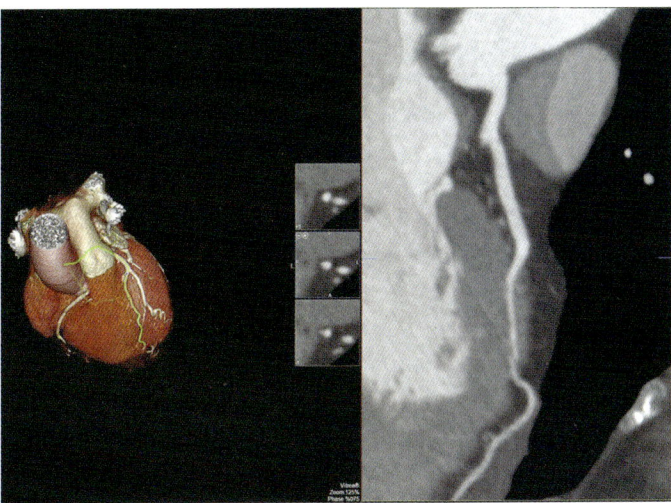

A. Sublingual nitroglycerin
B. Digoxin
C. Adenosine
D. Beta blockers

4   How many coronary artery bypass grafts were placed in this patient on this image?

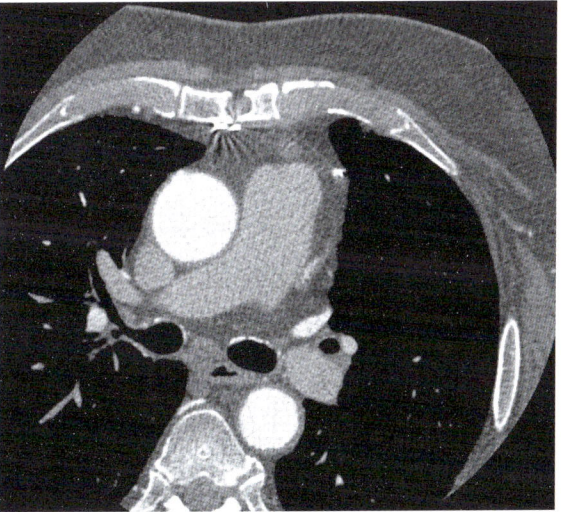

A. None
B. At least 1
C. At least 2
D. At least 3

5   What statement is correct regarding the patency of bypass grafts at 10 years?

A. LIMA > SVG
B. LIMA < SVG
C. LIMA = SVG
D. Indeterminate

6 A coronary CTA is ordered for a 72-year-old patient with shortness of breath. As part of the examination, a calcium score is performed and the below image is obtained. (Total calcium score is calculated at 2,286 Agatston units.) Which of the following conclusions is accurate?

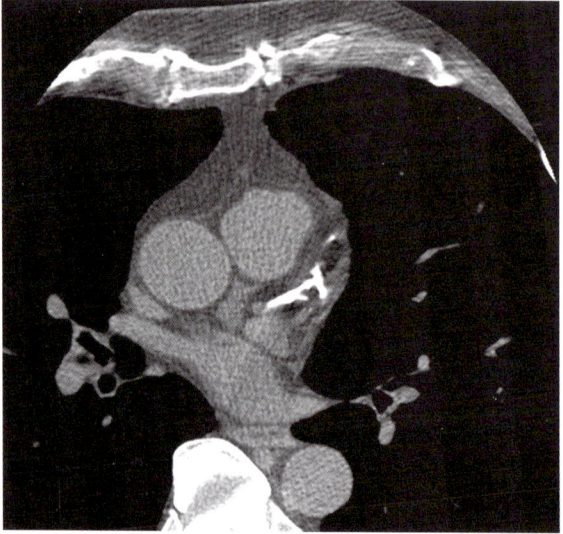

A. The patient has atherosclerotic plaque.
B. High-grade stenosis is likely.
C. The patient is at low risk for a coronary event.
D. Aortic stenosis is likely.

7 The following scan parameters were used to obtain the image in a patient with a heart rate of 60 beats per minute: kVp = 120; mA = 700; gantry rotation speed = 320 msec; contrast volume = 80 mL; contrast rate = 6.5 mL/sec; and slice width = 0.625 mm. The poor image quality in this case is most likely from

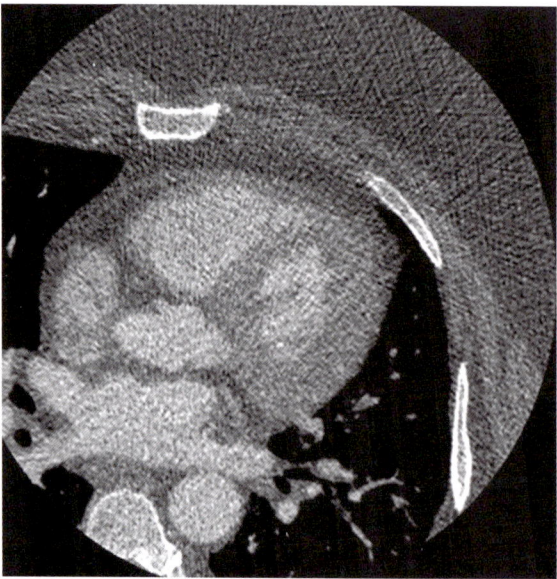

A. Poor temporal resolution
B. Increased body mass index
C. Incorrect contrast timing
D. Too high spatial resolution

8   A 66-year-old patient is status post myocardial infarction 2 days ago. Which of the following conclusions can be made?

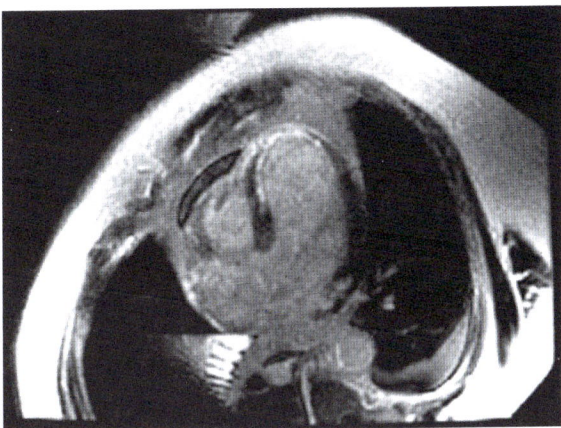

A. There is thrombus at the apex.
B. The septal myocardium is viable.
C. The lesion was most likely in the left circumflex coronary artery.
D. The septum is normokinetic.

9   A 50-year-old male with no past medical history presents for coronary CTA. What is the treatment of choice for the lesion in the left main coronary artery?

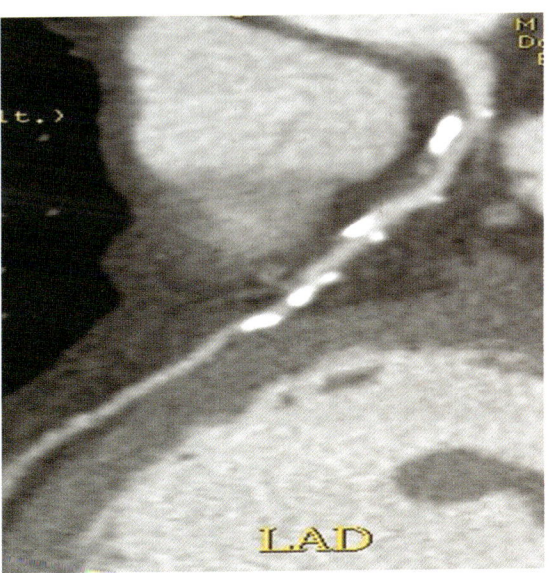
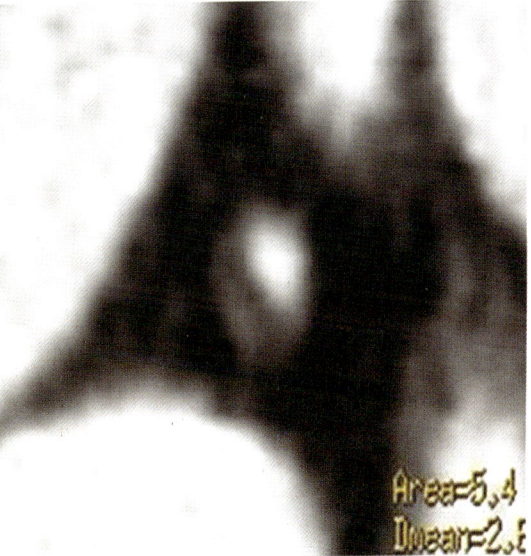

A. Angioplasty
B. Stenting
C. Bypass grafting
D. Lifestyle modification and statin therapy

10 Which of the following statements is correct regarding the area of low signal in the anterior wall on this delayed enhancement sequence?

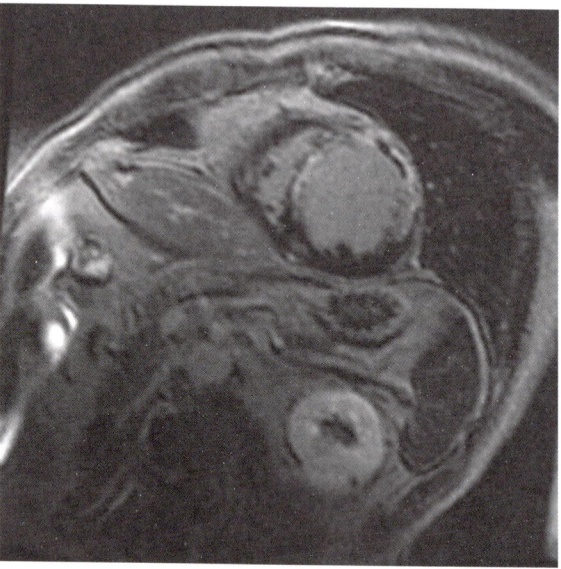

A. It is an area of normal nulled myocardium.
B. It represents an area without reflow and carries a less favorable prognosis.
C. It represents hibernating myocardium.
D. It indicates that a suboptimal inversion time was used during acquisition.

11 Which of the following clinical scenarios is an appropriate indication for coronary CTA based on current Appropriateness Criteria Guidelines?

A. Acute myocardial infarction with ST elevation
B. Preoperative clearance for orthopedic surgery in a 70-year-old male with diabetes
C. Persistent symptoms (chest pain) with a normal ECG stress test
D. Coronary CTA in a patient with a known 2.0-mm stent in the LAD to assess disease

12 A 40-year-old female patient presents to the ER with chest pain, negative cardiac enzyme tests and a normal EKG. A review of the medical record reveals she presented 2 months prior with similar symptoms. At that time, she underwent a coronary CTA, which was normal. What is the next step?

A. Repeat coronary CTA
B. Admission and stress test
C. Catheter angiography
D. Evaluate for possible noncardiac causes of chest pain.

13 A 39-year-old male with no past medical history presents to the ER with chest pain. The workup reveals a normal ECG and negative cardiac enzymes. He undergoes a coronary CTA angiogram (shown below). Based on the images and clinical trials, which of the following is a reasonable plan of disposition?

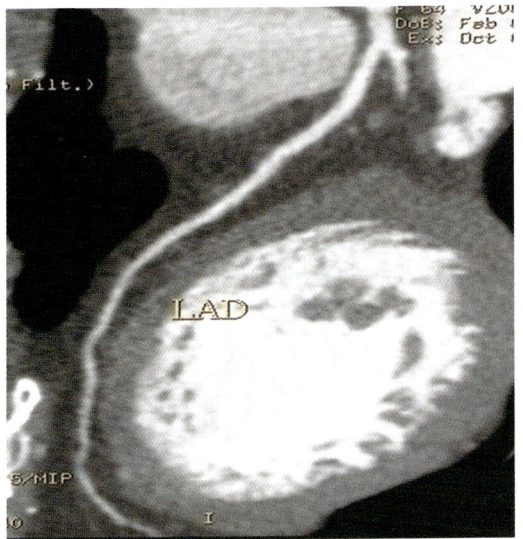
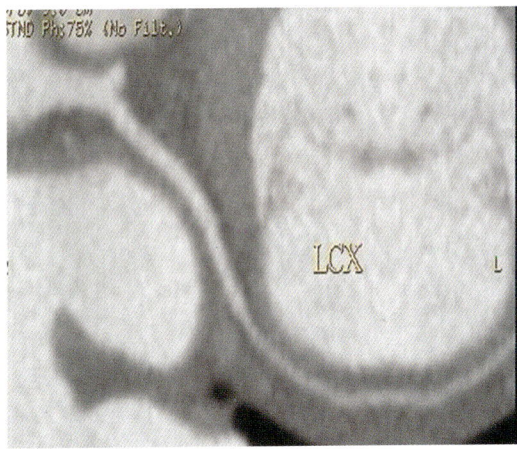
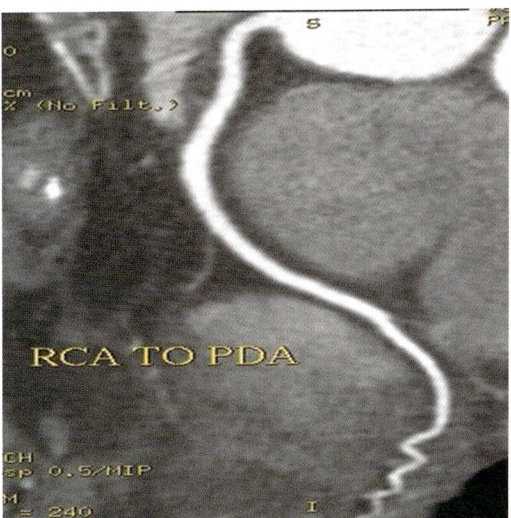

A. Discharge to home
B. Admit to telemetry
C. Stress test
D. Cardiology consult for possible catheterization

14 A patient presents for cardiac MRI 3 days following myocardial infarction. On admission, catheterization reveals severe stenosis in the left anterior descending and right coronary arteries. On admission day 2, new-onset mitral regurgitation is discovered, and the patient develops right upper lobe pulmonary edema. What complication of infarction should be considered?

A. Aneurysm formation
B. Thrombus formation
C. Papillary muscle infarction
D. Pericardial effusion

15 Which of the following features of the plaque shown deem it high risk for development of an acute coronary syndrome?

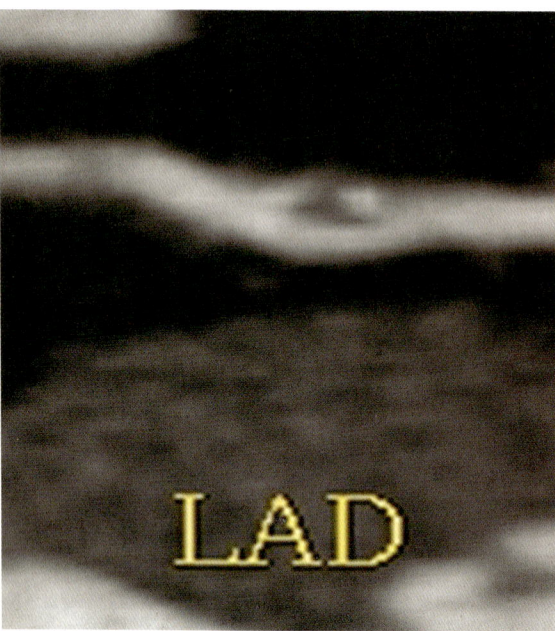

   A. Positive remodeling
   B. Dense calcification
   C. High attenuation centrally
   D. Thick fibrinous cap

16 The image on the right (short axis) was obtained by prescribing a plane in what orientation through the image on the left (four-chamber view)?

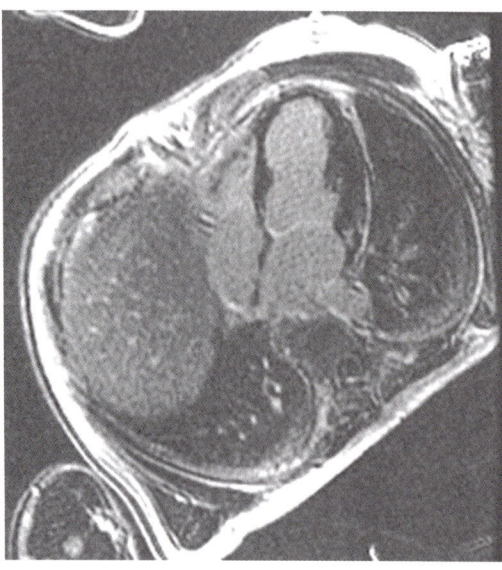 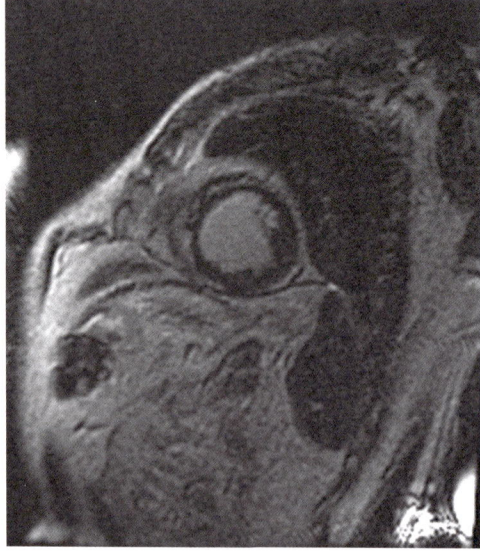

   A. Perpendicular to the LV apex
   B. Perpendicular to the mitral valve
   C. Perpendicular to the left ventricular outflow tract
   D. Perpendicular to the septum and parallel to the mitral valve

17 As time from injection of gadolinium increases during a delayed enhancement sequence, what adjustment, if any, must be made to the inversion time to preserve quality of myocardial nulling?

   A. Increase the inversion time.
   B. Decrease the inversion time.
   C. No change necessary

18 The images below are taken from the same patient. The findings should be reported as

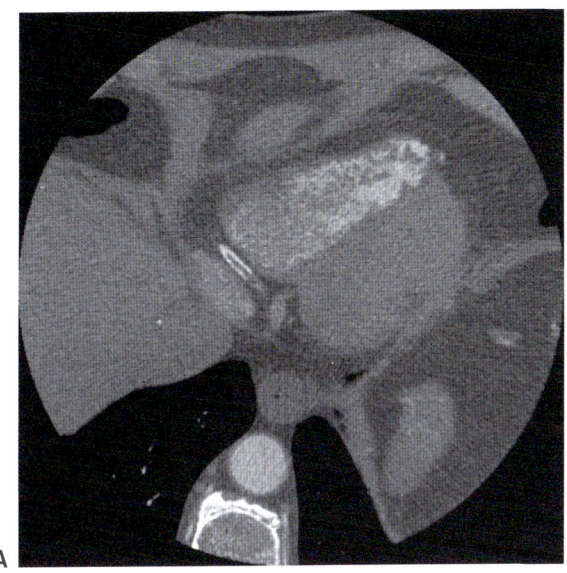
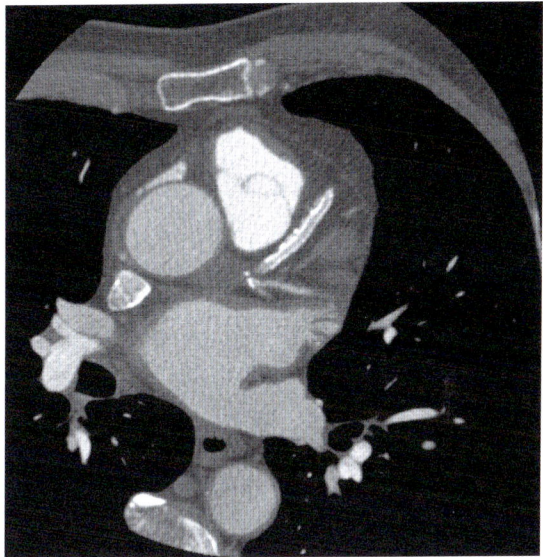

   A. Patent LAD stent and RCA stent
   B. Occluded LAD and RCA stent
   C. Patent LAD stent and occluded RCA stent
   D. Occluded LAD stent and patent RCA stent

19 Stent thrombosis after percutaneous intervention can be due to the failure to comply with which of the following prescribed regimen?

   A. Statin therapy
   B. Inotropic therapy
   C. Beta-blocker therapy
   D. Dual antiplatelet therapy

20 Which stent diameter does sensitivity significantly decrease as it related to the efficacy of coronary CT to detect stent occlusion/stenosis?

   A. 3 mm
   B. 4 mm
   C. 5 mm
   D. 6 mm

21 The placement of the cardiac support devices in the chest radiograph is most often associated with which clinical parameters?

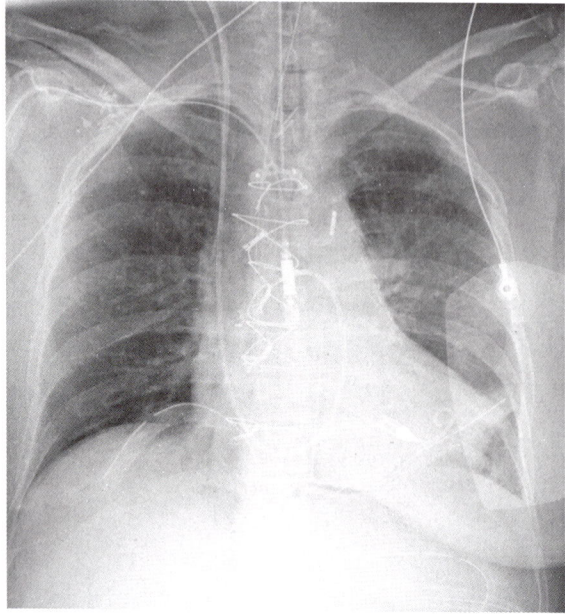

A. Atrial fibrillation
B. Isolated left bundle branch block
C. Acute myocardial infarction with cardiogenic shock
D. Placement of a stent in a patient with stable angina

22 Which of the following statements is correct regarding the left ventricle in this patient post myocardial infarction?

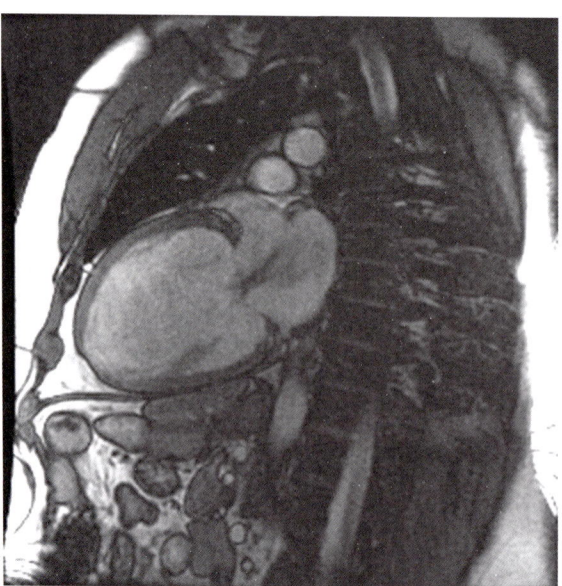

A. Diffuse calcifications in the left ventricle
B. Mitral regurgitation
C. Diffuse fatty deposition in the left ventricle
D. Increased trabeculation in the left ventricle

23 Approximately what percent of dilated cardiomyopathy cases are due to ischemic heart disease?
    A. 0.5% to 1%
    B. 5% to 7%
    C. 15% to 20%
    D. 25% to 30%

24 Suboptimal image quality in this study was most likely secondary to

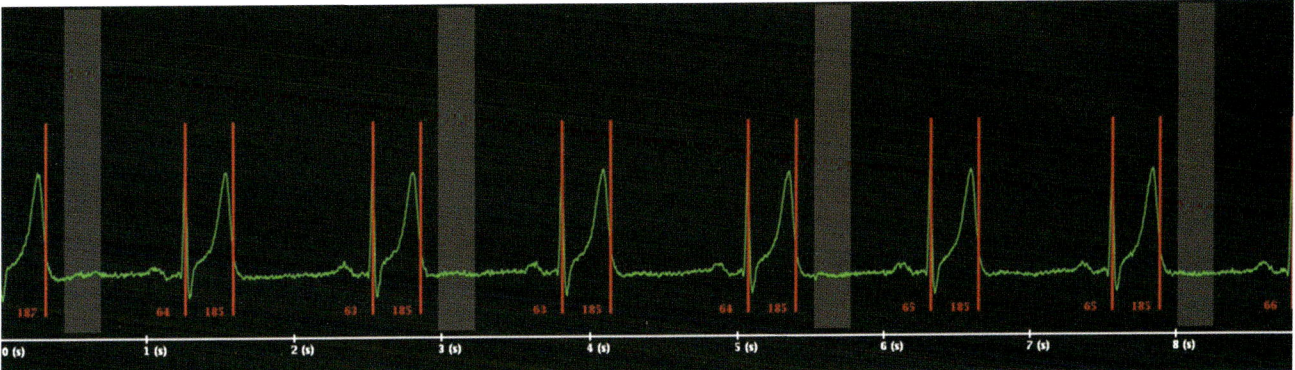

    A. Ventricular bigeminy
    B. Improper triggering
    C. Tachyarrhythmia
    D. Low voltage ECG

25 What is the dose of adenosine typically given for adenosine stress perfusion MRI?
    A. 25 µg/kg/min
    B. 50 µg/kg/min
    C. 100 µg/kg/min
    D. 140 µg/kg/min

26 Percutaneous coronary intervention (PCI) in symptomatic patients with stable coronary artery disease receiving optimal medical therapy has which of the following benefit?
    A. It improves survival.
    B. It decreases future myocardial infarctions (MI).
    C. It improves angina.
    D. It decreases survival.

27 Which of the following patient is best suited for coronary CTA?
    A. 35-year-old female with atypical chest pain during emotion stress
    B. 47-year-old male with history of smoking, family history of CAD, and atypical chest pain
    C. 55-year-old female with history of smoking, atrial fibrillation, and atypical chest pain
    D. 76-year-old male with history of smoking and angina

28a A 47-year-old female with chest pain and no prior cardiac history. Labs show elevated troponin. What is the most likely diagnosis?

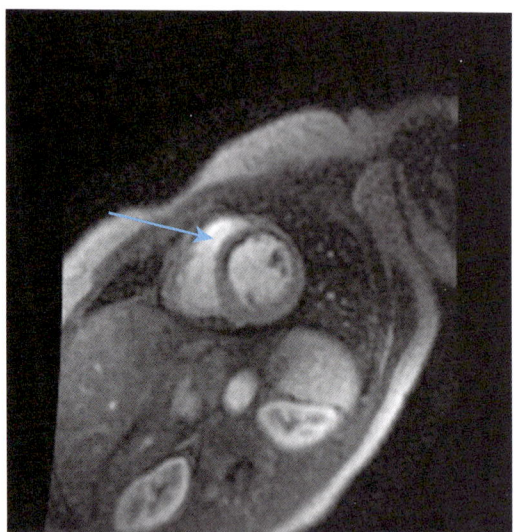
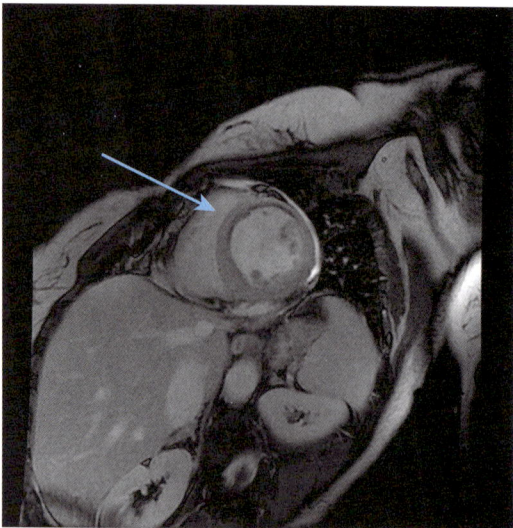
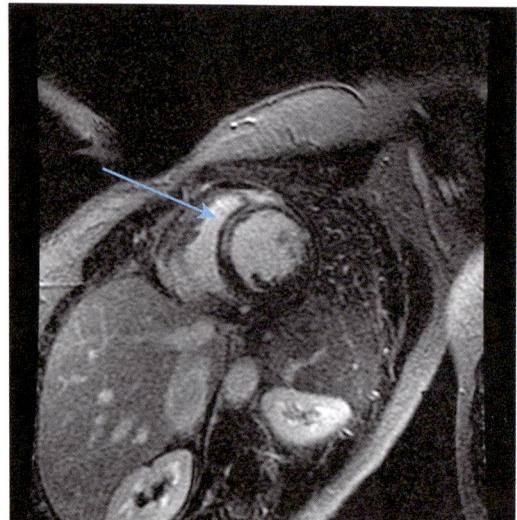

    A. Myocarditis
    B. Acute infarct
    C. Cardiac amyloid
    D. Sarcoid
    E. Noncompaction cardiomyopathy

28b What vascular territory does this abnormality involve?
    A. LAD
    B. LCX
    C. PDA
    D. PLV

28c Compared to a regular infarct, what is the prognosis of infarct with microvascular obstruction?
    A. It is worse than regular infarct.
    B. It is better than a regular infarct.
    C. It is the same as a regular infarct.

ANSWERS AND EXPLANATIONS

1 Answer B. The curved multiplanar reformat of the RCA (right-dominant system) demonstrates mixed plaque within the proximal vessel resulting in severe (roughly 80%) stenosis. A more proximal lesion consisting of noncalcified plaque causes 40% to 50% stenosis. A lesion is considered hemodynamically significant if it causes >70% stenosis. This is based on myocardial blood flow studies. The lateral wall is perfused by the circumflex, not the RCA. Contrast is noted throughout the lumen indicating partial patency. STEMI is caused by acute plaque rupture and acute total occlusion.

Reference: Uren NG, Melin JA, De Bruyne B, et al. Relation between myocardial blood flow and severity of coronary-artery stenosis. *N Engl J Med* 1994;330(25):1782–1788.

2 Answer B. During coronary CTA, sublingual nitroglycerin (SL NTG) is given for coronary artery dilation. Use of phosphodiesterase inhibitors serves as a contraindication for SL NTG administration because of possible hypotension. A review of the patient's medication list is mandatory prior to performing coronary CTA.

Reference: http://www.ctisus.com/learning/pearls/cardiac/patient-prep:-beta-blockers,-iv-contrast,-etc

3 Answer D. The curved multiplanar reformat of the LAD shows a long-segment intramyocardial bridge in the mid LAD. This is the most common site for bridging. Studies show that there is increased likelihood of ischemia with increasing depth and length of the bridge. Initial treatment is with beta blockers to unload the left ventricle. Refractory cases may be referred to surgery for unroofing.

References: Nakanishi R, et al. Myocardial bridging on coronary CTA: an innocent bystander or a culprit in myocardial infarction? *JCCT* 2012;6:3–13.

Vliegen HW, Jukema JW, Bruschke AVG. *Congenital coronary artery anomalies. Anatomy, diagnosis, and management*. Leiden, The Netherlands: TTMA B.V., 2012.

4 Answer C. The image shows a "nubbin" from an occluded vein graft arising from the aorta. Additionally, the left internal mammary artery (LIMA) is not along the chest wall like the right one, indicating that the LIMA has been used as a graft to (most likely) the LAD.

Reference: Frazier A, et al. Coronary artery bypass grafts: assessment with multidetector CT in the early and late postoperative settings. *Radiographics* 2005;25:881–896.

5 Answer A. Graft at 10 years was 61% for saphenous vein grafts compared with 85% for internal mammary artery grafts ($p < 0.001$).

Reference: Goldman, et al. *J Am Coll Cardiol* 2004;44(11):2149–2156.

6 Answer A. Coronary artery calcification occurs in proportion to underlying plaque burden but not degree of stenosis. While it has been shown that a calcium score of >100 AU carries a 5× increased risk of a coronary event than a score <100, the presence of high-grade stenosis cannot be accurately determined on a calcium score image alone, as this does not account for occult noncalcified plaque. Additionally, it is possible that calcium is mostly intramural and does not cause significant luminal narrowing.

References: Guerci AD, et al. Relation of coronary calcium score by electron beam computed tomography to arteriographic findings in asymptomatic and symptomatic adults. *Am J Cardiol* 1997;79:128–133.

Yadon, et al. *J Am Coll Cardiol* 2005;46(1):158–165.

7 Answer B. All scan parameters listed above are within reasonable protocol limits. The body habitus in this patient, however, is causing significant attenuation of the x-ray and increased image noise. BMI > 39 can potentially lead to nondiagnostic studies and is a relative contraindication.

Reference: Raff, et al. SCCT guidelines on the use of coronary computed tomographic angiography for patients presenting with acute chest pain to the emergency department: A Report of the Society of Cardiovascular Computed Tomography Guidelines Committee. *J Cardiovas Comput Tomogr* 2014;8:254 e271.

8 Answer B. Infarcted tissue demonstrates subendocardial enhancement or (when extensive) transmural enhancement. If less than 50% of the affected wall demonstrates scarring/enhancement, it is deemed viable, and revascularization has been shown to improve postinfarction ejection fraction and clinical outcome.

References: Cummings, et al. A pattern based approach to assessment of delayed enhancement in nonischemic cardiomyopathy at MR imaging. *Radiographics* 2009;29:89-103.

Kim R, et al. The use of contrast enhanced magnetic resonance imaging to identify reversible myocardial dysfunction. *NEJM* 2000;343(2):1445-1453.

9 Answer C. The curved multiplanar reformat of the left main and LAD shows mixed plaque within the LM resulting in greater than 50% stenosis. A lesion is considered hemodynamically significant if it causes >50% stenosis in the left main. This is based on myocardial blood flow studies. A greater than 50% lesion in the left main is an indication for coronary artery bypass grafting.

References: Uren NG, Melin JA, De Bruyne B, et al. Relation between myocardial blood flow and severity of coronary-artery stenosis. *N Engl J Med* 1994;330(25):1782-1788.

Eagle KA, et al. ACC/AHA guidelines for coronary artery bypass graft surgery: executive summary and recommendations: a report of the American College of Cardiology/American Heart Association Task Force on Practice Guidelines (Committee to revise the 1991 guidelines for coronary artery bypass graft surgery). *Circulation* 1999;100(13): 1464-1480.

10 Answer B. Microvascular obstruction (MVO), also known as no-reflow phenomenon is a focus of infarcted myocardium where obstruction of the microvasculature does not allow contrast to perfuse the tissue. Following infarction, administered contrast resides in the interstitium and creates the scar seen on delayed enhancement images. In areas where the microvasculature is obstructed, the contrast never reaches the interstitium, and this tissue appears as very dark signal surrounded by an enhancing scar on both sides. MVO is recognized as a poor prognostic indicator and marker of subsequent adverse LV remodeling.

Reference: Wu K. CMR of microvascular obstruction and hemorrhage in myocardial infarction. *JCMR* 2012;14:68.

11 Answer C. Coronary CTA has a negative predictive value greater than 95% and is an excellent test to exclude coronary artery disease. In particular, it has been shown to be of value when evaluating low risk patients with atypical chest pain, low risk patients with negative or equivocal stress testing an in the emergency room setting to evaluate patients with acute chest pain who are of low- to medium-risk (shown in ACRIN-PA and ROMICAT-II clinical trials).

Reference: Taylor, et al. ACCF/SCCT/ACR/AHA/ASE/ASNC/NASCI/SCAI/SCMR 2010 Appropriate use criteria for cardiac computed tomography. Evaluation of graft patency after CABG has an appropriateness score of 8/9 in a symptomatic patient. *Circulation* 2010;122: e525-e555.

12 Answer D. Long-term data is now available for patients who underwent coronary CTA in the emergency room. Current data suggests that a normal CTA in a low-risk patient presenting to the ER has a "warranty period" of up to 2 years meaning a rescan is not necessary as there has been no recorded incident of ACS within 2 years in this population.

Reference: Schlett, et al. Prognostic value of CT angiography for major adverse cardiac events in patients with acute chest pain from the emergency department. *JACC Cardiovas Img* 2011;4(5):481–491.

13 Answer A. Several clinical trials such as ACRIN-PA, CT-STAT, and ROMICAT have demonstrated the utility of coronary CTA for low-risk emergency room patients presenting with chest pain. Current data supports the position that a CCTA-based strategy for low- to intermediate-risk patients presenting with a possible acute coronary syndrome allows for the safe, expedited discharge home rather than admission and continued monitoring.

Reference: Litt HI, et al. CT angiography for safe discharge of patients with possible acute coronary syndromes. *N Engl J Med* 2012;366:1393–1403.

14 Answer C. Myocardial infarction carries many associated complications that include apical aneurysm formation, decreased ejection fraction, ventriculoseptal defect formation and papillary muscle infarction.

In one study, the incidence of rupture of the papillary muscle was found to be 0.9%. The clinical features usually occur during the first week after infarction. More common is slight mitral regurgitation without pulmonary edema from papillary muscle dysfunction.

Reference: Clements, et al. Ruptured papillary muscle, a complication of myocardial infarction: clinical presentation, diagnosis, and treatment. *Clin Cardiol* 1985;8:93–103.

15 Answer A. Current interest in cardiac CTA centers on determining which plaque can be considered "high risk" for rupture and can lead to acute coronary syndrome. Certain morphologic features of plaque (even if it is not considered flow limiting) are considered adverse. These include low attenuation (fatty composition), positive remodeling, spotty calcifications, and plaque ulceration.

References: Motoyama, et al. Coronary CT angiography and high-risk plaque morphology. *Cardiovas Interv Ther* 2013;28(1):1–8.

Voros S, Rinehart S, Qian Z, et al. Coronary atherosclerosis imaging by coronary CT angiography: current status, correlation with intravascular interrogation and meta-analysis. *J Am Coll Cardiol Img* 2011;4(5):537–548. doi: 10.1016/j.jcmg.2011.03.006.

16 Answer D. Knowledge of cardiac imaging planes is crucial to performing a proper cardiac MRI examination to evaluate the myocardium axial; two-, three-, and four-chamber; and short-axis views are core planes used to evaluate function, wall motion, edema and scar. The short axis image is used to measure function, evaluate wall motion and identify scar on delayed enhanced images. The short axis image is obtained by prescribing a plane parallel to the mitral valve and perpendicular to the interventricular septum.

Reference: Ginat D, et al. Cardiac imaging: Part 1, MR pulse sequences, imaging planes, and basic anatomy. *AJR Am J Roentgenol* 2011;197(4):808–815.

17 Answer A. Selecting the appropriate TI or inversion time is extremely important for obtaining accurate imaging results. The TI is chosen to "null" normal myocardium (normal myocardium will not retain gadolinium whereas injured myocardium will retain gadolinium). In principle, the optimal TI at which normal myocardium is nulled (black) must be determined by imaging iteratively with different inversion times. As time progresses after gadolinium administration normal myocardium will have increased signal and a longer inversion time must be chosen to null its signal.

Reference: Kim R, et al. How we perform delayed enhancement imaging. *J Cardiovas Magnet Reson* 2003;5(3):505-514.

18 **Answer C.** Image A shows low attenuation within the distal RCA stent placed remotely. The low attenuation material is secondary to thrombus, which has developed over time. Image B shows two patent stents in the LAD. In general, stents greater than 3.0 mm in size are readily evaluable, while stents measuring less than 2.5 mm can be difficult to evaluate.

References: Hong C, Chrysant GS, Woodard PK, et al. Coronary artery stent patency assessed with in-stent contrast enhancement measured at multi-detector row CT angiography: initial experience. *Radiology* 2004;233(1):286-291.

Martine R-J, Rémy J. *Integrated cardiothoracic imaging with MDCT*. Berlin, Germany: Springer Verlag, 2009.

19 **Answer D.** After a successful procedure, coronary stents can fail to maintain vessel patency due to stent thrombosis or stent restenosis. Stent thrombosis can occur early, late or very late following stent placement and is more common with bare metal stent placment. The incidence of thrombosis has decreased following the development and use of drug eluting stents and anticoagulation therapy. Current guidelines for bare-metal stents require dual antiplatelet therapy for 1 month and for 1 year following placement of a drug-eluting stent.

Reference: Cutlip, et al. Antithrombotic therapy for elective percutaneous coronary intervention: General use. Uptodate.com.

20 **Answer A.** The sensitivity for detecting stent patency increases from 54% in stents with a diameter of ≤3 mm to 86% in stents >3 mm. As a result, knowning stent size can be a key factor in determinig if the exam will be successful.

References: Gilard M, et al. Assessment of coronary artery stents by 16 slice computed tomography. *Heart* 2006;92(1):58-61.

Mahnken A, et al. CT Imaging of coronary stents: past present and future. *ISRN Cardiol* 2012; 2012(1):286-291. Article ID 139823.

21 **Answer C.** The image demonstrates an endotracheal tube and nasogastric tube and bilateral chest tubes. An intra-aortic balloon pump is noted along with a percutaneous left ventricular assist device. These circulatory support devices are placed in the setting of acute myocardial infarction with shock requiring hemodynamic support.

References: Delgado D, et al. Mechanical circulatory assistance state of the art. *Circulation* 2002;106:2046-2050.

Naidu SS. Novel percutaneous cardiac assist devices: the science of and indications for hemodynamic support. *Circulation* 2011;123(5):533-543. doi: 10.1161/CIRCULATIONAHA. 110.945055. Review.

22 **Answer B.** The image demonstrates a dilated left ventricle. There is also secondary poor coaptation of the mitral valve leaflets and concurrent mitral regurgitation. The mitral regurgitation is shown as dephasing artifact (low signal) in the left atrium. A dilated left ventricle is defined by an enlarged left ventricular diastolic dimension (>112% of expected LV size given age and body surface area) and diminished left ventricular ejection fraction.

Reference: Chatterjee K, Massie B. Systolic and diastolic heart failure: differences and similarities. *J Card Fail* 2007;13:569-576.

23 Answer B. The majority of heart failure cases have no clear origin and are idiopathic. Ischemic cardiomyopathy accounts for 5% of cases.

References: Elliott P. Diagnosis and management of dilated cardiomyopathy. *Heart* 2000;84: 106–112.

Michael Felker G, Thompson RE, Hare JM, et al. Underlying causes and long-term survival in patients with initially unexplained cardiomyopathy. *NEJM* 2000;342:1077–1084.

24 Answer B. Optimal imaging of the coronary arteries is performed at approximately 60 to 80% of the R–R interval. Normal ECG tracing entails the highest voltage within the R wave. In the setting of high-voltage T waves, the scan may trigger incorrectly by interpreting the high T wave as another R wave. The resultant apparent heart rate will also be falsely elevated. This problem can be corrected by increasing the trigger threshold so that the higher R wave can serve as the only peak to register or changing leads so that the R wave is higher than the T wave. (It is important to ensure no underlying pathology is an organic cause of high T wave voltage. In the right clinical setting, the referring physician may need to be alerted.)

References: Lee V. *Cardiovascular MRI: Physical principles to practical protocols.* Philadelphia, PA: Lippincott Williams & Wilkins, 2005:302.

Shuman et al. Prospective versus retrospective ECG Gating for 64-detector CT of the coronary arteries: comparison of image quality and patient radiation dose. *Radiology* 2008;248(2).

25 Answer D. Recent advances in cardiac MRI now allow perfusion imaging in addition to delayed enhancement imaging for scar. Perfusion imaging has the added advantage of showing cardiac wall motion and ejection fraction during stress. Wall motion abnormalities indicating ischemia may only manifest during stress. Perfusion scanning requires both a stress and a rest phase, and adenosine is given during the study at a dose of 140 μg/kg/min infusion.

References: Kramer C, et al. Standardized cardiovascular magnetic resonance imaging (CMR) protocols, society for cardiovascular magnetic resonance: board of trustees task force on standardized protocols. *J Cardiovas Magn Reson* 2008;10:35.

Vogel-Claussen J, et al. Comprehensive adenosine stress perfusion MRI defines the etiology of chest pain in the emergency room: comparison with nuclear stress test. *J Magn Reson Img* 2009;30(4):753–762.

26 Answer C. Percutaneous coronary intervention (PCI) in symptomatic patients with stable CAD receiving optimal medical therapy has only been shown to improve angina. It has not been proven to improve survival nor decrease future myocardial infarctions. PCI in patients with stable CAD is only recommended if patients have unacceptable symptoms or cannot tolerate optimal medical therapy.

Reference: Kureshi F, Jones PG, Buchanan DM, et al. Variation in patients' perceptions of elective percutaneous coronary intervention in stable coronary artery disease: cross sectional study. *BMJ* 2014;349:g5309. doi: 10.1136/bmj.g5309.

27 Answer B. Coronary CTA should be done in patients with low to moderate pretest probability for coronary artery disease. Of the choices given, the 47-year-old male with smoking and family history of coronary artery disease best fits this category. The 35-year-old female would have very low probability for coronary artery disease. The 55-year-old female could potentially be a good candidate but has atrial fibrillation, which is not ideal for coronary CTA. A 76-year-old with angina has high probability of coronary artery disease so should just get a cardiac catheterization.

Reference: American College of Cardiology Foundation Task Force on Expert Consensus Documents; Mark DB, Berman DS, Budoff MJ, et al. ACCF/ACR/AHA/NASCI/SAIP/SCAI/SCCT 2010 expert consensus document on coronary computed tomographic angiography: a report of the American College of Cardiology Foundation Task Force on Expert Consensus Documents. *Circulation* 2010;121(22):2509–2543. doi: 10.1161/CIR.0b013e3181d4b618.

28a Answer B. Perfusion image shows subendocardial perfusion abnormality in the anteroseptal region. On the b-SSFP image, there is persistent hypoperfusion in the anterior septal endocardium. On the late gadolinium enhancement image, there is evidence for microvascular obstruction with a subendocardial area of nonenhancement due to microvascular obstruction and enhancement of the infarct in the mid wall indicating mycoardial infarction.

28b Answer A. The anteroseptal region indicates the left anterior descending coronary artery territory.

28c Answer A. Infarcts with microvascular obstruction has worse prognosis than infarcts without microvascular obstruction.

Reference: Hamirani YS, Wong A, Kramer CM, et al. Effect of microvascular obstruction and intramyocardial hemorrhage by CMR on LV remodeling and outcomes after myocardial infarction: a systematic review and meta-analysis. *JACC Cardiovas Img* 2014;7(9):940-952. doi: 10.1016/j.jcmg.2014.06.012.

5 Cardiomyopathy

QUESTIONS

1. Which of the following is a major/minor criterion for arrhythmogenic right ventricular dysplasia?
   A. Normalized RV end-diastolic volume of 90 mL/m^2
   B. Fatty infiltration of the ventricular wall
   C. Right ventricular ejection fraction of 50%
   D. Dyssynchronous RV wall motion

2. A 26-year-old patient with fever, weight loss, and blood cultures positive for *Staphylococcus* infection.

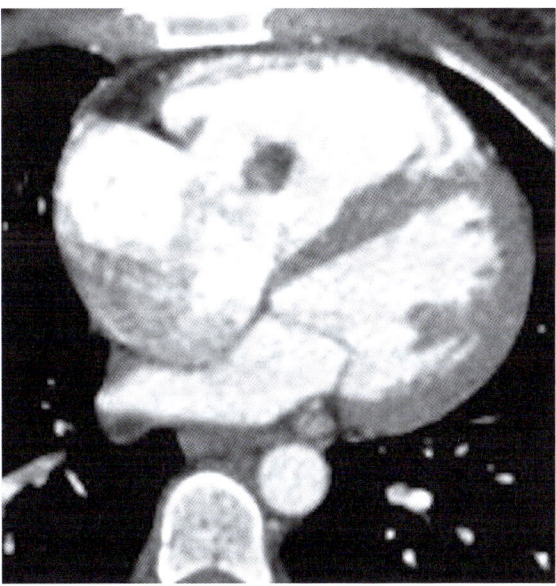

Given the history and imaging findings, which is the most likely etiology?
   A. HOCM
   B. Myxomatous mitral valve
   C. Paradoxical embolus
   D. Infective endocarditis

3 Which process best characterizes the imaging findings?

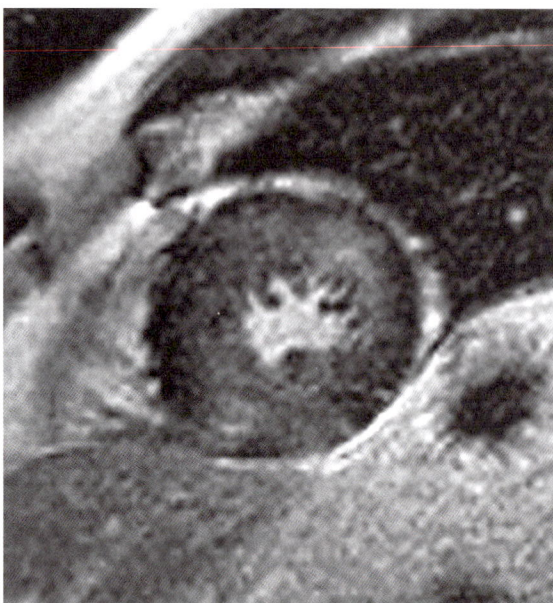

A. Myocardial infarction
B. Hypertrophic cardiomyopathy
C. Myocarditis
D. Arrhythmogenic right ventricular dysplasia

4 What is the most likely diagnosis of the condition shown in the figure below?

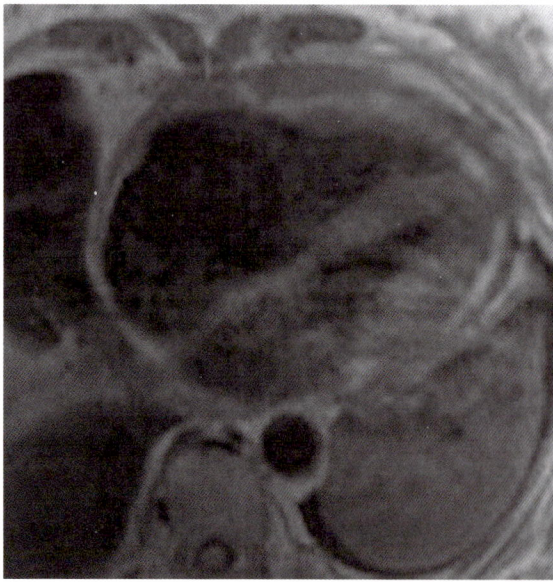

A. Restrictive cardiomyopathy
B. Constrictive pericarditis
C. Hypertrophic cardiomyopathy
D. Left ventricular noncompaction

5. Patient is a 26-year-old with worsening heart failure. Given the imaging findings, what is the most likely explanation for the patient's condition?

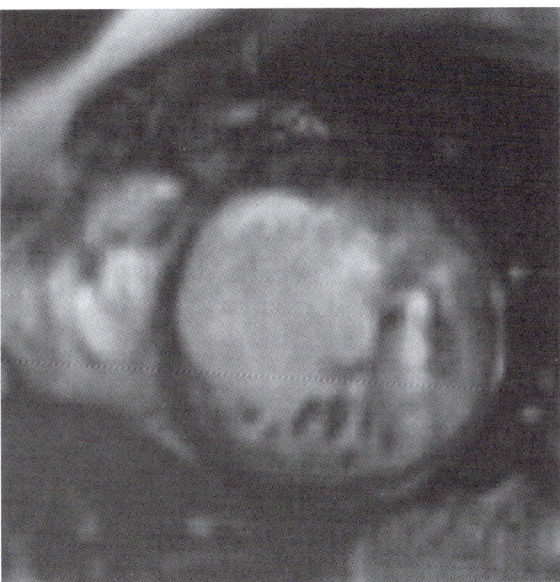

A. Restrictive cardiomyopathy
B. Constrictive pericarditis
C. Hypertrophic cardiomyopathy
D. Left ventricular noncompaction

6. Patient is referred for atypical chest pain and exercise intolerance over the last few months. No personal or family history of cardiac disease is otherwise noted. Given the imaging findings, what is the most likely etiology of the patient's condition?

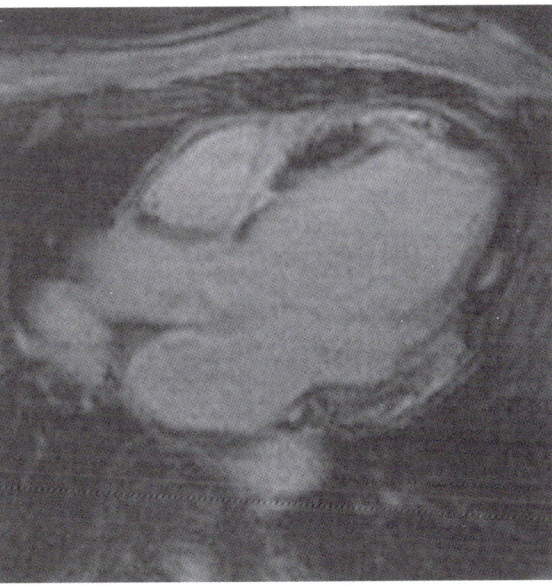

A. Myocardial infarction
B. Hypertrophic cardiomyopathy
C. Myocarditis
D. Arrhythmogenic right ventricular dysplasia

7 Patient is referred for cardiac MR for decreased systolic function and decreased exercise tolerance. Given the imaging findings, what is the most likely cause of the patient's condition?

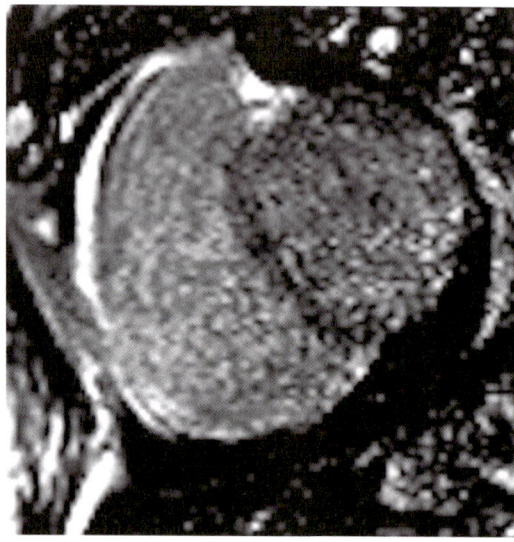
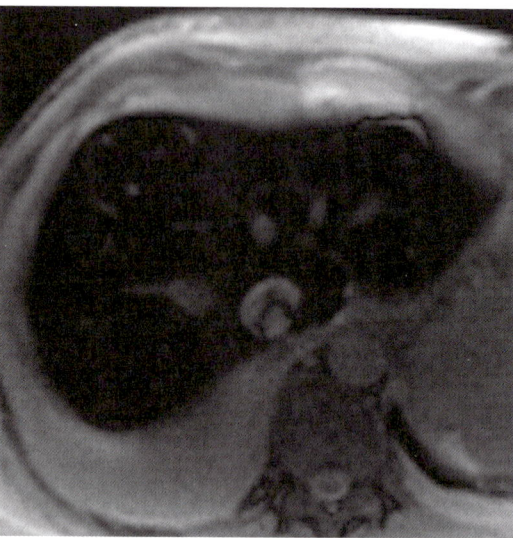

A. Myocardial infarction
B. Hypertrophic cardiomyopathy
C. Myocarditis
D. Hemochromatosis

8 A 36-year-old woman presents with acute chest pain and elevated troponins. Apart from mild hypertension, she has no significant past medical history. Emergency cardiac catheterization shows no obstructive coronary artery disease, and the left ventriculogram demonstrates apical hypokinesis at end systole (below).

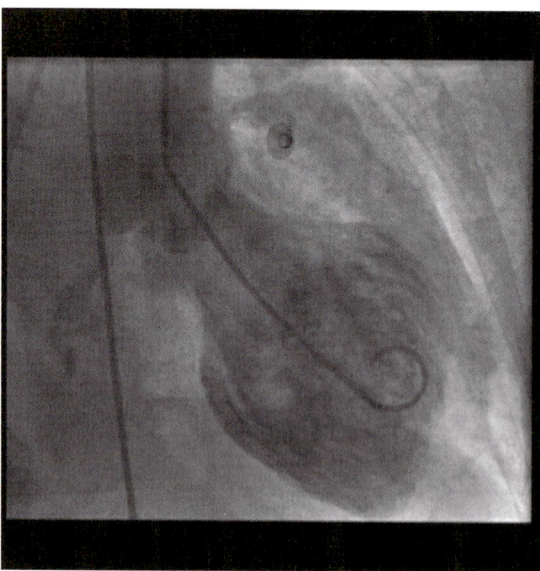

Given the clinical presentation and imaging, which of the following is the most likely etiology?

A. Dilated cardiomyopathy due to alcohol
B. Hypertrophic cardiomyopathy
C. Stress-induced cardiomyopathy
D. Ischemic cardiomyopathy

9   Which of the following entities can cause hypertrophy of the basal septum?

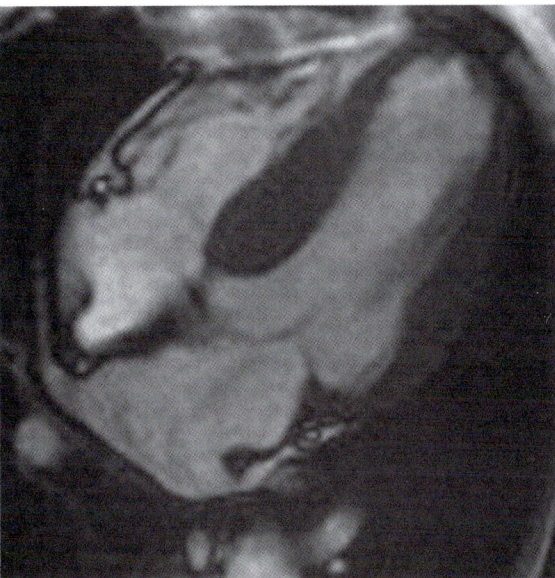

A. Ventricular noncompaction
B. Severe aortic stenosis
C. Uhl anomaly
D. Annuloaortic ectasia

10 A 27-year-old male has a syncopal episode while playing soccer. He was resuscitated by medical personnel in the field and brought to the emergency department. On review of family history, he notes that he had an uncle who unexpectedly died at the same age playing basketball. Cardiac MR demonstrates the following:

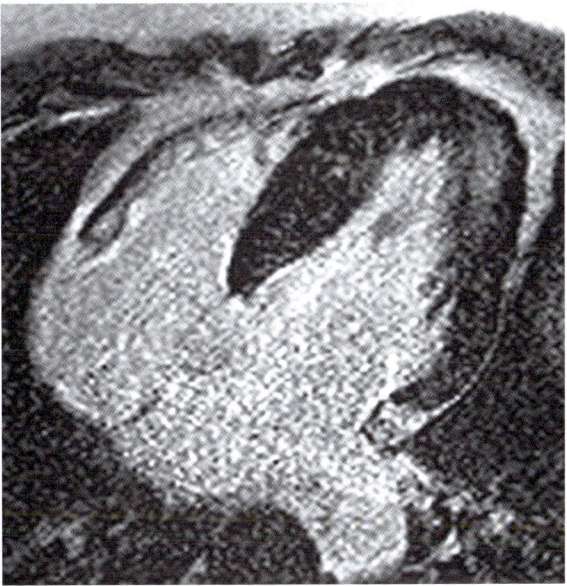

Given the clinical presentation and the imaging findings, what treatment recommendation would you suggest?

A. Beta blockers
B. ICD
C. ACE inhibitors
D. Steroid therapy

11 A patient with cardiomyopathy and peripheral eosinophilia presents with the following imaging findings:

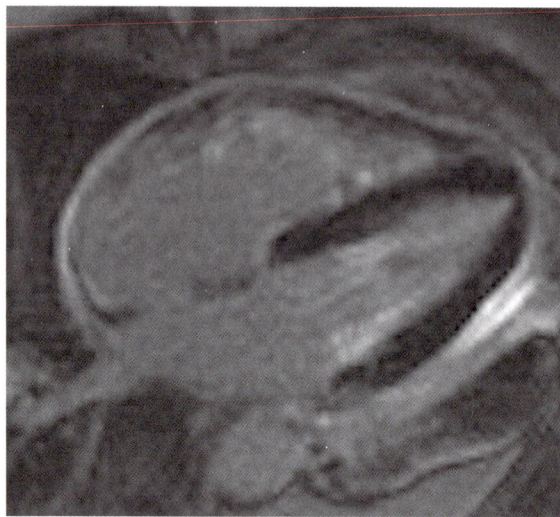

Which abnormality most likely reflects the underlying cardiomyopathy?

A. Loeffler endocarditis
B. Myocardial infarction
C. Cardiac sarcoidosis
D. Amyloidosis

12 A 68-year-old patient with was found to have moderate decreased left ventricular function and severe diastolic dysfunction. Cardiac MR reveals biatrial enlargement, bilateral pleural effusions, and both systolic and diastolic dysfunction (below).

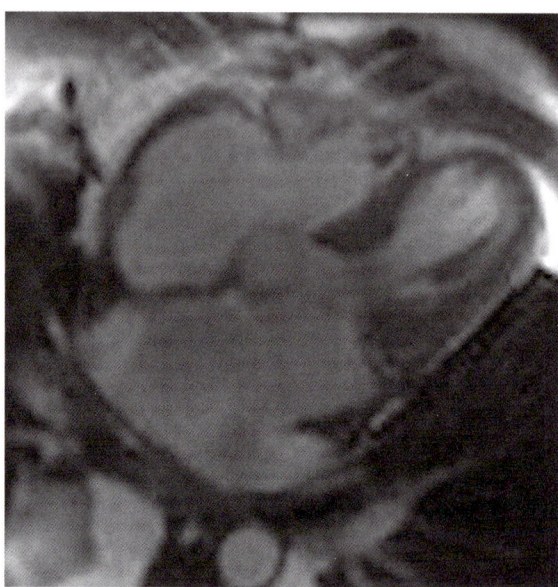

Given the clinical picture and imaging findings, which etiology would explain the patient's condition?

A. Restrictive cardiomyopathy
B. Ischemic cardiomyopathy
C. Dilated cardiomyopathy
D. Inflammatory cardiomyopathy

13 A 47-year-old patient with worsening heart failure presents for evaluation by cardiac MR. A representative image is noted below. Which of the following is most closely associated with the MR finding?

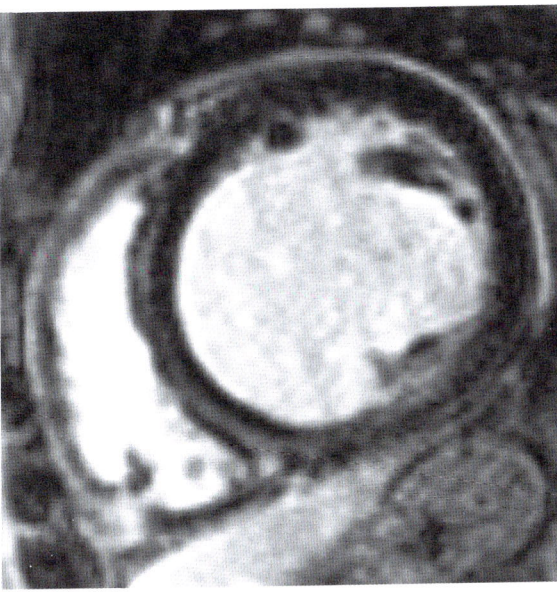

A. Nonischemic dilated cardiomyopathy
B. Sarcoid cardiomyopathy
C. Arrhythmogenic right ventricular cardiomyopathy
D. Ischemic cardiomyopathy with septal infarct

14 A 77-year-old male with multiple myeloma has worsening dyspnea with global ventricular hypertrophy and decreased left ventricular function by echocardiography. Cardiac MR was ordered for further evaluation.

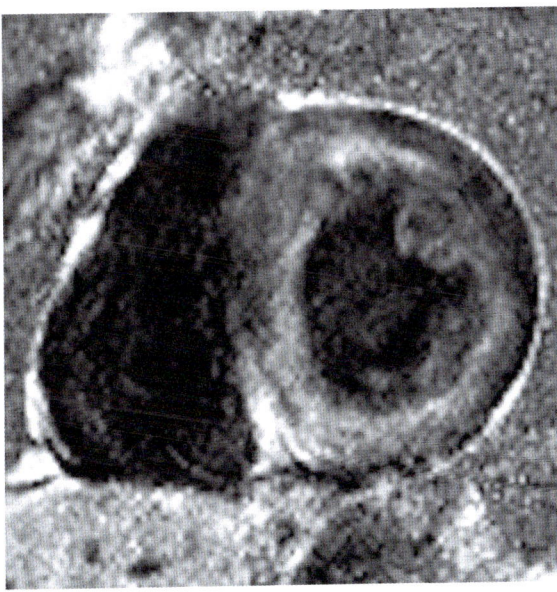

Given the clinical history and imaging findings, which of the following diagnoses best characterize the underlying cardiomyopathy?

A. Amyloidosis
B. Dilated cardiomyopathy
C. Hypertrophic cardiomyopathy
D. Iron overload cardiomyopathy

15 What is the most common etiology of dilated cardiomyopathies (DCM)?
   A. Ischemic
   B. Familial
   C. Inflammatory
   D. Idiopathic

16a A 27-year-old patient presents with atypical chest pain for the last 2 days. Patient is otherwise healthy without significant past medical history. Review of systems reveals recent upper respiratory infection and fever for which he took over-the-counter medication. Echocardiography notes small pericardial effusion but otherwise normal.

Given the clinical picture, which would be the most likely etiology of the patient's condition?
   A. Myocardial infarction
   B. Myocarditis
   C. Restrictive cardiomyopathy
   D. Constrictive pericarditis

16b Considering the previous question, the MR protocol for the diagnosis includes an inversion recovery sequence for late gadolinium enhancement. What additional MR sequence should be included in the evaluation of myocarditis?
   A. Chemical shift imaging
   B. Pre- and early postgadolinium enhancement
   C. CSPAMM myocardial tagging
   D. Contrast-enhanced MR angiography

17a A 27-year-old male without any prior medical history presents to his primary physician with progressive dyspnea and difficulty with exercise over the last couple of months. A cardiac MR reveals decreased left ventricular function and the following imaging findings:

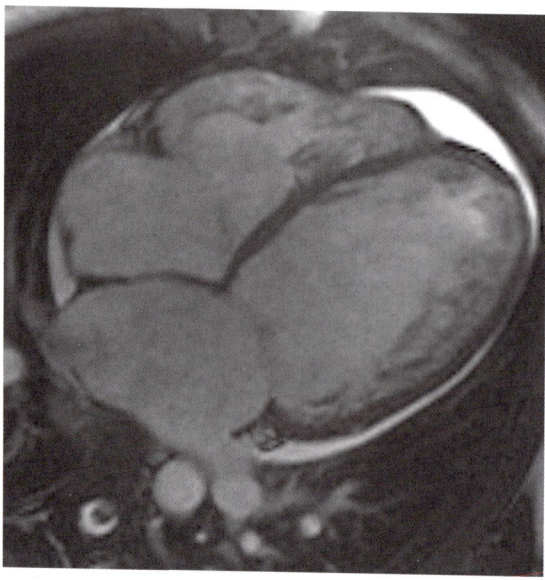

Given the clinical history and imaging, which of the following best characterizes the patient's cardiomyopathy?
   A. Dilated cardiomyopathy
   B. Inflammatory cardiomyopathy (myocarditis)
   C. Ventricular noncompaction
   D. Chronic hypertensive changes

17b Which of the following is a complication of the previous abnormality?

  A. Conduction abnormalities
  B. Left ventricular hypertrophy
  C. Ventricular aneurysms
  D. Valvular stenosis

18 A patient with acute myelogenous leukemia presents for a CT of the chest as a result of abnormal findings on echocardiogram. An infiltrating mass is observed in the septum and RV apex.

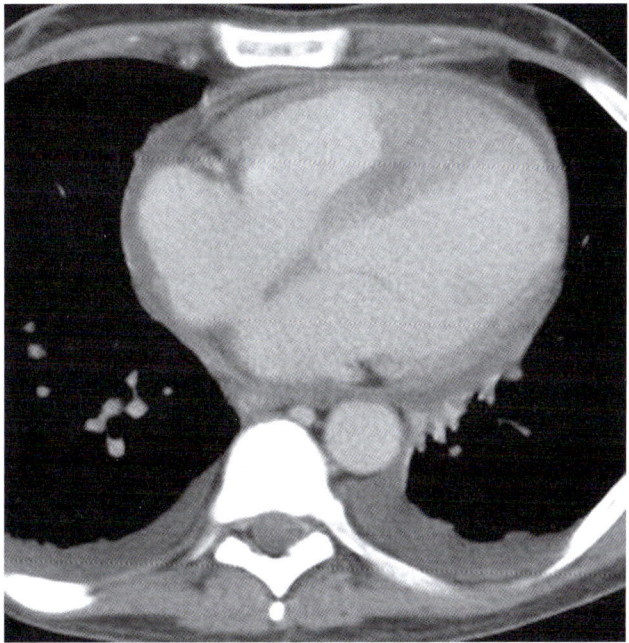

Given the clinical picture and imaging findings, which of the following entities should be considered?

  A. Primary angiosarcoma
  B. Granulocytic sarcoma
  C. Papillary fibroelastoma
  D. Primary cardiac lymphoma

19 In restrictive cardiomyopathy, what is the relationship of ventricular compliance and diastolic volume?

  A. Increased ventricular compliance with reduced diastolic volume
  B. Decreased ventricular compliance with increased reduced diastolic volume
  C. Increased ventricular compliance with increased diastolic volume
  D. Decreased ventricular compliance and reduced diastolic volume

20 Which MR sequence quantifies the severity of iron deposition in iron overload cardiomyopathies?

  A. T2 (star)
  B. Late gadolinium enhancement
  C. Chemical shift imaging
  D. T1

21 Which best describes the following MR sequence?

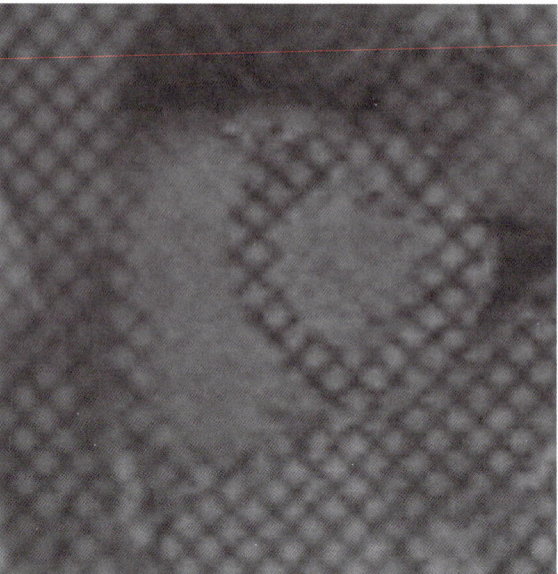

A. T1 mapping
B. Time of flight
C. Phase contrast
D. SPAMM tagging

22a A 66-year-old female presents with premature ventricular complexes (PVCs). The abnormality seen in the right ventricular wall is most often seen in what type of patients?

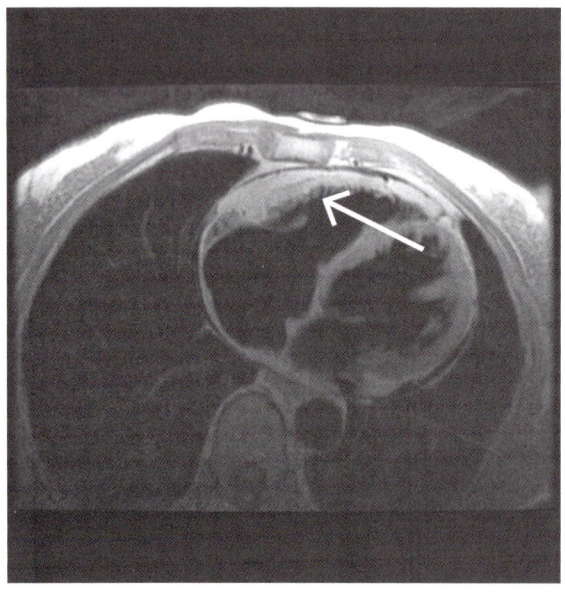
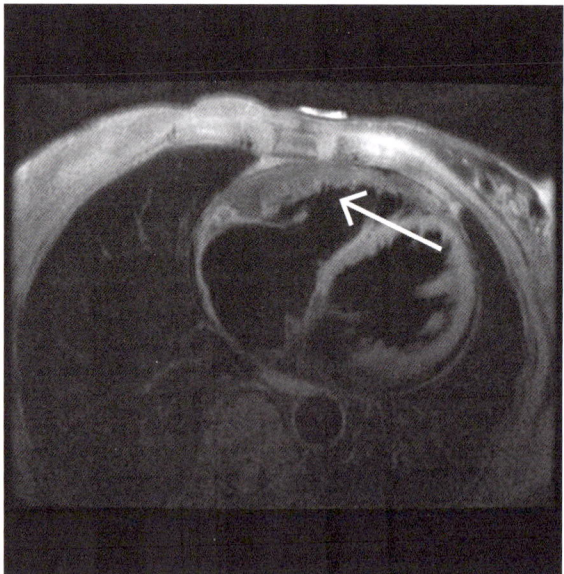

A. Young males with sudden cardiac death
B. Young females with dilated aorta
C. Old obese females
D. Old thin males

Cardiomyopathy

22b In this patient, the right ventricular ejection fraction (RVEF) is calculated to be 67% and the right ventricular end-diastolic volume index (RVEDVI) is calculated at 81 mL/m². There were also no RV wall motion abnormalities. What criterion can be given for the diagnosis of arrhythmogenic right ventricular dysplasia (ARVD)?

A. No criterion is given for the diagnosis of ARVD.
B. Minor criterion can be given for the diagnosis of ARVD.
C. Major criterion can be given for the diagnosis of ARVD.
D. Major and minor criterion can be given for the diagnosis of ARVD.

23a A 35-year-old patient presents with history of Chagas infection now presenting with increasing shortness of breath. CT imaging reveals the following:

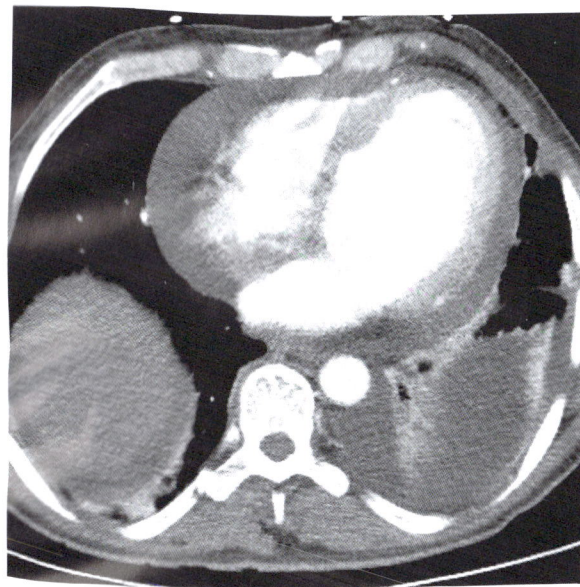

Which phase of Chagas involvement is most characterized by pericardial effusions and myocarditis?

A. Acute
B. Indeterminate
C. Chronic
D. End stage

23b What is a common extracardiac finding in chronic Chagas heart disease?

A. Esophageal strictures
B. Megacolon
C. Violaceous erythema
D. Pulmonary aneurysms

24 A 27-year-old woman presents with dyspnea, edema, and palpitations. She has no prior medical history and gave birth to a healthy newborn child 2 months ago, but still complains of progressive symptoms. An echocardiogram was performed and reports a dilated left ventricle with an EF of 35% and no other wall motion abnormalities.

Which form of cardiomyopathy is most likely?

A. Postpartum
B. Amyloidosis
C. Hypertrophic
D. ARVD

25. The ratio of early (E-wave) and late (A-wave) transmitral velocities is one parameter of diastolic ventricular filling. Which of the following E/A ratios is most consistent with a restrictive cardiomyopathy?

    A. >2.0
    B. 1.5 to 1.9
    C. 1.0 to 1.4
    D. <1.0

26. A 22-year-old male with a history of mental retardation and skeletal myopathy presents with worsening heart failure. Short-axis images of the left ventricle are presented below.

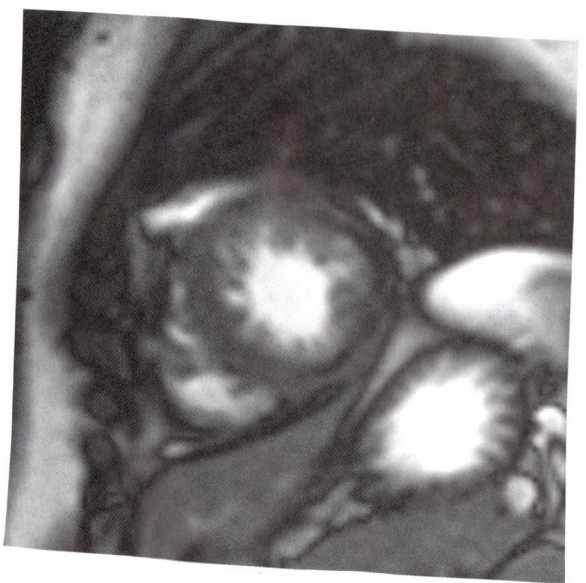
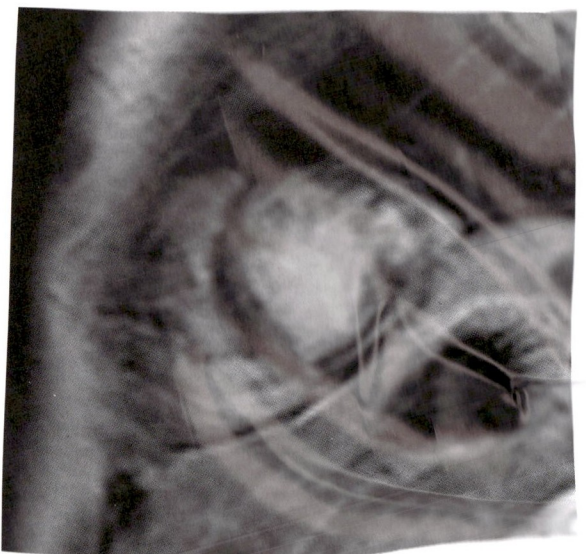

Given the combination of clinical history and imaging, what is the most likely diagnosis?

    A. Danon disease
    B. Friedreich Ataxia
    C. Fabry disease
    D. Amyloidosis

27. Patient with a history of pulmonary sarcoidosis recently presents to the hospital with third-degree heart block. The diagnosis of cardiac sarcoidosis was made during the hospitalization.

    FDG-PET images from the initial presentation demonstrate lateral wall activity. Follow-up PET imaging 6 months after therapy demonstrates no metabolic activity in the previous area.

    Which of the following best explains the PET findings?

    A. Previous inflamed myocardium no longer inflamed
    B. Previous perfused myocardium now ischemic
    C. Previous edematous myocardium no longer edematous
    D. Previous hibernating myocardium is no longer viable

28 A 54-year-old female presents with premature ventricular complexes (PVCs). Study was done to assess for ARVD. Images below are in end diastole and end systole. The bulge seen in systole in the RV wall near the apex represents what?

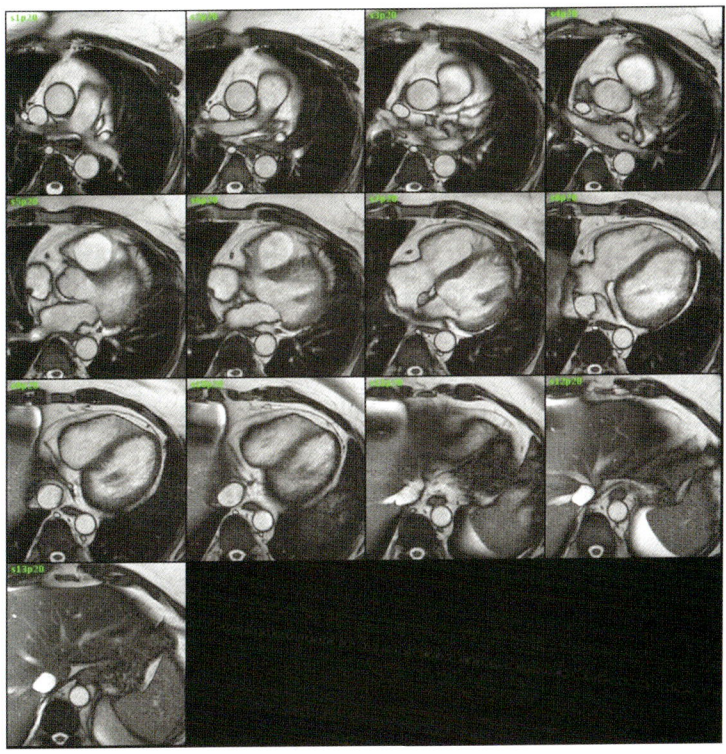

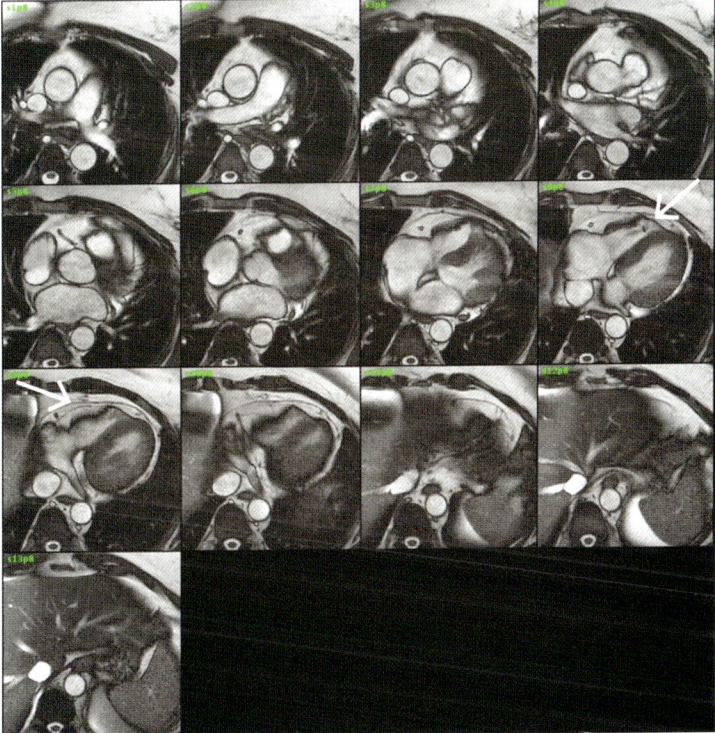

A. Normal finding in isolation of other RV wall motion abnormalities
B. Abnormal finding consistent with minor criterion for ARVD
C. Abnormal finding consistent with major criterion for ARVD

29 A patient with thalassemia major was started on chelation therapy for iron overload cardiomyopathy. Which of the following MR findings are most consistent with improvement on therapy?

  A. Increase in myocardial T1
  B. Decrease in myocardial T2*
  C. Increase in myocardial T2*
  D. Decrease in myocardial T1

30 A 57-year-old male with multiple myeloma presents with progressive heart failure symptoms. He is referred for CMR to rule out amyloidosis. Which of the following MR findings would be consistent with the diagnosis?

  A. Dilated thinned walled ventricles on precontrast GRE sequences
  B. Asymmetric septal hypertrophy on postcontrast T1 sequences
  C. Dyskinetic right ventricular wall motion on cine SSFP sequences
  D. Poor nulling of the myocardium on postcontrast inversion recovery

31 Which of the following cardiomyopathies has relative contraindications to heart transplantation?

  A. Hypertrophic
  B. Amyloidosis
  C. Idiopathic dilated
  D. Hemochromatosis

ANSWERS AND EXPLANATIONS

1. **Answer D.** Arrhythmogenic right ventricular dysplasia (ARVD) is a genetic cardiomyopathy with an incidence of the familial form of ARVD that is estimated between 15% and 50%. ARVD is difficult to diagnose.

   The diagnosis is based on clinical and nonclinical criteria, including family history, which are subdivided into major and minor criteria. A "definite" diagnosis consists of two major criteria or one major and two minor criteria, or else four minor criteria. A "borderline" diagnosis consists of one major and one minor criterion or three minor criteria. Finally, a "possible" diagnosis consists of one major or two minor criteria.

   The original criteria were revised in 2010 to include specific abnormalities that may be detected on MRI and echocardiography. Primary imaging criteria on MRI include a combination of

   a. Regional RV akinesia, dyskinesia, or dyssynchronous RV contraction
   b. Findings of right ventricular dysfunction, of which severity determines whether a major or minor criteria is reached:
      i. RV end-diastolic volume index ≥ 110 mL/m^2 (male) or ≥ 100 mL/m^2 (female)
         Or RV ejection fraction $\leq 40\%$, which in combination with (a) would fulfill a Major criteria
      ii. $100 \leq$ RV end-diastolic volume (EDV) < 110 mL/m^2 (male) or $90 \leq$ EDV < 100 mL/m^2 (female)
         Or $40\% <$ RV ejection fraction $\leq 45\%$, which in combination with a) would fulfill a Major criteria

   Other morphologic abnormalities such as fat infiltration and delayed enhancement images are detectable by MRI, but have not been considered sensitive enough to be considered in the diagnostic criteria.

   References: Marcus FI, McKenna WJ, Sherrill D, et al. Diagnosis of arrhythmogenic right ventricular cardiomyopathy/dysplasia proposed modification of the task force criteria. *Circulation* 2010;121(13):1533–1541.

   Tavano A, Maurel B, Gaubert J-Y, et al. MR imaging of arrhythmogenic right ventricular dysplasia: what the radiologist needs to know. *Diagn Interv Imaging* 2015;96(5):449–460.

2. **Answer D.** Contrast-enhanced CT demonstrates a large vegetation on the septal tricuspid leaflet consistent with infective endocarditis (IE).

   The risk for IE among IV drug abusers is severalfold greater than that for patients with rheumatic heart disease or prosthetic valves. 65% to 80% of such cases of IE occur in men aged 27 to 37 years. IE is located on the tricuspid valve in 46% to 78%, mitral valve in 24% to 32%, and aortic valve in 8% to 19%; as many as 16% of patients have infection at multiple sites.

   IE is a rare complication of hypertrophic cardiomyopathy. It is estimated that incidence is 1.4 per 1,000 person/year in all patients and it increases to 3.8 per 1,000 person/year in patients with left ventricular outflow obstruction and left atrial enlargement.

   Mitral valve prolapse (MVP) is the most common cause of isolated mitral regurgitation requiring surgical treatment in the United States and the most common cardiac condition predisposing patients to infective endocarditis. However, the frequency of mitral valve prolapse in IE is not entirely a direct reflection of relative risk but rather a function of the frequency of the lesion in the general population. Risk factors for infective endocarditis in patients with MVP include the presence of mitral regurgitation or thickened mitral leaflets and account for 7% to 30% of native-valve endocarditis not related to drug abuse or nosocomial infection.

Risk of infective endarteritis in patients with patent ductus arteriosus seems to have declined during the last 30 to 40 years, and cases of patent ductus arteriosus complicated by infective endarteritis are now very rare.

References: Karchmer CM. Infectious endocarditis. In: Bonow RO, Braunwald E (eds). *Braunwald's heart disease: A textbook of cardiovascular medicine*. Philadelphia, PA: Saunders, 2012:1540-1560.

Louahabi T, Drighil A, Habbal R, et al. Infective endocarditis complicating hypertrophic obstructive cardiomyopathy. *Eur Heart J Cardiovas Imaging* 2006;7(6):468-470.

Sadiq M, Latif F, ur-Rehman A. Analysis of infective endarteritis in patent ductus arteriosus. *Am J Cardiol* 2004;93(4):513-515.

3 Answer B. Short-axis view of the heart demonstrating marked hypertrophy of the left ventricle. The MR sequence is an inversion recovery technique with an inversion time to null the myocardium and assess for late gadolinium enhancement. In this case, there is patchy enhancement within the midmyocardium with more focal fibrosis in anterolateral and inferoseptal segments. Findings are consistent with hypertrophic cardiomyopathy.

The pattern of enhancement is atypical for infarction, which should primarily be subendocardial. Left ventricular hypertrophy and patchy enhancement can be seen with amyloidosis. However, the nulling of the myocardium is characteristically difficult because of the T1 properties of the amyloid protein and diffusely increased extracellular volume.

Hypertrophic cardiomyopathy (HCM) is a genetic disorder characterized by left ventricular hypertrophy (wall thickness >12 to 15 mm) but is also heterogeneous in presentation, prognosis, and treatment strategies. Pathologic hallmarks of HCM include myocyte disarray and interstitial fibrosis.

Several recognized imaging phenotypes are recognized (e.g., asymmetric [septal] HCM, apical HCM, symmetric HCM [concentric HCM], and midventricular HCM). Increased LV wall thickness may result in narrowing of the left ventricular outflow tract (LVOT). Systolic anterior motion of the anterior mitral leaflet may also be observed, which can increase LVOT obstruction and decreased coronary and systemic outflow.

LV wall thickness, presence of underlying perfusion abnormalities, and fibrosis as evidenced by late gadolinium enhancement are important imaging markers pointing to increased risk for sudden death in HCM patients.

References: Hoey ETD, Teoh JK, Das I, et al. The emerging role of cardiovascular MRI for risk stratification in hypertrophic cardiomyopathy. *Clin Radiol* 2014;69(3):221-230.

Maron BJ. Hypertrophic cardiomyopathy: a systematic review. *JAMA* 2002;287(10):1308-1320.

4 Answer B. T1-weighted axial image demonstrates significant near-circumferential thickening of the pericardium (in this case, measuring >1 cm in max thickness). Findings are consistent with constrictive pericarditis.

Constrictive pericarditis (CP) is characterized by fibrous or calcific thickening of the pericardium, which prevents normal diastolic filling of the heart. Historically, tuberculosis was the most common cause of CP and was frequently associated with extensive pericardial calcification. In the modern era, tuberculous pericarditis is rare, and important causes are increasingly previous mediastinal irradiation and cardiac surgery.

Patients commonly present with signs and symptoms of right-sided heart failure that are disproportionate to the severity of left ventricular dysfunction or valvular disease. Both restrictive and constrictive diseases exhibit an abrupt reduction in filling, increased backpressure, and impaired stroke volume. It is important to distinguish between constrictive pericarditis and restrictive cardiomyopathy because treatment for the former condition is surgical, and treatment for the latter is medical.

Classically, the pericardium in patients with CP will be diffusely thicker than 4 mm; however, the diagnosis of should not be completely disregarded if thickening is not present. Cardiac chambers will be within normal limits in size. Superior and inferior vena cava as well as hepatic veins may be dilated. The influence of respiration on filling contributes important diagnostic information, both for imaging and for catheterization. The restriction in CP creates discordance with reduced left ventricular filling, which corresponds to increased right ventricular filling. This manifests as a variance in the septal curvature during diastolic filling and a characteristic "septal bounce."

Restrictive cardiomyopathy is characterized by a marked decrease in ventricular compliance and results from a number of etiologies, including hypertrophic cardiomyopathy. Imaging often reveals thickening of the ventricles with biatrial enlargement.

Left ventricular noncompaction (VNC) is a congenital myocardial abnormality that can present in either childhood or adulthood with congestive heart failure, arrhythmia, or thromboembolism. VNC occurs due to persistence of noncompacted endocardium characteristic of the early fetal period before myocardial compaction is complete. The left ventricle is usually affected, and it may be either dilated or hypertrophied.

References: Hughes S. Cardiomyopathies. In: Suvarna SK (ed.). *Cardiac pathology*. London, UK: Springer, 2013:183–200.

Ling LH, Oh JK, Schaff HV, et al. Constrictive pericarditis in the modern era evolving clinical spectrum and impact on outcome after pericardiectomy. *Circulation* 1999;100(13):1380–1386.

5. **Answer D.** Midventricular short-axis SSFP image of the heart demonstrates significant increased trabeculation of the left ventricular cavity relative to normal compacted myocardium. This appearance is compatible with left ventricular noncompaction (VNC). Note that the papillary muscles are often not well formed in the setting of VNC.

Left ventricular noncompaction, also known as spongiform cardiomyopathy, is a congenital myocardial abnormality that can present in either childhood or adulthood. VNC occurs due to persistence of noncompacted endocardium characteristic of the early fetal period before myocardial compaction is complete. The left ventricle is usually affected, and it may be either dilated or hypertrophied.

Echocardiography or MRI is the diagnostic method of choice for detecting VNC cardiomyopathy and is characterized by prominent trabeculations associated with deep intertrabecular recesses. Diagnostic clues include ≥3 trabeculations in one imaging plane located apically from the insertion of the papillary muscles and a ratio of noncompacted myocardium to compacted myocardium of more than 2.3:1 (sensitivity, 86%; specificity, 99%).

Patients with VNC have high morbidity and mortality as a result of heart failure, ventricular arrhythmias, and systemic embolism. Sudden death by arrhythmia is most often the cause of death. Unfortunately, there is no specific therapy for VNC with the only definitive treatment is cardiac transplant.

References: Petersen SE, Selvanayagam JB, Wiesmann F, et al. Left ventricular non-compaction: insights from cardiovascular magnetic resonance imaging. *J Am Coll Cardiol* 2005;46(1):101–105.

Zenooz NA, Zahka KG, Siwik ES, et al. Noncompaction syndrome of the myocardium: pathophysiology and imaging pearls. *J Thorac Imaging* 2010;25(4):326–332.

6. **Answer C.** Inversion recovery sequence demonstrating nulling of the myocardium and multifocal areas of late gadolinium enhancement in mid- and epicardial distribution. The findings are most compatible with myocarditis. The epicardial distribution is not compatible with infarction. Hypertrophic cardiomyopathy typically has asymmetric thickening and a familial association. Arrhythmogenic right ventricular cardiomyopathy typically demonstrates abnormality in myocardial nulling.

Myocarditis (inflammatory cardiomyopathy) is inflammation of the heart caused by a variety of pathogens and triggers (e.g., viral, bacterial, fungal infections, drug toxicity, or postradiation). Despite the etiology, the inflammation culminates in leukocytic cell infiltration, nonischemic degeneration, myocyte necrosis, and cardiac dysfunction.

Presence of late gadolinium enhancement (LGE) is an indication of irreversible myocardial necrosis and fibrosis. The pattern is classically subepicardial in distribution, although midinterventricular and focal transmural patterns are also possible. T2-weighted and early gadolinium enhancement imaging techniques are well validated to detect edema and hyperemia, respectively. In addition to LGE, these imaging features comprise the three "Lake Louise Consensus Criteria," recommended for diagnosing myocarditis. When two or more of these tissue characterization sequences are positive, pooled diagnostic accuracy for myocarditis is 78%; if only delayed enhancement is performed, diagnostic accuracy is 68%.

Quantitative T2 mapping offers the potential for increased accuracy in the detection of myocardial edema. Moreover, T1 mapping promises to overcome the limitation of needing large areas of necrosis to get a sufficient T1 contrast for LGE imaging.

References: Ferreira VM, Piechnik SK, Dall'Armellina E, et al. T1 mapping for the diagnosis of acute myocarditis using CMR. *JACC Cardiovas Imaging* 2013;6(10):1048-1058.

Friedrich MG, Sechtem U, Schulz-Menger J, et al. Cardiovascular magnetic resonance in myocarditis: a JACC white paper. *J Am Coll Cardiol* 2009;53(17):1475-1487.

Yilmaz A, Ferreira V, Klingel K, et al. Role of cardiovascular magnetic resonance imaging (CMR) in the diagnosis of acute and chronic myocarditis. *Heart Fail Rev* 2013;18(6):747-760.

7 **Answer D.** Inversion recovery sequence on the left demonstrates patchy late gadolinium enhancement consistent with fibrosis. Axial SSFP image on the right shows characteristic dark appearance of the liver compatible with iron deposition and signal loss due to susceptibility. The other etiologies do not demonstrate these changes.

Iron overload cardiomyopathy (IOC) is a secondary form of cardiomyopathy resulting from the accumulation of iron in the myocardium. IOC may result from hereditary disorders of iron metabolism (e.g., cardiomyopathy in hemochromatosis, thalassemia) or may be secondary due to multiple transfusions or abnormalities of hemoglobin synthesis leading to aberrant erythropoiesis.

Two main imaging phenotypes are generally noted—infiltration of the ventricular myocardium resulting in a restrictive cardiomyopathy, common in primary hemochromatosis, and a dilated cardiomyopathy with severe diastolic dysfunction in the early stages of secondary hemochromatosis. Echocardiography may not be able to distinguish IOC from idiopathic dilated cardiomyopathy. Deposition of iron in the myocardium causes a decrease in T2* relaxation time, which can be detected by multiecho gradient sequences on cardiac MRI. T2* values associated with IOC are typically less than 20 msec. The iron load is considered severe if the value is less than 10 msec. Varying amounts of delayed enhancement may also be observed depending on the severity of fibrosis.

References: Anderson L. Cardiovascular T2-star (T2*) magnetic resonance for the early diagnosis of myocardial iron overload. *Eur Heart J* 2001;22(23):2171-2179.

Kremastinos DT, Farmakis D. Iron overload cardiomyopathy in clinical practice. *Circulation* 2011;124(20):2253-2263.

8 **Answer C.** Given the symptoms of chest pain and elevated troponins, the primary concern would be the presence of an obstructive coronary lesion and need for immediate coronary intervention. The absence of coronary disease and the characteristic appearance of apical dilation on the ventriculogram are compatible with a stress-induced cardiomyopathy, also called Takotsubo cardiomyopathy.

22b Answer A. No imaging criterion is given for the diagnosis of ARVD. There is normal RV size and function without wall motion abnormalities. According to the 2010 Task Force Criteria for ARVD, fat is only diagnosed by tissue pathology and not imaging; in addition, this type of fat is considered a benign variant and not the fibrofatty infiltration seen in ARVD. In cases of ARVD with fibrofatty infiltration, the wall is thin, and there should be RV enlargement and motion abnormalities with decreased function. The diagnosis of ARVD cannot be excluded by imaging alone and should always be correlated with other findings.

Reference: Marcus FI, McKenna WJ, Sherrill D, et al. Diagnosis of arrhythmogenic right ventricular cardiomyopathy/dysplasia: proposed modification of the task force criteria. *Circulation* 2010;121(13):1533-1541.

23a Answer A. Chagas disease, caused by the parasite *Trypanosoma cruzi*, is responsible for a greater disease burden than any other parasitic disease in the Western hemisphere. While primarily prevalent in Latin America, the epidemiologic profile of Chagas disease has changed due to successful control in its transmission in endemic areas and new patterns of immigration leading to the urbanization and globalization of the disease. The Centers for Disease Control and Prevention estimates that there are more than 300,000 people infected with *Trypanosoma cruzi* in the United States, and a calculated total of 30,000 to 45,000 individuals likely have undiagnosed Chagas cardiomyopathy.

Severe acute disease occurs in <1% of patients, and the clinical manifestations include an acute myocarditis, pericardial effusion, and/or meningoencephalitis. Once the acute phase subsides, patients may be completely free of clinical signs and symptoms of the disease, sometimes for several years. This indeterminate form of the disease has an excellent prognosis, with affected patients having a life expectancy similar to individuals without the disease.

One-third of patients will ultimately develop chronic and symptomatic disease within two decades after the initial infection and can have cardiac or digestive symptoms or a combination of the two. The earliest manifestations of Chagas heart disease are usually conduction system abnormalities. Dilated cardiomyopathy is a severe and late manifestation of Chagas disease and is further complicated by heart failure, ventricular arrhythmias, heart blocks, thromboembolic phenomena, and sudden death.

References: Bern C, Montgomery SP. An estimate of the burden of chagas disease in the United States. *Clin Infect Dis* 2009;49(5):e52-e54.

Nunes MCP, Dones W, Morillo CA, et al. Chagas disease. *J Am Coll Cardiol* 2013;62(9):767-776.

23b Answer B. Manifestations of acute Chagas disease resolve spontaneously in about 90% of infected individuals even if the infection is not treated with trypanocidal drugs. About 60% to 70% of these patients will develop the intermediate form of the disease and will never manifest clinically apparent disease. The remaining 30% to 40% of patients will subsequently develop chronic disease with clinical presentations related to the pathologic involvement of specific organs—particularly the heart, esophagus, or colon. Gastrointestinal dysfunction (mainly megaesophagus, megacolon, or both) develops in about 10% to 15% of chronically infected patients.

References: Nunes MCP, Dones W, Morillo CA, et al. Chagas disease. *J Am Coll Cardiol* 2013;62(9):767-776.

Rassi A Jr, Rassi A, Marin-Neto JA. Chagas disease. *Lancet* 2010;375(9723):1388-1402.

24 Answer A. Peripartum/postpartum cardiomyopathy (PPCM) is a disorder associated with pregnancy distinguished by ventricular dilation and decreased systolic function, leading to symptoms of heart failure. PPCM is diagnosed when the following three criteria are met:

1. Heart failure develops in the last month of pregnancy or within 5 months of delivery.
2. Reduced systolic function, with an ejection fraction (EF) less than 45%.
3. No other cause for heart failure with reduced EF can be found.

Most patients (80%) present within 3 months of delivery, with the minority presenting in the last month of pregnancy (10%) or 4 to 5 months postpartum (10%). Because there is a significant overlap between symptoms related to pregnancy, especially toward the end of the third trimester or after delivery, and heart failure, the diagnosis may be initially missed or delayed.

Reference: Givertz MM. Peripartum cardiomyopathy. *Circulation* 2013;127(20):e622–e626.

25 Answer A. The E peak arises due to early diastolic filling. Most filling (70% to 75%) of the ventricle occurs during this phase, and it is influenced by the pressure gradient between the LA and LV. The A peak arises due to atrial contraction, forcing approximately 20% to 25% of stroke volume into the ventricle. It is influenced by LV stiffness and LA contractility.

With normal function, early passive filling of the left ventricle predominates with the peak velocity of the E wave being approximately 1 to 1.5 times greater than the velocity of the A wave.

As diastolic function deteriorates, LV end-diastolic pressure increases, which then in turn causes increased left atrial pressure. With mild abnormalities in ventricular relaxation (impaired relaxation), the E wave is reduced and prolonged resulting in greater dependency on atrial contraction (A wave becomes dominant over the E wave; E/A < 1.0). Further diastolic dysfunction leads to even greater left atrial pressure. Paradoxically, this improves early ventricular filling with a return of E-wave predominant velocities (pseudonormalization). In severe cases, and notable for restrictive cardiomyopathies, left atrial pressure becomes so high that all ventricular filling occurs in the early phase. The E-wave peak velocity becomes much greater than A-wave velocity with E/A ratios being greater than 2 (restrictive filling).

Reference: Ryding A. *Diastolic function and dyssynchrony*. In: Essential echocardiography, 2013:44–56.

26 Answer A. Danon disease is a rare X-linked disorder originally described as a type of glycogen storage disease, but now known to be a primary deficiency of lysosome-associated membrane protein 2. Affected men typically present with a triad of heart failure, skeletal myopathy, and mental retardation. In female carriers, the disease predominantly affects the cardiac myocytes. Skeletal myopathy occurs in most men and about half of affected women. The weakness typically occurs in the muscles of the upper arms, shoulders, neck, and upper thighs. Ophthalmic abnormalities or Wolff-Parkinson-White syndrome have also been reported.

Cardiac symptoms begin during adolescence, and patients die of severe heart failure in their third decade. Unlike HCM, in which LGE is midepicardial and patchy, Danon disease has subendocardial LGE. The value of cardiac transplantation has not been established, because very few patients live long enough (they die at very young ages) to undergo transplantation.

Amyloidosis, Fabry disease (FD), and Friedrich ataxia (FA) can all present with ventricular hypertrophy and fibrosis. Of these, only Friedrich ataxia is associated

Takotsubo cardiomyopathy (TTC) is a rapidly reversible form of acute heart failure reported to be triggered by stressful events and associated with a distinctive left ventricular (LV) contraction pattern. TTC mimics acute coronary syndrome in clinical presentation in the absence of angiographically significant coronary artery stenosis.

Variants of TTC include apical, midventricular, basal, or biventricular "ballooning". The most common form is severe anteroapical akinesis and hypercontractility of the basal segments ("apical ballooning"). There is typically an absence of late enhancement on delayed contrast sequences, which differentiates Takotsubo cardiomyopathy from anterior myocardial infarction.

Many studies report a good long-term prognosis; however, the acute phase of TTC can truly be life threatening. Complications, which may occur in the acute setting, include heart failure, arrhythmia, cardiogenic shock, LVOT obstruction, mitral regurgitation, ventricular thrombus, and cardiac rupture.

Treatment of TTC during the acute phase is mainly symptomatic treatment. Patients with TTC usually have a good prognosis, and almost perfect recovery is observed in 96% of the cases.

References: Eitel I, Schuler G, Gutberlet M, et al. Biventricular stress-induced (takotsubo) cardiomyopathy with left midventricular and right apical ballooning. *Int J Cardiol* 2011;151(2):e63-e64.

Virani SS, Khan AN, Mendoza CE, et al. Takotsubo cardiomyopathy, or broken-heart syndrome. *Tex Heart Inst J* 2007;34(1):76-79.

9 Answer B. Although commonly seen in the setting of hypertrophic cardiomyopathy, basal septal hypertrophy (BSH) can be seen independently of HCM, being more prevalent in the elderly and in the presence of systemic hypertension. One study identified over 3,500 patients with isolated septal hypertrophy in the Framingham Heart Study, where BSH was characterized as septal thickness greater than 1.4 cm in the absence of septal abnormalities. The presence of BSH was not associated with an increased risk of cardiovascular disease or mortality.

Based on autopsy series and echocardiographic data, about 10% of patients with hemodynamically significant AS show asymmetric thickening of the septum. Recent studies have demonstrated that hypertrophic heart disease from valvular aortic stenosis implicates a poor prognosis early and late after aortic valve replacement. However, it is still controversial whether directed therapy such as myotomy or alcohol ablation should be considered concomitant to aortic valve repair.

Noncompaction, Uhl anomaly and annuloaortic ectasia are not associated with this phenomenon.

References: Di Tommaso L, Stassano P, Mannacio V, et al. Asymmetric septal hypertrophy in patients with severe aortic stenosis: the usefulness of associated septal myectomy. *J Thoracic Cardiovas Surg* 2013;145(1):171-175.

Diaz T, Pencina MJ, Benjamin EJ, et al. Prevalence, clinical correlates, and prognosis of discrete upper septal thickening on echocardiography: the Framingham Heart Study. *Echocardiography* 2009;26(3):247-253.

Kelshiker MA, Mayet J, Unsworth B, et al. Basal septal hypertrophy. *Curr Cardiol Rev* 2013;9(4):316-324.

10 Answer B. Horizontal long axis demonstrates marked left ventricular thickening with mild asymmetric thickening of the septum, consistent with hypertrophic cardiomyopathy (HCM). Patchy late gadolinium enhancement is also observed near the LV apex, compatible with areas of myocardial fibrosis.

HCM is a clinically and genetically heterogeneous disorder, characterized most commonly by left ventricular (LV) hypertrophy. HCM has a range of potential outcomes including heart failure and sudden cardiac death, but also survival to normal life expectancy.

The estimated prevalence of HCM of 1 in 500 is based on data originally collected almost 20 years ago. However, advances in HCM, including enhanced understanding of the underlying molecular and genetic substrate, contemporary family screening, and more sensitive diagnostic cardiac imaging, suggest that the prevalence of HCM may be underestimated. Although many patients remain asymptomatic with a benign natural history, sudden death (SD) can occur as the initial manifestation of the disease in otherwise asymptomatic or mildly symptomatic young (<25 years of age) patients.

Conventional risk factors for SD in HCM include family history HCM-related sudden death; one of more episodes of unexplained recent syncope; LV hypertrophy >30 mm; nonsustained ventricular tachycardia on 24 hour electrocardiography; and hypotensive blood pressure response to exercise. Cardiac magnetic resonance (CMR) imaging has emerged as a precise diagnostic tool and powerful adjunct in assessing risk of SD with HCM. CMR provides characterization of morphologic phenotypes of LV wall thickening, often not reliably visualized with standard echocardiographic cross-sectional planes. The presence of late gadolinium enhancement (LGE) in HCM patients has been shown to have a sevenfold increased risk for potential lethal ventricular tachyarrhythmias compared with those without LGE. Although large prospective studies validating its utility are still emerging, many experts consider the presence of LGE as influential in the decision of placing an ICD in HCM patients currently classified as intermediate risk.

References: Efthimiadis GK, Pagourelias ED, Gossios T, et al. Hypertrophic cardiomyopathy in 2013: current speculations and future perspectives. *World J Cardiol* 2014;6(2):26-37.

Hoey ETD, Teoh JK, Das I, et al. The emerging role of cardiovascular MRI for risk stratification in hypertrophic cardiomyopathy. *Clin Radiol* 2014;69(3):221-230.

Semsarian C, Ingles J, Maron MS, et al. New perspectives on the prevalence of hypertrophic cardiomyopathy. *J Am Coll Cardiol* 2015;65(12):1249-1254.

11 **Answer A.** Horizontal long-axis image of the heart demonstrates subendocardial late gadolinium enhancement involving both ventricles. The remaining myocardium nulls appropriately. Although infarction is classically subendocardial, the distribution of the abnormality does not follow a vascular distribution. The unremarkable nulling of the remaining myocardium is atypical in amyloid. Cardiac sarcoidosis is usually mid- to epicardial in its involvement.

Eosinophil-mediated myocarditis can occur in association with parasitic infection (tropical endomyocardial fibrosis) or Churg-Strauss syndrome (a necrotizing small vessel vasculitis) or can occur as an idiopathic entity (termed Loeffler endocarditis or hypereosinophilic syndrome). Classically, three clinicohistologic stages have been described:

1. Acute necrotic stage—characterized by subendocardial necrosis as well as constitutional symptoms, pulmonary infiltrates, atrioventricular valve regurgitation, and biventricular failure
2. Subacute thrombotic stage—characterized by thrombosis, splinter hemorrhages, and more severely resulting in cerebral, splenic, renal, and coronary infarctions
3. Late fibrotic stage—characterized by late-stage fibrosis of the endomyocardial surface of either or both left and right ventricles

Cardiac MR is instrumental in identifying markers of eosinophilic involvement including myocardial inflammation, mural thrombi, and endocardial fibrosis. The use of first-pass perfusion MRI allows differentiation of perfused and enhancing myocardium from poorly vascularized and hypoenhancing thrombus or eosinophilic infiltrate. Late gadolinium enhancement images typically show intense global subendocardial enhancement that is not limited to a vascular territory. Nonenhancing thrombi may also be observed in left and right ventricular apices.

Endomyocardial fibrosis and especially cardiac thromboembolic events originating from mural thrombus may cause potentially fatal complications or irreversible neurologic defects if not appropriately treated without delay. Follow-up MRI can help document therapeutic improvement with reduction of left ventricular mass and improved contractile function along with simultaneous improvement of clinical symptoms.

References: Kleinfeldt T, Ince H, Nienaber CA. Hypereosinophilic syndrome: a rare case of Loeffler's endocarditis documented in cardiac MRI. *Int J Cardiol* 2011;149(1):e30-e32.

Mannelli L, Cherian V, Nayar A, et al. Loeffler's endocarditis in hypereosinophilic syndrome. *Curr Probl Diagn Radiol* 2012;41(4):146-148.

Perazzolo Marra M, Thiene G, Rizzo S, et al. Cardiac magnetic resonance features of biopsy-proven endomyocardial diseases. *JACC Cardiovas Img* 2014;7(3):309-312.

12 **Answer A.** Horizontal long axis demonstrates biatrial enlargement and relative normal appearance of both ventricles. Whereas both constrictive pericarditis and restrictive cardiomyopathy can present with similar clinical signs, restrictive cardiomyopathy classically demonstrates biatrial enlargement and constrictive pericarditis classically has normal appearance to the cardiac chambers. This results from decreased ventricular compliance. Ventricular enlargement can be seen ischemic, inflammatory, or dilated cardiomyopathies.

Generally, restrictive cardiomyopathy (CMP) refers to a group of primary or secondary infiltrative disorders characterized by normal left ventricular cavity size and systolic function but with increased myocardial stiffness and decreased ventricular compliance. Primary restrictive cardiomyopathies include endomyocardial fibrosis, Loeffler endomyocarditis, and idiopathic primary restrictive CMP. Secondary types of restrictive CMP are more common and are typically due to conditions where the heart is affected as part of a multisystem disorder (e.g., amyloidosis, hemochromatosis).

The morphologic appearance in restrictive CMP often demonstrates atrial enlargement and ventricular thickening. The RV may also enlarge if pulmonary hypertension coexists. Cardiac MRI is a fundamental diagnostic tool because it helps in the differentiation between restrictive CMP and constrictive pericarditis, which have different therapeutic approaches. The presence of late gadolinium enhancement is consistent with fibrosis in myocardium.

Diastolic function is severely disturbed and could easily be assessed by studying the ventricular filling pattern on cine or phase contrast images. The characteristic features of restrictive left ventricular filling are short isovolumic relaxation time, dominant early diastolic filling with short deceleration time, and small or absent late diastolic filling component.

References: Belloni E, De Cobelli F, Esposito A, et al. MRI of cardiomyopathy. *Am J Roentgenol* 2008;191(6):1702-1710.

Gupta A, Singh Gulati G, Seth S, et al. Cardiac MRI in restrictive cardiomyopathy. *Clin Radiol* 2012;67(2):95-105.

Hughes S. Cardiomyopathies. In: Suvarna SK (ed.). *Cardiac pathology*. London: Springer, 2013:183-200.

13 **Answer A.** Short-axis inversion recovery sequence after contrast demonstrates linear late gadolinium enhancement in the midwall of the interventricular septum.

A linear midwall septal stripe of late gadolinium enhancement has been described in approximately 30% of patients with nonischemic dilated cardiomyopathies. The location of the stripe does not follow a pattern consistent with ischemic disease. The abnormality is thought to develop secondary to replacement fibrosis, which has been reported in pathologic samples and may be related to subclinical foci of myocardial ischemia. This linear abnormality has been suggested as a marker for increased risk of sudden cardiac death, since the fibrosis may predispose to electrical instability.

Reference: Cummings KW, Bhalla S, Javidan-Nejad C, et al. A pattern-based approach to assessment of delayed enhancement in nonischemic cardiomyopathy at MR imaging. *Radiographics* 2009;29(1):89-103.

14 Answer A. Short-axis image of the left ventricle demonstrates diffusely abnormal nulling of the myocardium on inversion recovery sequences. Classically, with the blood pool containing the largest concentration of gadolinium, the inversion time of the blood pool occurs before nulling of the myocardium. In this case, subendocardial myocardium has traversed its null point before the blood pool, and the remaining myocardium reaches its null point near the same time as the blood pool. This gross aberration of late gadolinium enhancement is almost exclusively seen in the setting of amyloid deposition.

Cardiac amyloidosis is the most common infiltrative type of secondary restrictive cardiomyopathies and is caused by the deposition of insoluble amyloid protein fibrils in the interstitium of the myocardium. Cardiac amyloidosis may be classified according to the type of amyloid fibril protein deposited. The most common type of amyloidosis to affect the heart is AL amyloidosis due to the deposition of amyloid fibrils complexed with monoclonal kappa and lambda immunoglobulin light chains. AL amyloidosis is principally associated with plasma cell dyscrasias (e.g., B-cell lymphoma, Waldenstrom macroglobulinemia, multiple myeloma). Mutations in the gene for transthyretin predominantly result in neurologic and heart disease, and with some mutations, amyloid deposits are exclusive to the myocardium. Fragments of serum amyloid A protein are responsible for AA (secondary) amyloidosis, which is associated with a variety of chronic inflammatory disorders, but rarely associated with cardiac involvement.

No single noninvasive test or abnormality is pathognomonic of cardiac amyloid; diagnosis of cardiac amyloid has usually relied on (1) echocardiographic assessment, especially measurement of LV wall thickness, subjective assessment of myocardial appearance, and evaluation of diastolic function/restrictive physiology, and (2) histopathologic findings of amyloid deposition on endomyocardial biopsy.

The high spatial resolution and signal-to-noise ratio of cardiac MR permit reproducible measurement of cardiac chamber volumes and mass, as well as LV and atrial septal wall thickness. The main feature of cardiac amyloidosis is diffuse myocardial thickening including the atria and valves. Biatrial dilation and restriction of diastolic filling may also be seen associated with depressed systolic ventricular function and reduced wall compliance, which in later stages can evolve to overt restrictive CMP.

Tissue characterization with LGE provides unique clinical value in further assessment of amyloid infiltration. The pattern of late gadolinium enhancement is characterized by a diffuse, heterogeneous subendocardial distribution that may resemble an incorrect myocardial signal suppression due to an inappropriate choice of inversion time.

References: Maceira AM. Cardiovascular magnetic resonance in cardiac amyloidosis. *Circulation* 2005;111(2):186–193.

Selvanayagam JB, Leong DP. MR imaging and cardiac amyloidosis: where to go from here? *JACC Cardiovas Imaging* 2010;3(2):165–167.

15 Answer D. Dilated cardiomyopathies (DCM) are a spectrum of heterogeneous myocardial disorders that are characterized by ventricular dilation and depressed myocardial contractility (typically ejection fraction less than 40%).

The cause is not well understood, and although up to 50% of cases are considered to be idiopathic, it is recognized that other cases of the disease may have ischemic, genetic or familial, viral, immune, or a toxic origin or can be secondary to cardiovascular diseases with myocardial dysfunction that is not explained by ischemic damage. About 20% to 35% cases of idiopathic DCM are familial in origin.

DCM is the most common cause of cardiomyopathy and cardiac transplantation in children and adults. The most common causes of infantile DCM include idiopathic, inborn errors of metabolism, and malformation syndromes. Myocarditis and neuromuscular disorders are the most common causes during childhood.

The most common determination among cardiomyopathies with a dilated phenotype is whether or not the etiology is related to underlying coronary disease (ischemic vs. nonischemic). Existing clinical studies suggest that the prognosis of patients with nonischemic dilated cardiomyopathy is better than patients with underlying ischemic heart disease.

References: Bozkurt B. Chapter 24—heart failure as a consequence of dilated cardiomyopathy. In: Mann DL (ed.) *Heart failure: a companion to Braunwald's heart disease*, 2nd ed. Philadelphia, PA: Saunders, 2011:372–394.

Jefferies JL, Towbin JA. Dilated cardiomyopathy. *Lancet* 2010;375(9716):752–762.

Towbin JA, Lowe AM, Colan SD, et al. Incidence, causes, and outcomes of dilated cardiomyopathy in children. *JAMA* 2006;296(15):1867–1876.

16a Answer B. Myocarditis (inflammatory cardiomyopathy) is defined as an inflammatory disorder of the myocardium, characterized by leukocytic cell infiltration, nonischemic degeneration, myocyte necrosis, and cardiac dysfunction.

Clinical presentation is variable in severity, ranging from asymptomatic to cardiogenic shock. Myocarditis is typically associated with other viral symptoms, 7 to 10 days after the onset of the systemic illness. Young adults are most commonly affected. The mean age of patients with giant-cell myocarditis (GCM) is 42 years, whereas the mean age of adult patients with other forms of myocarditis has been reported to range from 20 to 51 years.

Currently, no single clinical or imaging finding confirms the diagnosis of myocarditis with absolute certainty. Rather, an integrated synopsis, including history, clinical assessment, and noninvasive test results, should be used to diagnose the disease and guide treatment. Most patients respond well to standard heart failure therapy, although, in severe cases, mechanical circulatory support or heart transplantation is indicated. More than 75% of patients with acute myocarditis gain spontaneous recovery, except in patients with giant-cell myocarditis. Persistent, chronic myocarditis usually has a progressive course but may respond to immunosuppression.

The standard Dallas pathologic criteria for the definition of myocarditis require that an inflammatory cellular infiltrate with or without associated myocyte necrosis be present on conventional endomyocardial biopsy. Noninvasive cardiac magnetic resonance imaging (MRI) may provide an alternative method for diagnosis without the risks of biopsy.

References: Cooper LT Jr. Myocarditis. *NEJM* 2009;360(15):1526–1538.

Maisch B, Pankuweit S. Current treatment options in (peri)myocarditis and inflammatory cardiomyopathy. *Herz* 2012;37(6):644–656.

16b Answer B. The expected tissue pathology in active myocarditis includes intracellular and interstitial myocardial edema, capillary leakage, hyperemia, and, in more severe cases, cellular necrosis and subsequent fibrosis.

The ability to characterize myocardial tissue with respect with these pathologic processes has made cardiac MR the primary tool in the noninvasive assessment of patients with suspected myocarditis. Myocardial edema appears as areas of high signal intensity on T2-weighted images. Contrast-enhanced fast spin-echo T1-weighted MR can be used to assess precontrast and early postcontrast gadolinium enhancement (EGE) of the myocardium, which correlates with inflammation, hyperemia, and capillary leak. Myocardial late gadolinium enhancement (LGE) specifically reflects myocardial injury (i.e., necrosis and fibrosis).

A consensus group evaluated the evidence for cardiac MR with respect to these techniques and determined that these three parameters (T2, EGE, and LGE) are most helpful in making the diagnosis of myocarditis. These "Lake Louise Criteria" were found to have a sensitivity of 67%, specificity of 91%, accuracy of 78%, positive predictive value of 91%, and negative predictive value of 69%, when any 2 of the 3 criteria were compared with clinical or histopathologic data. Interval decrease in edema and hyperemia at follow-up compared with baseline scan can help distinguish acute from chronic myocarditis.

Chemical shift imaging and myocardial tagging do not contribute to the sensitivity of making the diagnosis.

Reference: Friedrich MG, Sechtem U, Schulz-Menger J, et al. Cardiovascular magnetic resonance in myocarditis: a JACC white paper. *J Am Coll Cardiol* 2009;53(17):1475-1487.

17a **Answer C.** SSFP, horizontal long-axis image demonstrates biventricular dilation and notable trabeculation involving both chambers, consistent with ventricular noncompaction. Also noted is the absence of well-formed papillary muscles.

Ventricular noncompaction (VNC), also known as spongiform cardiomyopathy, is a congenital myocardial abnormality that can present in either childhood or adulthood. VNC occurs due to persistence of noncompacted endocardium characteristic of the early fetal period before myocardial compaction is complete.

Echocardiography is usually the first modality obtained for the assessment of VNC cardiomyopathy and characteristically demonstrates prominent trabeculations associated with deep intertrabecular recesses. Noncompacted segments are usually hypokinetic and global ventricular function is commonly decreased. RV involvement has been described but rarely in isolation.

With the advent of ECG gating, computed tomography has expanded its role in identification of the disorder. It has better spatial resolution, allows for better visualization of trabeculations than echo, and is not limited by acoustic windows. Cardiac MR is the most robust modality with the capability of multiplanar imaging of the heart, evaluation of ventricular function, and tissue characterization of the myocardium.

References: Petersen SE, Selvanayagam JB, Wiesmann F, et al. Left ventricular non-compaction: insights from cardiovascular magnetic resonance imaging. *J Am Coll Cardiol* 2005;46(1):101-105.

Zenooz NA, Zahka KG, Siwik ES, et al. Noncompaction syndrome of the myocardium: pathophysiology and imaging pearls. *J Thorac Imaging* 2010;25(4):326-332.

17b **Answer A.** The triad of heart failure symptoms, arrhythmias and embolic events is the major clinical manifestation in patients with left ventricular noncompaction (VNC). A substantial percentage of these patients have a dilated left ventricle with systolic dysfunction, mimicking dilated cardiomyopathy. Criteria suggesting the diagnosis of VNC include ≥3 trabeculations in one imaging plane and a ratio of noncompacted myocardium to compacted myocardium of more than 2.3:1.

In adults, various forms of congenital heart disease are associated with left VNC, particularly stenotic lesions of the left ventricular outflow tract, Ebstein anomaly, and tetralogy of Fallot. VNC is rarely associated with muscular dystrophies, unclassified myopathies, or neuropathies. One particular association, Barth syndrome, is an X-linked recessive disorder that is typically characterized by cardiomyopathy, skeletal myopathy, growth retardation, and neutropenia.

There is no specific therapy for VNC. Because of a high incidence of thromboembolic events, all patients should receive systemic anticoagulation. Heart failure is treated with conventional therapies. Since the main causes of death are arrhythmias, antiarrhythmic medications should be considered for all VNC patients, whether symptomatic or not. Also, in some patients, implantation of a defibrillator may be necessary.

References: Jefferies JL, Towbin JA. Dilated cardiomyopathy. *Lancet* 2010;375(9716):752-762.

Stähli BE, Gebhard C, Biaggi P, et al. Left ventricular non-compaction: prevalence in congenital heart disease. *Int J Cardiol* 2013;167(6):2477-2481.

Udeoji DU, Philip KJ, Morrissey RP, et al. Left ventricular noncompaction cardiomyopathy: updated review. *Ther Adv Cardiovasc Dis* 2013;7(5):260-273.

Zenooz NA, Zahka KG, Siwik ES, et al. Noncompaction syndrome of the myocardium: pathophysiology and imaging pearls. *J Thorac Imaging* 2010;25(4):326-332.

18 Answer B. Axial image from a contrast-enhanced CT demonstrates an infiltrating mass in the apical septum of the LV.

Metastatic disease is commonly considered whenever a cardiac mass is discovered, since tumors giving rise to cardiac metastasis are by far the most common cardiac tumors. In descending order of frequency, the malignancies most strongly associated with metastasis to the heart include lung cancer, breast cancer, melanoma, and hematologic malignancies (leukemia and lymphoma). Infiltrative masses can have the appearance of focal or diffuse cardiomyopathies.

Granulocytic sarcoma (GS) is an invasive tumor mass composed of immature cells of the granulocytic series, occurring before, concomitantly, or after the overt development of acute or chronic myelogenous leukemia. Most cases of GS occur in childhood in association with acute myelogenous leukemia.

The majority of primary cardiac tumors are benign. Papillary fibroelastomas are the second most common primary cardiac tumor after myxoma, accounting for 10% of tumors. They most commonly occur on valve leaflets and are most frequently found on the aortic valve. Primary malignant tumors of the heart are rare and are represented by sarcomas, primary lymphomas, and malignant pericardial tumors. Primary cardiac angiosarcoma is the most common cardiac sarcoma, accounting for 33% of cases. Angiosarcomas tend to occur on the right side, most commonly the right atrium. The tumors are large, hemorrhagic, and infiltrative. Primary cardiac lymphoma is defined as a lymphoma confined to the heart and pericardium. It is very rare and accounts for only 1% of primary cardiac tumors. Primary cardiac lymphomas are almost invariably non-Hodgkin lymphomas of B-cell type. The most common primary cardiac lymphoma is diffuse large B-cell lymphoma, which accounts for 80% of cases.

References: Burke A, Jeudy J, Virmani R. Cardiac tumours: an update. *Heart* 2008;94(1):117–123.

Jankovic M, Bonacina E, Masera G, et al. Cardiac relapses in myeloid leukemia: case report and review of the literature. *Pediatr Hematol Oncol* 1987;4(3):237–245.

Makaryus AN, Tung F, Liu W, et al. Extensive neoplastic cardiac infiltration in a patient with acute myelogenous leukemia: role of echocardiography. *Echocardiography* 2003;20(6):539–544.

Rassl DM, Davies SJ. Cardiac tumors. In: Suvarna SK (ed.). *Cardiac pathology*. London, UK: Springer, 2013:201–221.

19 Answer D. Both restrictive and constrictive diseases exhibit an abrupt reduction in filling, increased backpressure, and impaired stroke volume. Restrictive cardiomyopathy is characterized by normal left ventricular cavity size and systolic function but with decreased diastolic volume and ventricular compliance. Imaging often reveals thickening of the ventricles with biatrial enlargement secondary to a differential of intracardiac chamber pressures.

Constrictive pericarditis is characterized by fibrous or calcific thickening of the pericardium, which leads to discordance in normal diastolic filling of the heart—reduced left ventricular filling, which corresponds to increased right ventricular filling. This manifests as a variance in the septal curvature during diastolic filling and characteristic "septal bounce." Intracardiac pressures are typically equal throughout the cardiac chambers.

While constrictive pericarditis is an extracardiac constraint, restrictive cardiomyopathy is an intrinsic myocardial disease of the ventricle. Respiratory variation of ventricular filling and ejection velocities may be modestly present in constriction but is absent in restrictive right ventricular disease.

It is important to distinguish between constrictive pericarditis and restrictive cardiomyopathy because treatment for the former condition is surgical and treatment for the latter is medical.

References: Henein MY, Sheppard M. Restrictive cardiomyopathy. In: Henein MY (ed.). *Clinical echocardiography*. London: Springer, 2012:203–212.

Henein MY, Sheppard M. Pericardial disease. In: Henein MY (ed.). *Clinical Echocardiography*. London, UK: Springer, 2012:251–266.

20 **Answer A.** Iron overload cardiomyopathy can occur either as a result of inappropriate excess iron absorption, as in the case of hemochromatosis or thalassemia major, or due to multiple transfusions. Myocardial iron content cannot be predicted from serum ferritin or liver iron, and conventional assessments of cardiac function can only detect those with advanced disease.

The measurement of T2* relaxation by cardiac MR is the most widely used technique for the direct assessment of myocardial iron because it is fast and robust, is reproducible, and is sensitive to iron deposition. T2* relaxation is the combined effect of T2 relaxation and the effect of magnetic field nonuniformities. Excess iron in the tissues induces a significant loss of signal due to changes in magnetic susceptibility, causing a shortening of T2* values. As iron accumulates in the normal storage form in the heart, the T2* falls, but there is minimal effect on cardiac function until a threshold is reached where the iron storage capacity is exhausted. Once this critical level is reached, rapid deterioration of cardiac function occurs. Thus, cardiac T2* is a powerful predictor of the subsequent development of heart failure. Iron clears more slowly from the heart than the liver, which may contribute to the high mortality of patients with established cardiomyopathy despite intensive chelation.

LGE is widely used to detect macroscopic fibrosis in a range of nonischemic cardiomyopathies, and the presence of LGE is associated with the development of cardiac events, including heart failure. LGE, however, is not specific for iron deposition. Additionally, macroscopic fibrosis, which is commonly identified in other pathologies, is less common in iron overload cardiomyopathies, particularly at early stages. Newer developing techniques such as T1 mapping may play a more critical role in the evaluation of early microscopic changes in the future.

References: Kirk P, Carpenter JP, Tanner MA, et al. Low prevalence of fibrosis in thalassemia major assessed by late gadolinium enhancement cardiovascular magnetic resonance. *J Cardiovas Magn Reson* 2011;13(1):8.

Kirk P, Roughton M, Porter JB, et al. Cardiac T2* magnetic resonance for prediction of cardiac complications in thalassemia major. *Circulation* 2009;120(20):1961-1968.

21 **Answer D.** Spatial modulation of magnetization (SPAMM) tagging is a robust, noninvasive technique that provides detailed and comprehensive evaluation of myocardial contractility, strain, and torsion.

MR SPAMM tagging has become the reference technique for evaluating early LV impairment and multidimensional cardiac strain evolution. Saturation bands or tags are created by perturbations of the magnetization field perpendicular to the imaging plane. The resulting tags follow myocardial motion during the cardiac cycle, thus reflecting the underlying myocardial deformation.

Abnormalities in regional strain can serve as a marker of subclinical cardiomyopathies and identify individuals who might benefit from targeted preventive interventions.

Reference: Shehata ML, Cheng S, Osman NF, et al. Myocardial tissue tagging with cardiovascular magnetic resonance. *J Cardiovasc Magn Reson* 2009;11(1):55.

22a **Answer C.** There is fat in the RV wall, which is thickened. This can be seen in obese older female patients, which is considered a benign variant of RV fat rather than the fibrofatty infiltration seen in ARVD. The fibrofatty infiltration of ARVD can be difficult to image but often occurs in setting of RV enlargement and dysfunction; there can be RV aneurysms/abnormal tethering.

Reference: Macedo R, Prakasa K, Tichnell C, et al. Marked lipomatous infiltration of the right ventricle: MRI findings in relation to arrhythmogenic right ventricular dysplasia. *AJR Am J Roentgenol* 2007;188(5).

22b Answer A. No imaging criterion is given for the diagnosis of ARVD. There is normal RV size and function without wall motion abnormalities. According to the 2010 Task Force Criteria for ARVD, fat is only diagnosed by tissue pathology and not imaging; in addition, this type of fat is considered a benign variant and not the fibrofatty infiltration seen in ARVD. In cases of ARVD with fibrofatty infiltration, the wall is thin, and there should be RV enlargement and motion abnormalities with decreased function. The diagnosis of ARVD cannot be excluded by imaging alone and should always be correlated with other findings.

Reference: Marcus FI, McKenna WJ, Sherrill D, et al. Diagnosis of arrhythmogenic right ventricular cardiomyopathy/dysplasia: proposed modification of the task force criteria. *Circulation* 2010;121(13):1533–1541.

23a Answer A. Chagas disease, caused by the parasite *Trypanosoma cruzi*, is responsible for a greater disease burden than any other parasitic disease in the Western hemisphere. While primarily prevalent in Latin America, the epidemiologic profile of Chagas disease has changed due to successful control in its transmission in endemic areas and new patterns of immigration leading to the urbanization and globalization of the disease. The Centers for Disease Control and Prevention estimates that there are more than 300,000 people infected with *Trypanosoma cruzi* in the United States, and a calculated total of 30,000 to 45,000 individuals likely have undiagnosed Chagas cardiomyopathy.

Severe acute disease occurs in <1% of patients, and the clinical manifestations include an acute myocarditis, pericardial effusion, and/or meningoencephalitis. Once the acute phase subsides, patients may be completely free of clinical signs and symptoms of the disease, sometimes for several years. This indeterminate form of the disease has an excellent prognosis, with affected patients having a life expectancy similar to individuals without the disease.

One-third of patients will ultimately develop chronic and symptomatic disease within two decades after the initial infection and can have cardiac or digestive symptoms or a combination of the two. The earliest manifestations of Chagas heart disease are usually conduction system abnormalities. Dilated cardiomyopathy is a severe and late manifestation of Chagas disease and is further complicated by heart failure, ventricular arrhythmias, heart blocks, thromboembolic phenomena, and sudden death.

References: Bern C, Montgomery SP. An estimate of the burden of chagas disease in the United States. *Clin Infect Dis* 2009;49(5):e52–e54.

Nunes MCP, Dones W, Morillo CA, et al. Chagas disease. *J Am Coll Cardiol* 2013;62(9):767–776.

23b Answer B. Manifestations of acute Chagas disease resolve spontaneously in about 90% of infected individuals even if the infection is not treated with trypanocidal drugs. About 60% to 70% of these patients will develop the intermediate form of the disease and will never manifest clinically apparent disease. The remaining 30% to 40% of patients will subsequently develop chronic disease with clinical presentations related to the pathologic involvement of specific organs—particularly the heart, esophagus, or colon. Gastrointestinal dysfunction (mainly megaesophagus, megacolon, or both) develops in about 10% to 15% of chronically infected patients.

References: Nunes MCP, Dones W, Morillo CA, et al. Chagas disease. *J Am Coll Cardiol* 2013;62(9):767–776.

Rassi A Jr, Rassi A, Marin-Neto JA. Chagas disease. *Lancet* 2010;375(9723): 1388–1402.

24 Answer A.
Peripartum/postpartum cardiomyopathy (PPCM) is a disorder associated with pregnancy distinguished by ventricular dilation and decreased systolic function, leading to symptoms of heart failure. PPCM is diagnosed when the following three criteria are met:

1. Heart failure develops in the last month of pregnancy or within 5 months of delivery.
2. Reduced systolic function, with an ejection fraction (EF) less than 45%.
3. No other cause for heart failure with reduced EF can be found.

Most patients (80%) present within 3 months of delivery, with the minority presenting in the last month of pregnancy (10%) or 4 to 5 months postpartum (10%). Because there is a significant overlap between symptoms related to pregnancy, especially toward the end of the third trimester or after delivery, and heart failure, the diagnosis may be initially missed or delayed.

Reference: Givertz MM. Peripartum cardiomyopathy. *Circulation* 2013;127(20):e622–e626.

25 Answer A.
The E peak arises due to early diastolic filling. Most filling (70% to 75%) of the ventricle occurs during this phase, and it is influenced by the pressure gradient between the LA and LV. The A peak arises due to atrial contraction, forcing approximately 20% to 25% of stroke volume into the ventricle. It is influenced by LV stiffness and LA contractility.

With normal function, early passive filling of the left ventricle predominates with the peak velocity of the E wave being approximately 1 to 1.5 times greater than the velocity of the A wave.

As diastolic function deteriorates, LV end-diastolic pressure increases, which then in turn causes increased left atrial pressure. With mild abnormalities in ventricular relaxation (impaired relaxation), the E wave is reduced and prolonged resulting in greater dependency on atrial contraction (A wave becomes dominant over the E wave; E/A < 1.0). Further diastolic dysfunction leads to even greater left atrial pressure. Paradoxically, this improves early ventricular filling with a return of E-wave predominant velocities (pseudonormalization). In severe cases, and notable for restrictive cardiomyopathies, left atrial pressure becomes so high that all ventricular filling occurs in the early phase. The E-wave peak velocity becomes much greater than A-wave velocity with E/A ratios being greater than 2 (restrictive filling).

Reference: Ryding A. *Diastolic function and dyssynchrony*. In: Essential echocardiography, 2013:44–56.

26 Answer A.
Danon disease is a rare X-linked disorder originally described as a type of glycogen storage disease, but now known to be a primary deficiency of lysosome-associated membrane protein 2. Affected men typically present with a triad of heart failure, skeletal myopathy, and mental retardation. In female carriers, the disease predominantly affects the cardiac myocytes. Skeletal myopathy occurs in most men and about half of affected women. The weakness typically occurs in the muscles of the upper arms, shoulders, neck, and upper thighs. Ophthalmic abnormalities or Wolff-Parkinson-White syndrome have also been reported.

Cardiac symptoms begin during adolescence, and patients die of severe heart failure in their third decade. Unlike HCM, in which LGE is midepicardial and patchy, Danon disease has subendocardial LGE. The value of cardiac transplantation has not been established, because very few patients live long enough (they die at very young ages) to undergo transplantation.

Amyloidosis, Fabry disease (FD), and Friedrich ataxia (FA) can all present with ventricular hypertrophy and fibrosis. Of these, only Friedrich ataxia is associated with neuromuscular abnormalities. However, mental retardation is not an associated finding in FA. FD and amyloidosis patients will have signs and symptoms related to protein deposition in different organ systems including peripheral neuropathies, cardiomyopathies, and renal damage. Amyloid patients reveal characteristic difficulty in nulling of the myocardium on MR.

Reference: Piotrowska-Kownacka D, Kownacki L, Kuch M, et al. Cardiovascular magnetic resonance findings in a case of Danon disease. *J Cardiovas Magn Reson* 2009;11(1):12.

27 Answer A. FDG-PET uptake assesses active inflammation, which is characterized by increased glucose metabolism, particularly by activated macrophages.

PET scanning protocols for cardiac sarcoidosis aim to suppress physiologic uptake of FDG by the myocardium and enable switch to free fatty acid metabolism. Areas of increased activity are compatible with inflamed and hypermetabolic myocardium. Patterns suggestive of active cardiac sarcoidosis are mainly focal areas of FDG uptake and focal on top of diffuse uptake. Whereas uptake on FDG-PET suggests an active inflammatory process, steroid treatment has been shown to decrease its size and intensity.

Reference: Skali H, Schulman AR, Dorbala S. 18F-FDG PET/CT for the assessment of myocardial sarcoidosis. *Curr Cardiol Reports* 2013;15(4).

28 Answer A. This bulge along the RV wall has been described as "apicolateral bulge" and is considered a benign variant in the absence of other RV wall motion abnormalities. This would not give any imaging criterion for the diagnosis of ARVD. Note the normal RV size in this patient.

Reference: Rastegar N, Burt JR, Corona-Villalobos CP, et al. Cardiac MR findings and potential diagnostic pitfalls in patients evaluated for arrhythmogenic right ventricular cardiomyopathy. *Radiographics* 2014;34(6):1553–1570.

29 Answer C. Iron overload cardiomyopathy (IOC) in the setting of thalassemia major is the result of recurrent blood transfusion. CMR $T2^*$ relaxation time is the current standard for noninvasive quantitative assessment of myocardial iron deposition. $T2^*$ values <20 msec are indicative of significant iron deposition, and values <10 msec are at increased risk for heart failure and arrhythmias.

Advances in the field of chelators have rendered iron overload efficiently treatable and IOC almost completely preventable. The improvement of $T2^*$ values correlates well to decrease of myocardial iron accumulation and is a powerful tool in guiding therapy.

References: Kremastinos DT, Farmakis D. Iron overload cardiomyopathy in clinical practice. *Circulation* 2011;124(20):2253–2263.

Pennell DJ, Porter JB, Cappellini MD, et al. Efficacy of deferasirox in reducing and preventing cardiac iron overload in beta-thalassemia. *Blood* 2010;115(12):2364–2371.

30 Answer D. Amyloidosis causes accumulation of an abnormal interstitial protein and expansion of extracellular space within the myocardium. As a consequence, suppression of myocardial signal using inversion recovery sequences becomes difficult due to the global abnormality of the myocardium. Diffuse subendocardial or transmural enhancement of the myocardium may be observed in a noncoronary distribution.

Reference: Pandey T, Jambhekar K, Shaikh R, et al. Utility of the inversion scout sequence (TI scout) in diagnosing myocardial amyloid infiltration. *Int J Cardiovasc Imaging* 2013;29(1):103–112.

31 Answer B. Cardiac amyloidosis, particularly with systemic involvement, has been considered a contraindication to heart transplantation (HT) because of the potential for recurrent disease in the donor organ and progression of disease in other organs.

Data from the United Network for Organ Sharing indicate that cardiac amyloid patients undergoing HT before 2008 had decreased post-HT survival compared with patients undergoing HT for all other diagnoses.

Modern patient selection strategies excluding amyloid patients at greatest risk for progression of disease and other post-HT complications related to amyloidosis have improved outcomes in this patient population in clinical trials.

Given more recent advances, transplantation may be considered only for amyloid patients without evidence of significant extracardiac disease and without traditional contraindications to HT.

References: Davis MK, Lee PHU, Witteles RM. Changing outcomes after heart transplantation in patients with amyloid cardiomyopathy. *J Heart Lung Transplant* 2015;34(5):658-666.

Mancini D, Lietz K. Selection of cardiac transplantation candidates in 2010. *Circulation* 2010;122(2):173-183.

6 Cardiac Masses

QUESTIONS

1a The abnormality is in

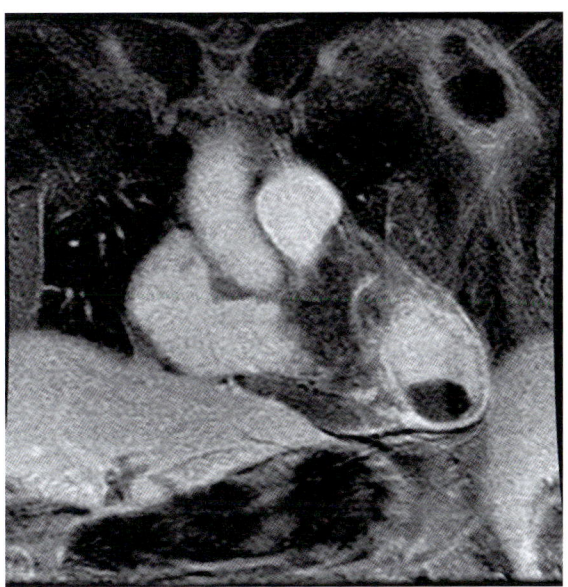

A. The left atrium
B. The left ventricle
C. The right atrium
D. The right ventricular outflow tract (RVOT)
E. The aorta

1b What is the best treatment for this lesion?

A. Surgical resection
B. Chemotherapy
C. No treatment
D. Anticoagulation

1c What is the most common type of mass seen in the heart?

   A. Myxoma
   B. Angiosarcoma
   C. Thrombus
   D. Rhabdomyoma
   E. Melanoma

2a Where is the abnormality?

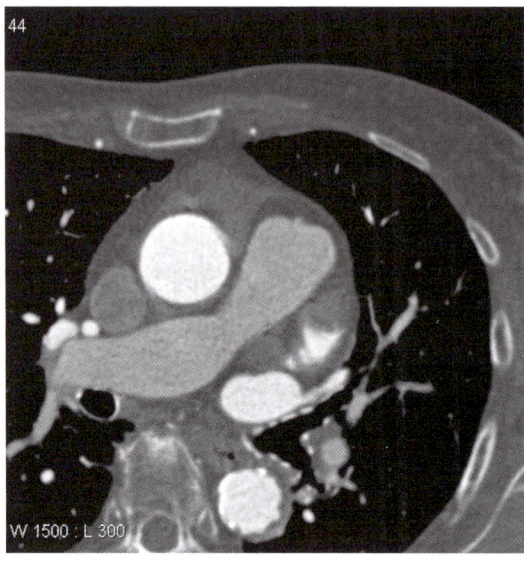

   A. Aorta
   B. Pulmonary artery
   C. Pulmonary vein
   D. Left atrium
   E. Left atrial appendage

2b This image was obtained immediately after the first image. What happened to the abnormality?

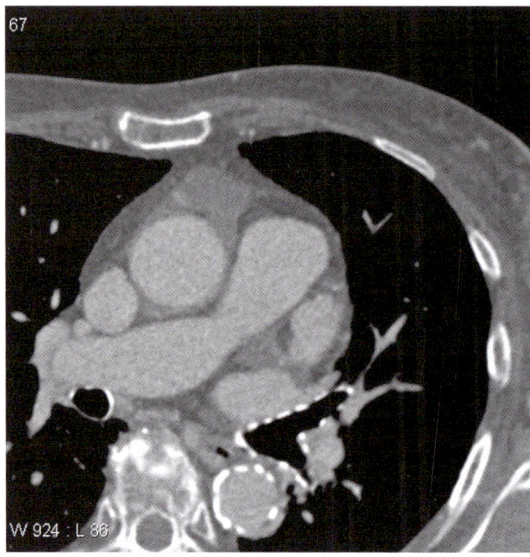

   A. It is still there.
   B. There is no abnormality.
   C. The abnormality embolized.

2c What modality is most often used to evaluate for left atrial appendage thrombus?
   A. CTA
   B. MRI
   C. Transesophageal echocardiogram
   D. Transthoracic echocardiogram

3 Left ventricular thrombus is most often seen in the setting of
   A. Hypercoagulable state
   B. Postinfarct
   C. Infective endocarditis
   D. Postsurgery

4 Left atrial appendage thrombus is most often associated with
   A. Lung cancer
   B. Hypercoagulable states
   C. Infarct
   D. Atrial fibrillation

5 This mass is most likely due to

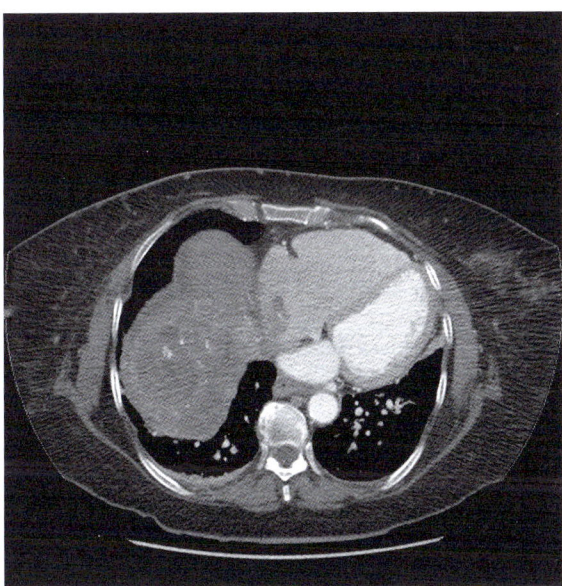

   A. Thrombus
   B. Metastasis
   C. Myxoma
   D. Infection
   E. Lymphoma

6 A 74-year-old male with a history of smoking and CAD. What is the best next step?

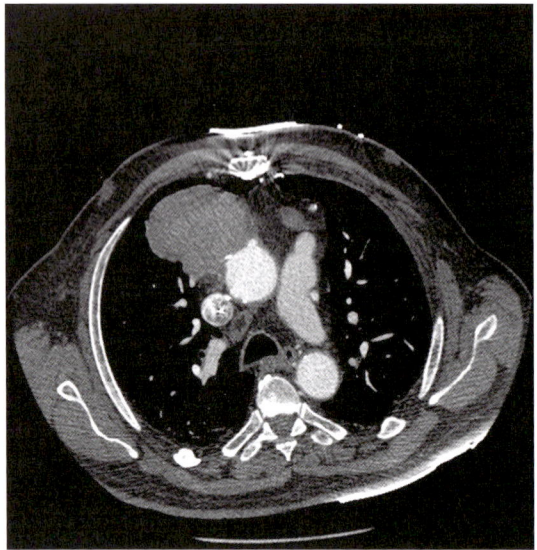
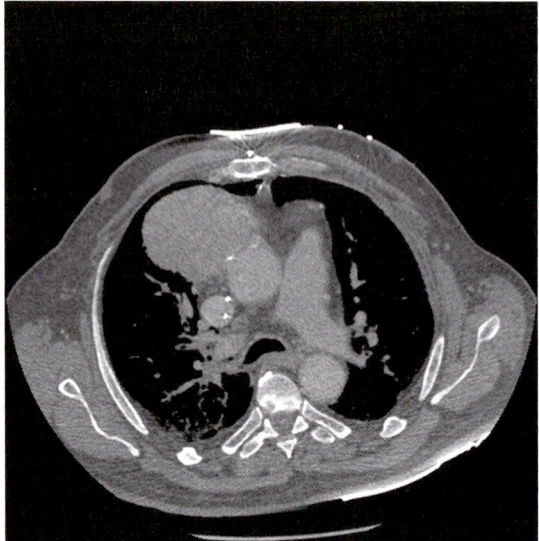

A. Catheter angiography
B. Biopsy
C. Surgical resection
D. CABG
E. Medical treatment/chemotherapy

7 An 18-year-old male presents with chest pain and history of febrile illness. What is the next step?

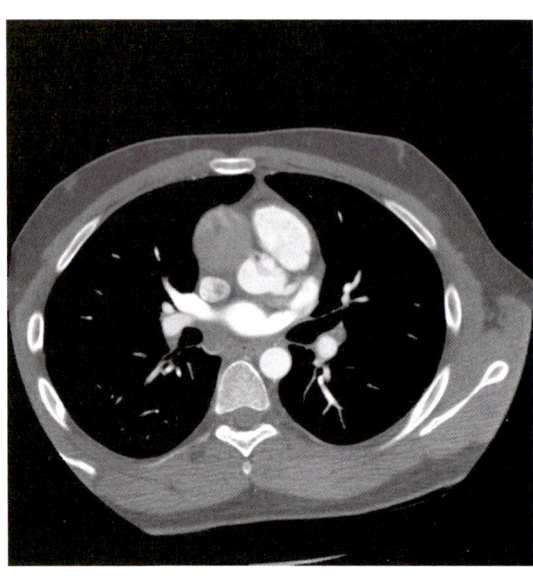
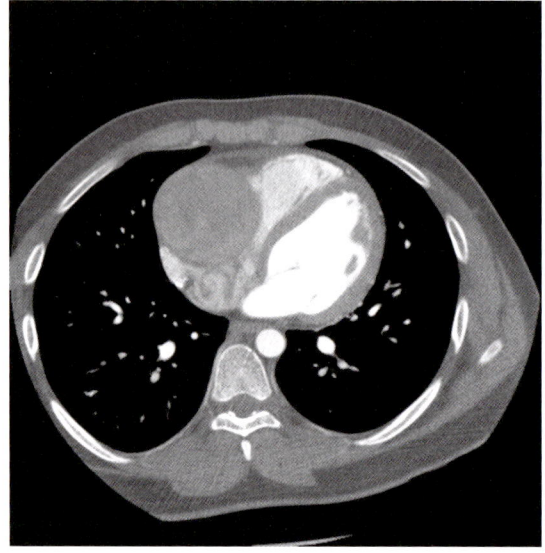

A. Catheter angiography
B. CT-guided biopsy
C. Chemotherapy
D. Cardiac MRI

8a A 50-year-old male presents with a history of chest pain. Where is the abnormality?

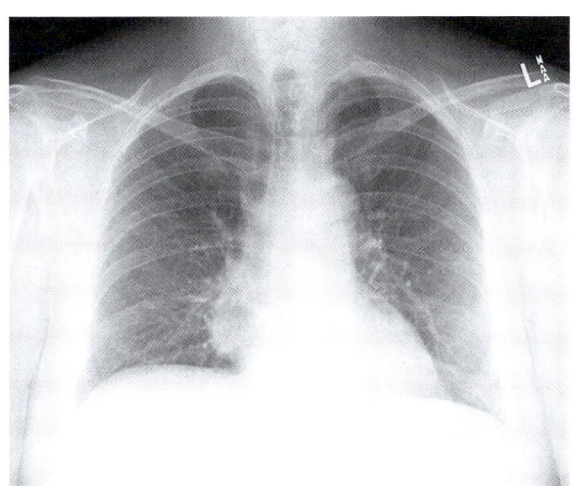
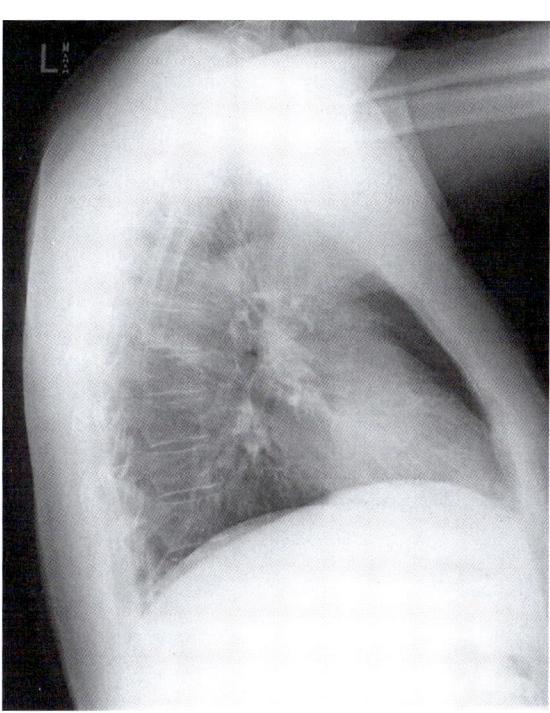

A. No abnormality
B. Right lower lobe
C. Ascending aorta
D. Right heart border
E. Left atrium

8b What is the treatment for this lesion?

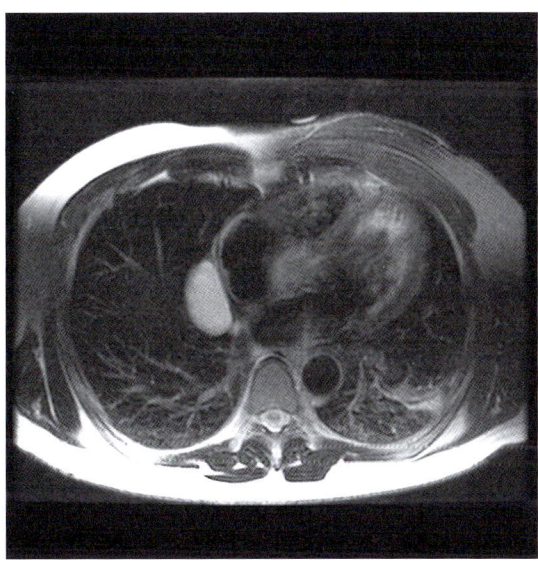
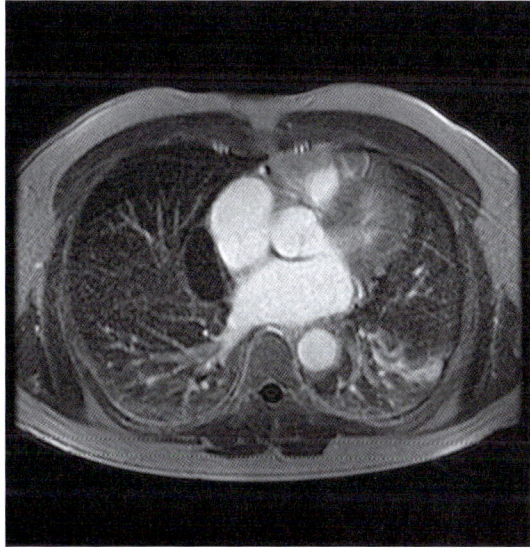

A. No treatment
B. Surgical resection
C. Serial MRI
D. Chemotherapy

9 What is the treatment for this patient?

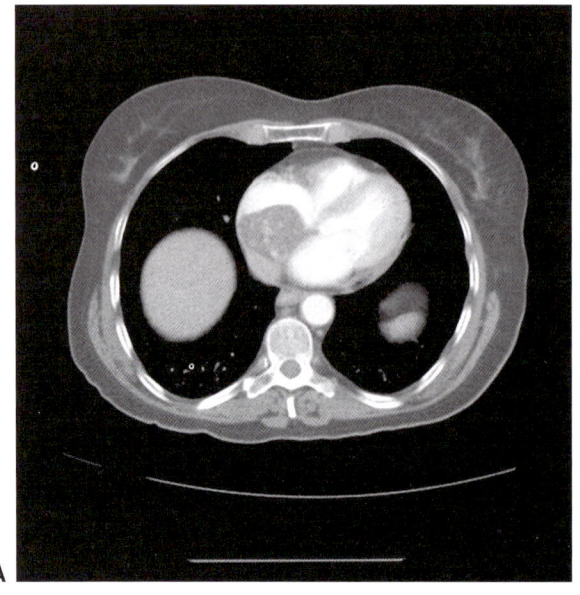
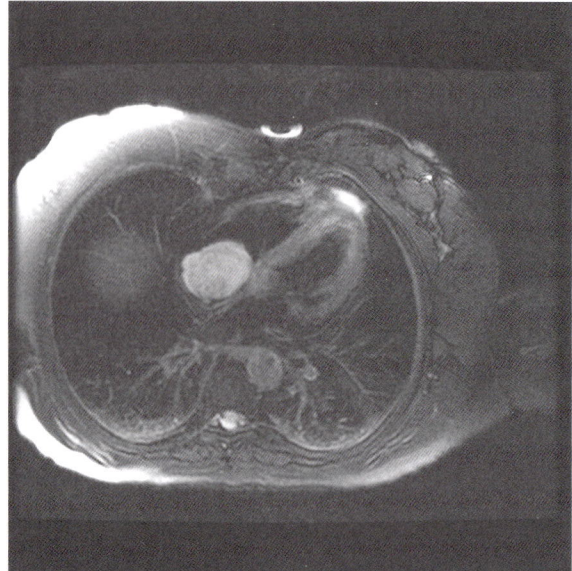
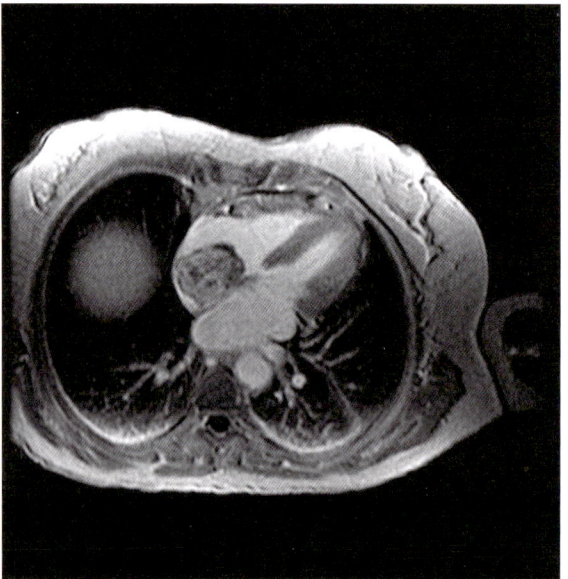

A. Anticoagulation
B. Chemotherapy
C. Surgery
D. Endovascular thrombolysis

10 What feature most suggests a benign lesion?

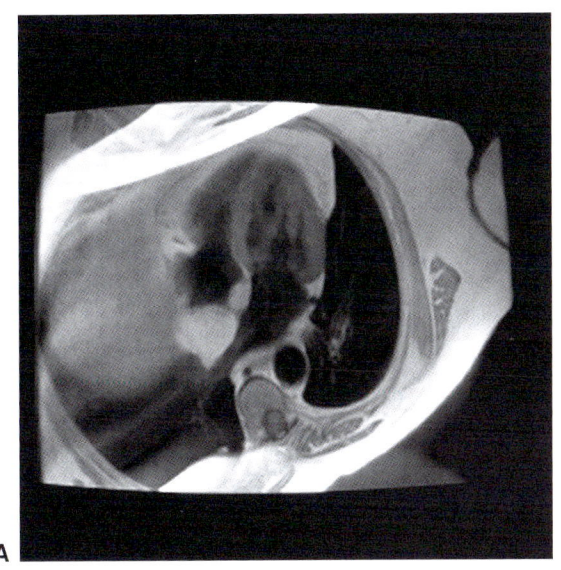 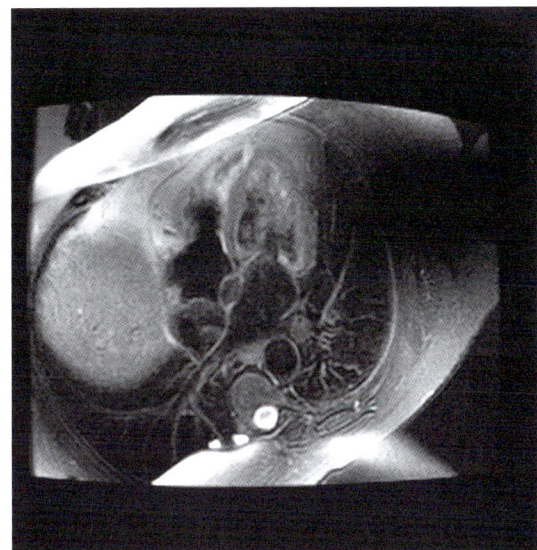

A. Right atrial location
B. Sparing of fossa ovalis
C. Fluid suppression
D. Lack of enhancement

11a What is the treatment for this lesion?

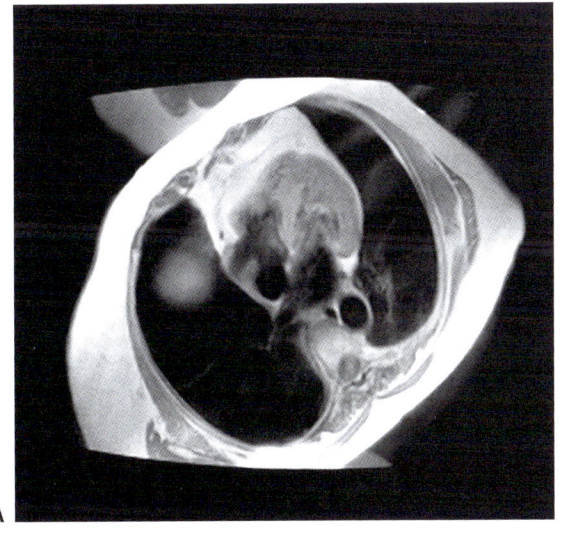 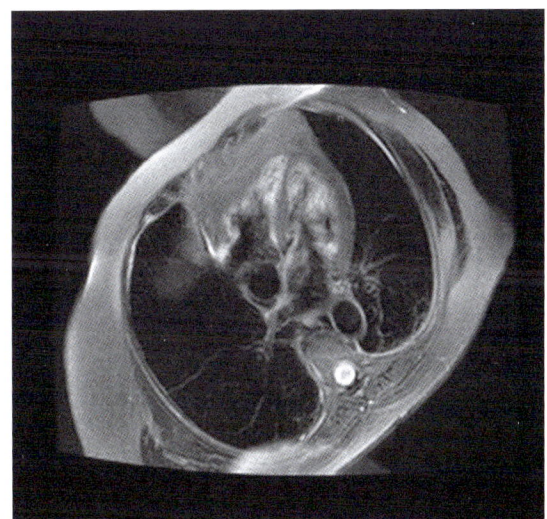

A. Surgery
B. Anticoagulation
C. Chemotherapy
D. No treatment is necessary.

11b What is an advantage of inversion recovery fat suppression over chemical fat suppression?

    A. It is specific for fat.
    B. It does not suppress contrast enhancement.
    C. It does not require high field strength.
    D. It is inherently high in signal.

12 Atrial and extracardiac myxomas can be seen in which condition?

    A. Tuberous sclerosis
    B. Von Hippel-Lindau
    C. Multiple endocrine neoplasia (MEN)
    D. Carney complex
    E. Gorlin syndrome

13a Which chamber of the heart abnormal based on this radiograph in a 3 year old boy?

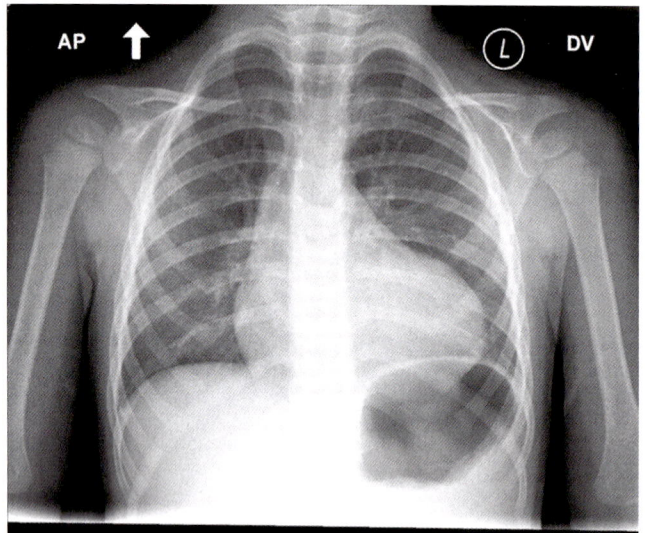
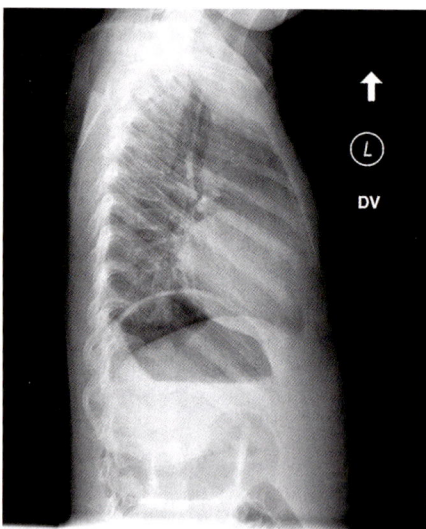

    A. Left atrium
    B. Left ventricle
    C. Right atrium
    D. Right ventricle

13b What is the most common type of primary cardiac tumor in a 3-year-old?

    A. Rhabdomyoma
    B. Myxoma
    C. Fibroma
    D. Teratoma

13c What is the best treatment for this tumor?

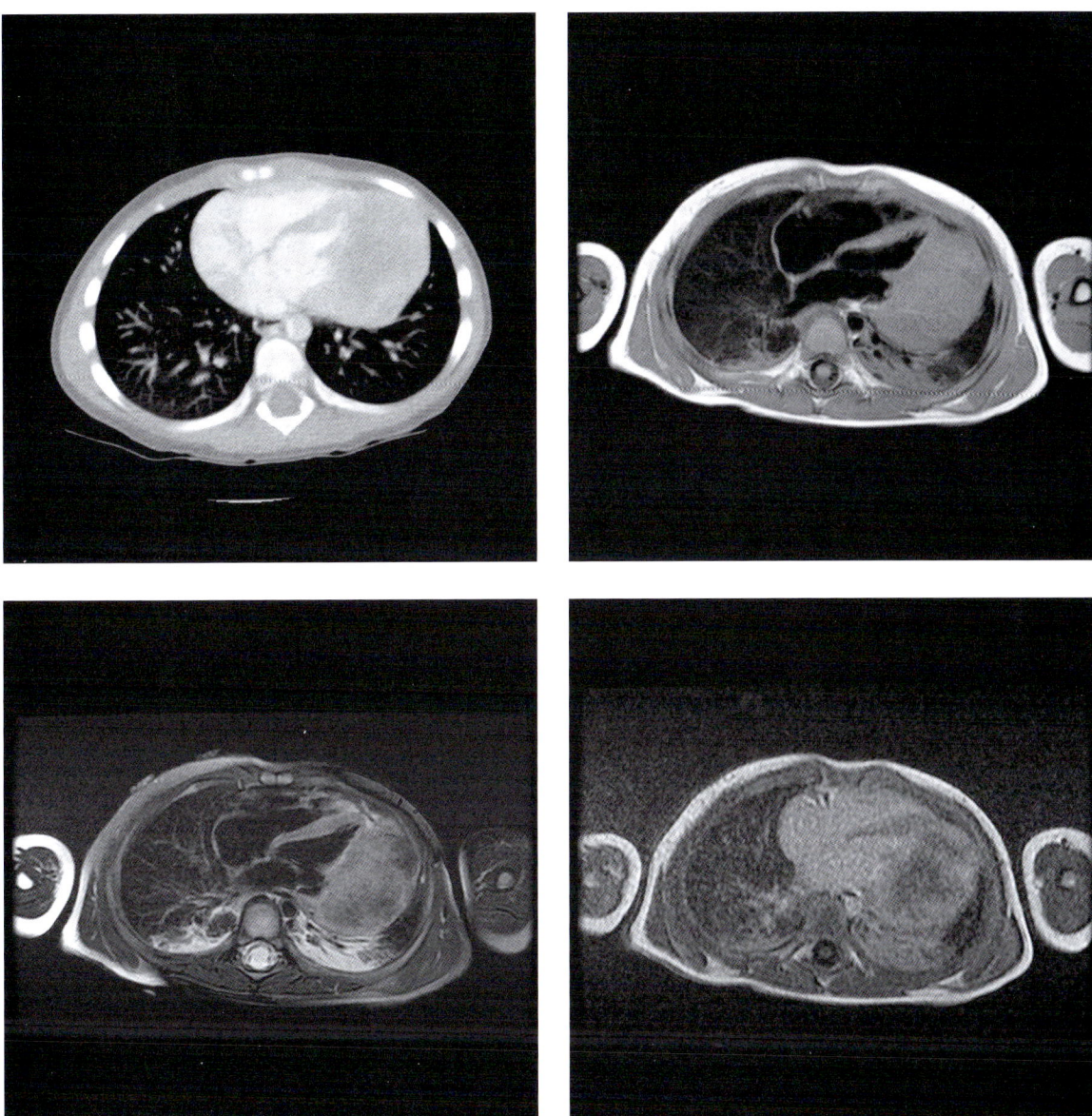

A. Surgical removal
B. Chemotherapy
C. Close follow-up
D. Alcohol ablation

14 If this patient were to undergo PET imaging, what part of the heart would most show abnormal activity?

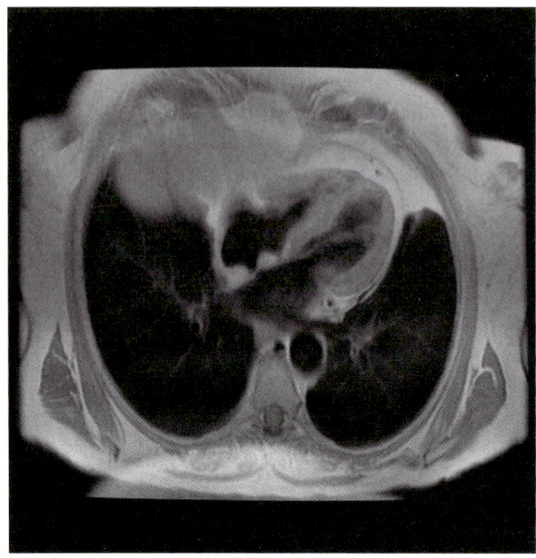
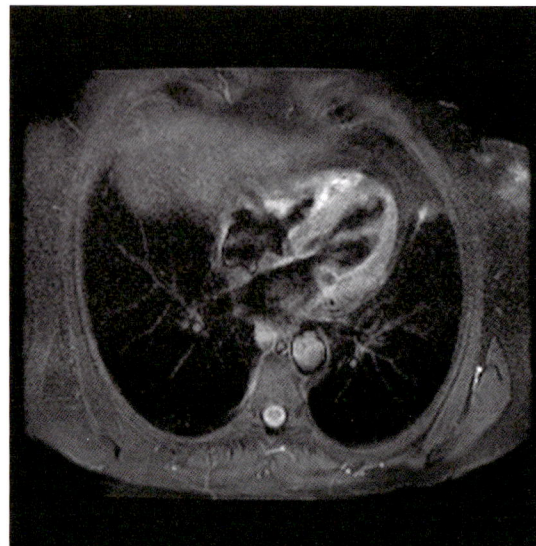

A. Right atrial wall
B. Right ventricular wall
C. Interatrial septum
D. Pericardial fat

15 A 55-year-old male presents with shortness of breath. What is the prognosis for this condition?

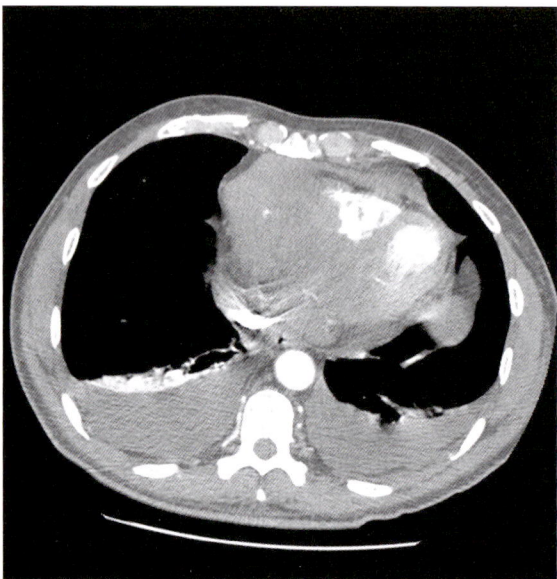

A. Good, it responds well to chemotherapy.
B. Fair, it can respond to radiation.
C. Poor, it typically does not respond to treatment.

16 What is the best next step for this patient?

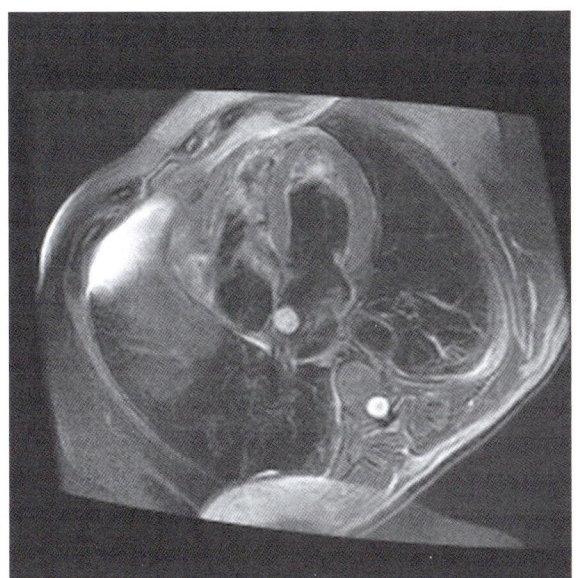
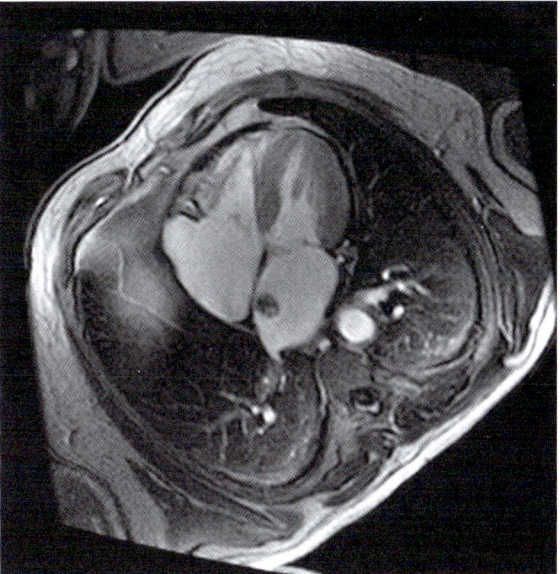
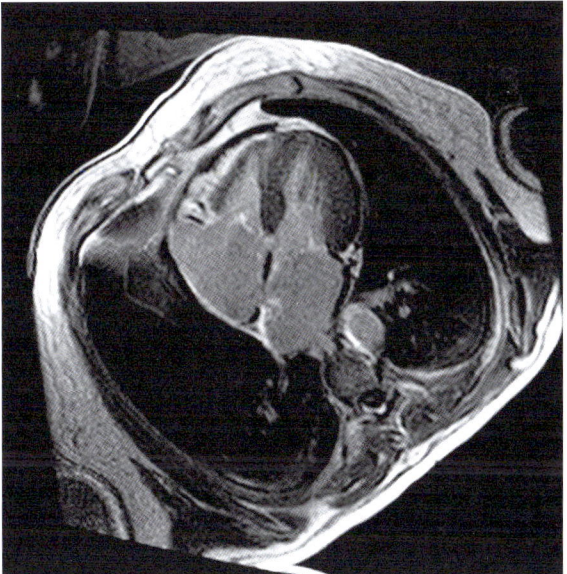

A. Anticoagulation
B. Surgery
C. Chemotherapy
D. Radiation
E. Close observation

17 A 60-year-old female has atrial fibrillation. Which of the following is the most likely diagnosis?

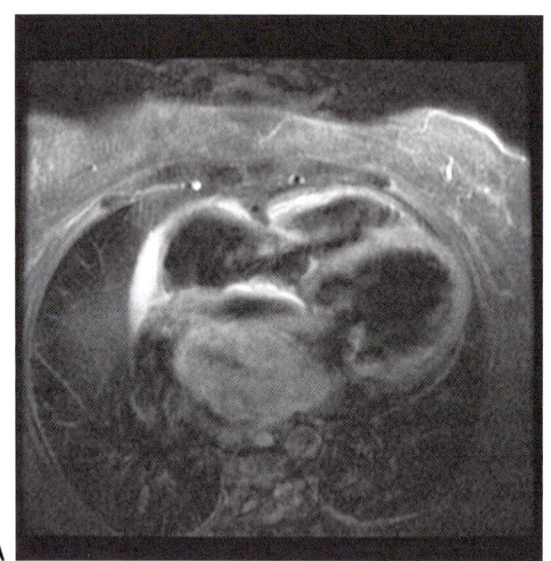
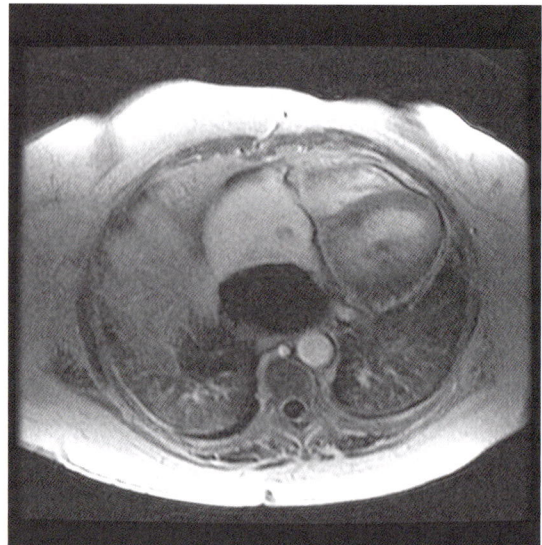

A. Myxoma
B. Fibroelastoma
C. Metastatic tumor
D. Thrombus
E. Fibroma

18a Where is the mass located?

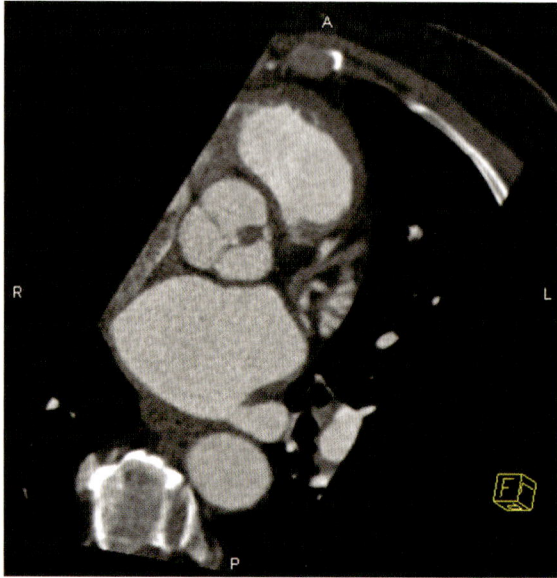

A. Between the noncoronary and right coronary cusp
B. Between the noncoronary and left coronary cusp
C. Between the right and left coronary cusp

18b The patient has no history endocarditis. However, the patient does have a history of transient ischemic attack. What is the best next step?

A. Anticoagulation
B. Antibiotics
C. Surgery
D. Observation

19 You have an infant who has been diagnosed with multiple cardiac rhabdomyomas. What else should you look for?

A. Renal cysts
B. Renal angiomyolipomas
C. Hepatic adenomas
D. Atrial myxomas

20 A 49-year-old male presents with a mass seen on echocardiography. What else should you look for in this patient?

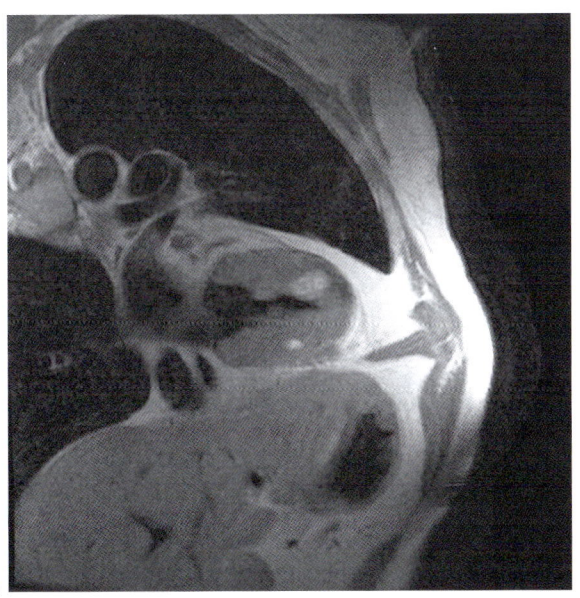
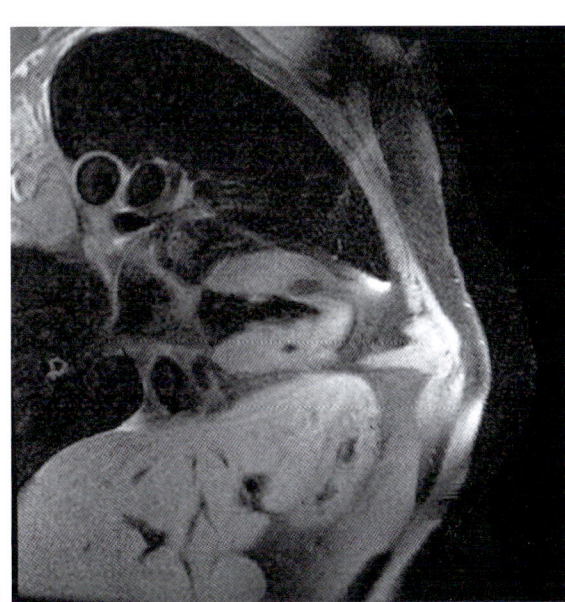

A. History of lymphoma
B. History of infarct
C. History of renal cysts
D. History of renal angiomyolipomas
E. History of echinococcosis infection

21 Metastatic tumors to the heart most often involve

A. Myocardium
B. Pericardium
C. Endocardium

22 An 80-year-old male presents with a cardiac mass. What history is most helpful in narrowing the differential?

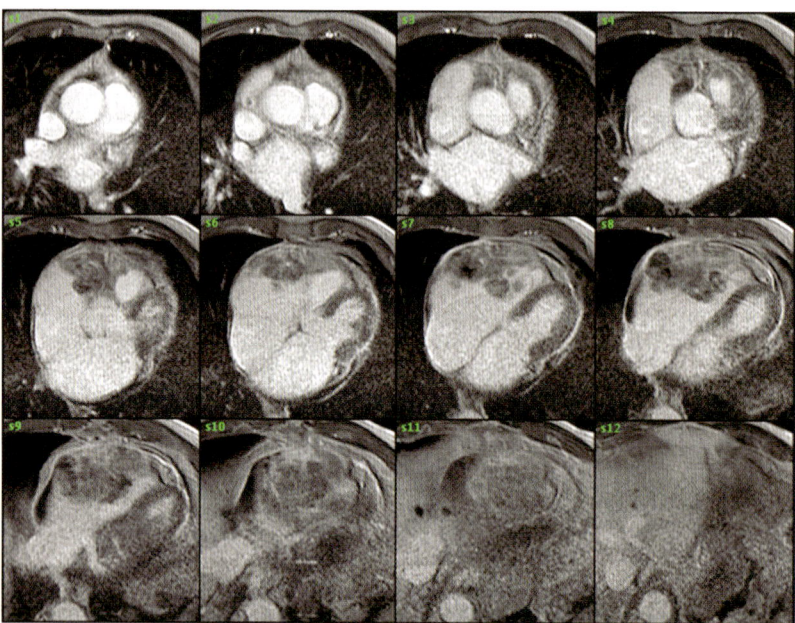

A. Patient has a history of echinococcosis.
B. Patient has a history of lymphoma.
C. Patient has a history of prior PET showing increased uptake in the right heart.
D. Patient has a history of endocarditis.

23a For the images below, select the most likely history. Each option may be used once, more than once, or not at all.

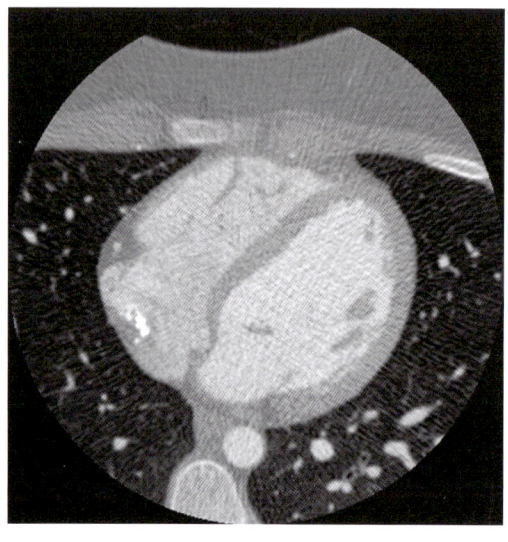
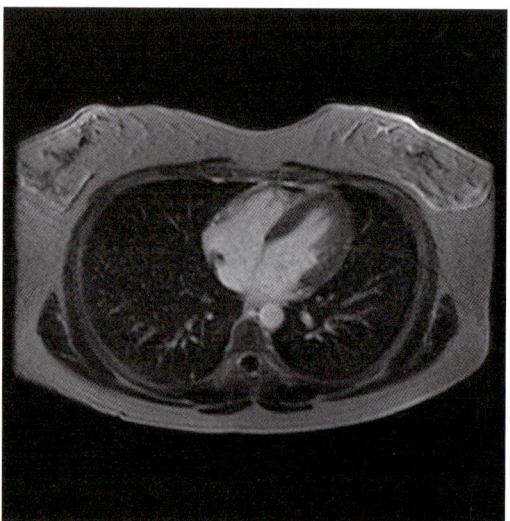

A. A 13-year-old with heart failure
B. A 24-year-old with history of central line placement
C. A 40-year-old with shortness of breath
D. A 45-year-old with unexplained hypertension and tachycardia
E. A 50-year-old with endocarditis
F. A 60-year-old, asymptomatic
G. A 77-year-old with history of echinococcus infection

23b For the images below, select the most likely history. Each option may be used once, more than once, or not at all.

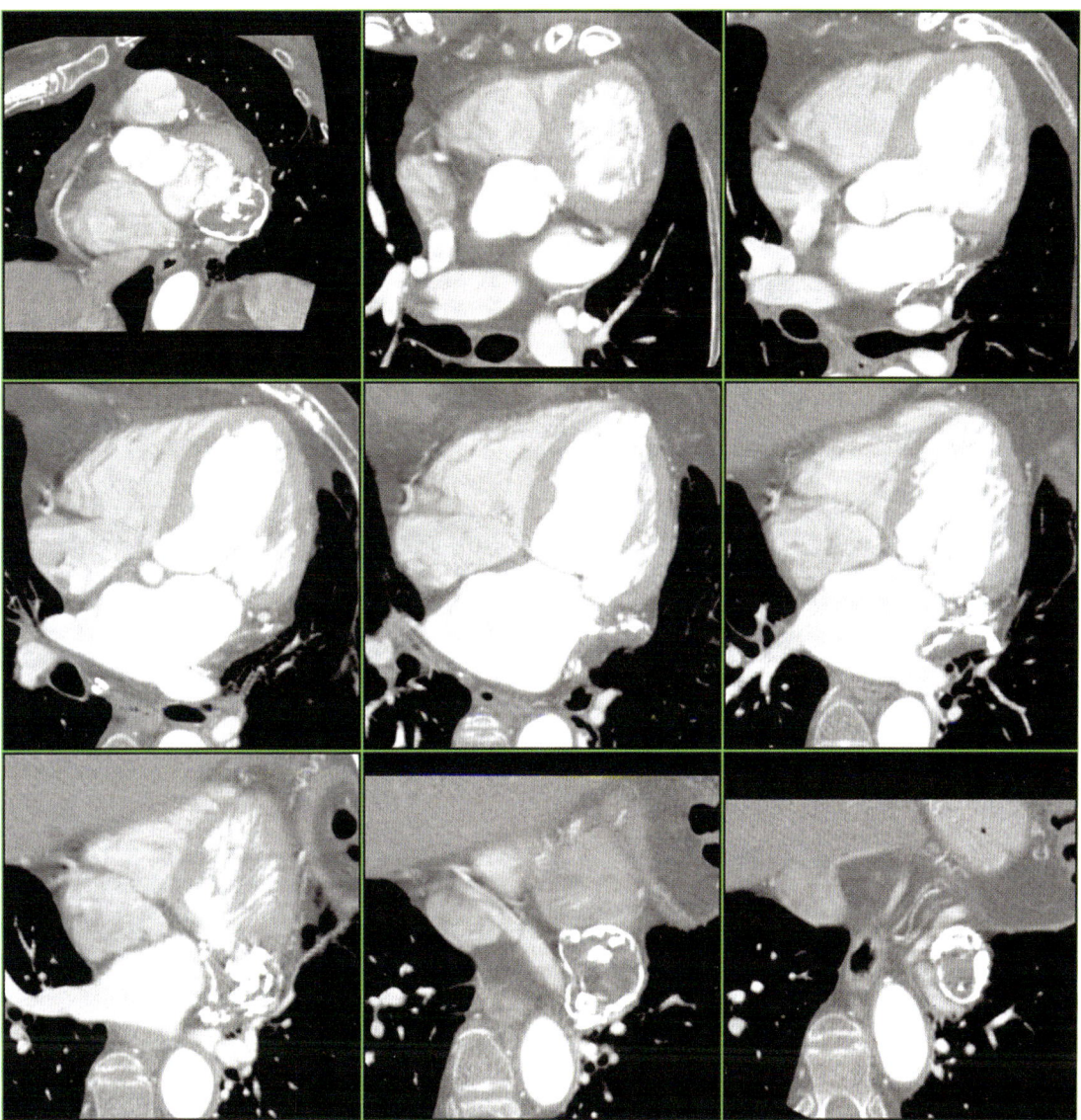

- A. A 13-year-old with heart failure
- B. A 24-year-old with history of central line placement
- C. A 45-year-old with shortness of breath
- D. A 40-year-old with unexplained hypertension and tachycardia
- E. A 50-year-old with endocarditis
- F. A 60-year-old, asymptomatic
- G. A 77-year-old with history of echinococcus infection

24a A 71-year-old male with an incidental mass. Based on the PET exam what should be the next step?

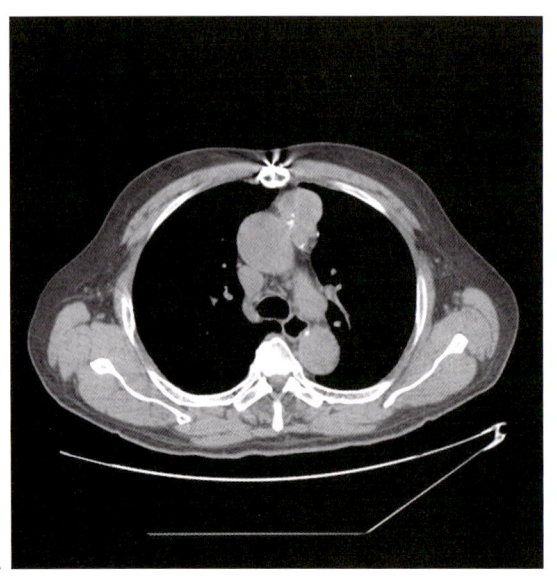
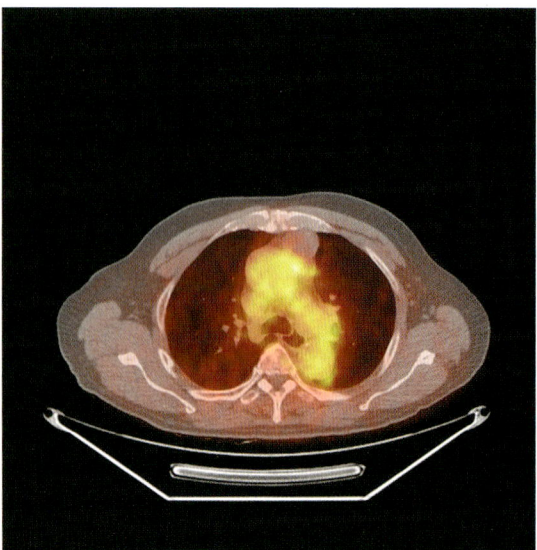

A. Biopsy for tissue diagnosis
B. Contrast-enhanced CTA for further evaluation
C. Chemotherapy/radiation
D. No further evaluation necessary, this is benign

24b A 71-year-old male has an incidental mass. This condition most commonly occurs in which vascular territory?

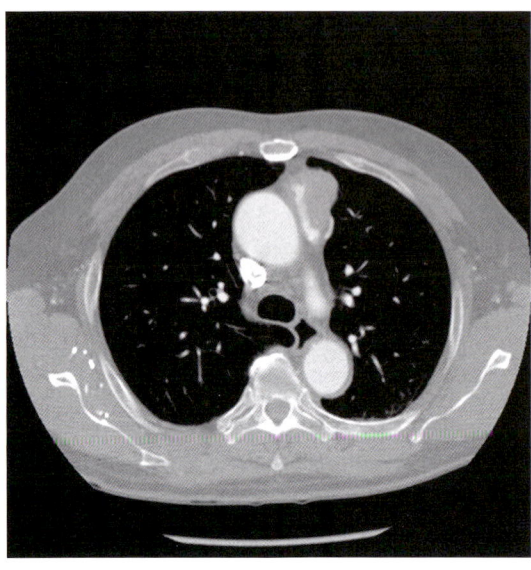
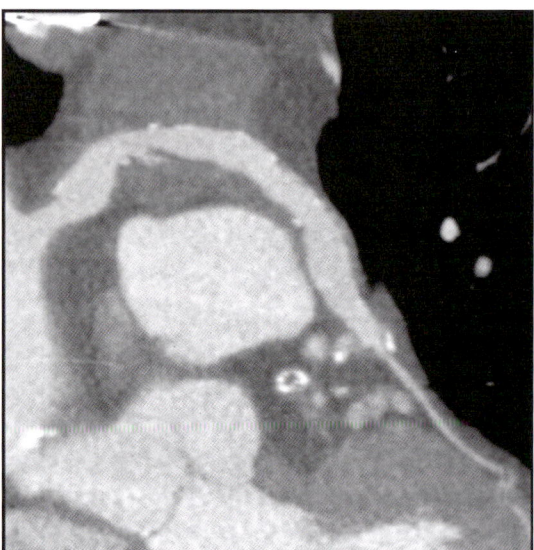

A. Right coronary artery
B. Left anterior descending artery
C. Left circumflex artery

25 An 18-year-old female with shortness of breath undergoes a CTA PE protocol with the abnormality shown. Subsequently, she got a cardiac MRI with the image shown after her symptoms resolved. What is the best explanation of the findings?

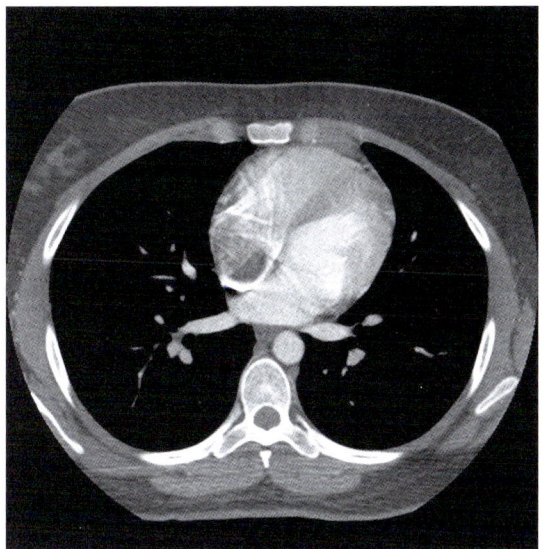
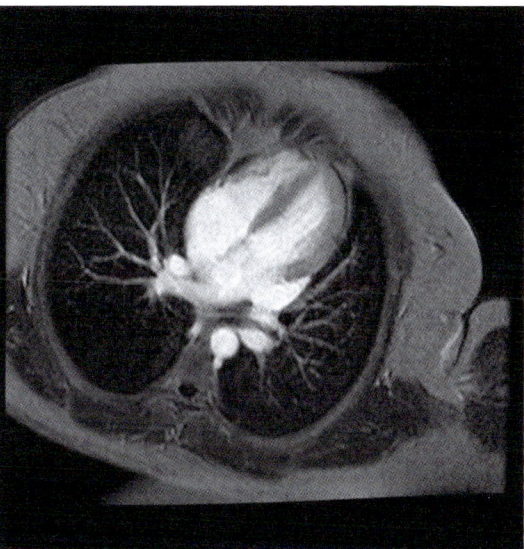

A. The pathology has embolized in the interval between the CT and MRI study.
B. This was a pseudomass caused by unopacified IVC venous return to the right atrium.
C. The mass shows equal enhancement relative to the blood pool on MRI.

ANSWERS AND EXPLANATIONS

1a Answer B. Coronal postcontrast image shows a mass along the inferior apical left ventricular cavity. Left atrium is not shown in this image. Right atrium appears grossly normal. RVOT is not fully seen but appears normal. Visualized ascending aorta appears normal.

1b Answer D. Left ventricular thrombus is most often associated with postinfarct wall motion abnormalities. Note the enhancement along the infarcted myocardium while there is no enhancement of the mass. Treatment of choice is anticoagulation. This is not a mass that requires surgical resection or chemotherapy. Treatment is necessary to prevent complications of thrombus embolization.

1c Answer C. The most common mass in the heart is thrombus. The most common benign cardiac tumor is myxoma. The most common malignant tumor is angiosarcoma. The most common tumor in children is rhabdomyoma. Melanoma can metastasize to the heart but is not the most common cause of cardiac mass.

References: Grebenc ML, Rosado de Christenson ML, Burke AP, et al. Primary cardiac and pericardial neoplasms: radiologic-pathologic correlation. *Radiographics* 2000;20(4):1073–1103; quiz 1110–1111, 1112. Review. PubMed PMID: 10903697.

Sparrow PJ, Kurian JB, Jones TR, et al. MR imaging of cardiac tumors. *Radiographics* 2005;25(5):1255–1276. Review. PubMed PMID: 16160110.

2a Answer E. Postcontrast gated coronary CTA shows a low-attenuation filling defect at the tip of the left atrial appendage. The aorta and pulmonary artery appear normal. Left atrium is only partially visualized along with the pulmonary veins, and they appear normal.

2b Answer B. The filling defect seen on the initial CTA at the tip of left atrial appendage is no longer identified on the delayed acquisition image. This is consistent with slow flow in the left atrial appendage, which can be seen in patients with atrial fibrillation and LA enlargement. Thrombus would have shown a persistent low-attenuation filling defect at the tip of the left atrial appendage with a border. It is unlikely that the thrombus could have embolized in the short amount of time between the initial CTA and the second acquisition.

2c Answer C. Left atrial appendage thrombus is most often evaluated by transesophageal echocardiogram (TEE). While CTA can visualize LA appendage thrombus, its specificity is not high given false positives can happen with slow flow. A delayed phase may be helpful but adds additional radiation. MRI can also visualize left atrial appendage thrombus but is not used routinely as TEE is more available and performed just prior to pulmonary vein ablation.

Reference: Saremi F, Channual S, Gurudevan SV, et al. Prevalence of left atrial appendage pseudothrombus filling defects in patients with atrial fibrillation undergoing coronary computed tomography angiography. *J Cardiovasc Comput Tomogr* 2008;2(3):164–171. doi: 10.1016/j.jcct.2008.02.012. Epub 2008 Mar 4. PubMed PMID: 19083941.

3 Answer B. Left ventricular thrombus is most often associated with postinfarct wall motion abnormalities. Treatment of thrombus is anticoagulation. Surgical resection is not indicated and thrombus does not enhance following contrast administration. Left ventricular thrombus can be seen in hypercoagulable state, endocarditis, and postsurgery but is most often due to wall motion abnormality.

Reference: Keren A, Goldberg S, Gottlieb S, et al. Natural history of left ventricular thrombi: their appearance and resolution in the posthospitalization period of acute myocardial infarction. *J Am Coll Cardiol* 1990;15(4):790–800. PubMed PMID: 2307788.

4 Answer D. Left atrial appendage thrombus is most often associated with atrial fibrillation. While LA thrombus can occur with lung cancer invasion, it usually will occur via pulmonary vein extension and not occur at the tip of left atrial appendage. Thrombus can also occur in setting of wall motion abnormality (postinfarct, mitral valve replacement). While hypercoagulable states can predispose one to thromboembolic disease, it is not the most often cause of LAA thrombus.

Reference: Romero J, Husain SA, Kelesidis I, et al. Detection of left atrial appendage thrombus by cardiac computed tomography in patients with atrial fibrillation: a meta-analysis. *Circ Cardiovasc Imaging* 2013;6(2):185–194. doi: 10.1161/CIRCIMAGING.112.000153. Epub 2013 Feb 13. Review. PubMed PMID: 23406625.

5 Answer B. While the most common type of mass in the heart is thrombus, in this case, there is evidence for metastatic disease (see liver lesions). This patient had hepatocellular carcinoma (HCC) with tumor invasion via the hepatic veins to the right atrium. Other tumors besides HCC with direct invasion to the right atrium include renal cell carcinoma and IVC sarcoma. Myxoma is within the differential and can be in the right atrium, but the liver lesions here make it more likely that this is a metastatic tumor. Endocarditis can cause masses in the valves, but they tend not to be this large. Lymphoma could also cause a mass in the heart but is not the best answer in this case given the liver findings.

References: Grebenc ML, Rosado de Christenson ML, Burke AP, et al. Primary cardiac and pericardial neoplasms: radiologic-pathologic correlation. *Radiographics* 2000;20(4):1073–1103; quiz 1110–1111, 1112. Review. PubMed PMID: 10903697.

Sparrow PJ, Kurian JB, Jones TR, et al. MR imaging of cardiac tumors. *Radiographics* 2005;25(5):1255–1276. Review. PubMed PMID: 16160110.

6 Answer E. This is a patient with metastatic lung cancer with likely vascular invasion (the mass appears to involve the aorta). The patient is already post-CABG (see sternotomy wires and bypass grafts). Saphenous graft aneurysm is also in the differential. However, note the heterogeneous enhancement of mass and irregular border, which would be more supportive of a mass such as lung cancer. Given that this is metastatic disease with likely vascular invasion, surgical intervention would not be indicated. While biopsy is a valid choice, if the differential includes saphenous aneurysm, then biopsy would not be a wise choice.

Reference: Gay SB, Black WC, Armstrong P, et al. Chest CT of unresectable lung cancer. *Radiographics* 1988;8(4):735–748. PubMed PMID: 3175085.

7 Answer A. This mass is most consistent with a large RCA aneurysm given the history suggesting Kawasaki disease. Catheter angiography is the best next step to better evaluate this aneurysm. One could argue for CABG right away if the diagnosis of giant RCA aneurysm was not in doubt. However, sometimes, the anatomy can be significantly distorted on CT that a catheter angiogram can show the aneurysm better than CT given the ability to directly inject the vessel. Biopsy would not be a wise choice for an aneurysm. Given this is not a tumor, medical treatment would not be helpful. CMR would not provide any more information given the findings are highly suggestive of giant RCA aneurysm already.

Reference: Díaz-Zamudio M, Bacilio-Pérez U, Herrera-Zarza MC, et al. Coronary artery aneurysms and ectasia: role of coronary CT angiography. *Radiographics* 2009;29(7):1939–1954. doi: 10.1148/rg.297095048. Review. PubMed PMID: 19926755.

8a Answer D. The contour abnormality is at the right heart border on the PA view. The lateral view shows it adjacent to the heart and not posterior in the right lower lobe.

8b Answer A.   This is right pericardial cyst along the right atrial border. It shows T2 prolongation on the T2W image. This mass shows no enhancement, septations, or nodules. Simple pericardial cysts do not require treatment or follow-up.

Reference: Restrepo CS, Vargas D, Ocazionez D, et al. Primary pericardial tumors. *Radiographics* 2013;33(6):1613–1630. doi: 10.1148/rg.336135512. Review. PubMed PMID: 24108554.

9 Answer C.   This is a right atrial mass showing T2 prolongation (Image B) and heterogeneous contrast enhancement (Image C). While thrombus is the most common mass in the right atrium, in this case, the contrast enhancement excludes thrombus. The T2 prolongation and enhancement is suggestive of a right atrial myxoma. The best treatment is therefore surgery.

Reference: Grebenc ML, Rosado-de-Christenson ML, Green CE, et al. Cardiac myxoma: imaging features in 83 patients. *Radiographics* 2002;22(3):673–689. Review. PubMed PMID: 12006696.

10 Answer B.   Proton density-weighted (Image A) and post fat-saturated T2W (Image B) images show lipomatous hypertrophy of the interatrial septum (LHIAS). There is a classic barbell shape of the fat in the interatrial septum sparing the fossa ovalis. The right atrial location does not indicate a benign lesion as malignant and metastatic tumors can occur in this chamber. Fat suppression is used here, not fluid suppression. The images are noncontrast images so nothing can be said about the lack or presence of enhancement.

Reference: Kimura F, Matsuo Y, Nakajima T, et al. Myocardial fat at cardiac imaging: how can we differentiate pathologic from physiologic fatty infiltration? *Radiographics* 2010;30(6):1587–1602. doi: 10.1148/rg.306105519. PubMed PMID: 21071377.

11a Answer D.   Proton density-weighted (Image A) and fat-saturated T2W (Image B) images show a right atrial wall mass that loses signal on fat suppression. There is suggestion of a thin capsule. This is most consistent with a right atrial lipoma. No treatment is necessary. This is not a tumor or thrombus that requires anticoagulation or chemotherapy or surgery. Lipomatous hypertrophy of the interatrial septum (LHIAS) can be positive on PET, but the lesion in this case does not involve the interatrial septum and appears to be a simple right atrial lipoma.

Reference: Kimura F, Matsuo Y, Nakajima T, et al. Myocardial fat at cardiac imaging: how can we differentiate pathologic from physiologic fatty infiltration? *Radiographics* 2010;30(6):1587–1602. doi: 10.1148/rg.306105519. PubMed PMID: 21071377.

11b Answer C.   Short tau inversion recovery (STIR) is not specific to fat as it will suppress anything with short T1 (including postcontrast T1 shortening). STIR imaging does not require a high field strength magnet. It will have lower signal due to the inversion pulse.

Chemical fat suppression is specific to fat and will not suppress contrast enhancement. However, it is susceptible to field inhomogeneity, which can cause incomplete fat saturation. With a higher-strength magnet, there is greater separation of the fat and water peaks making fat suppression easier.

Reference: Delfaut EM, Beltran J, Johnson G, et al. Fat suppression in MR imaging: techniques and pitfalls. *Radiographics* 1999;19(2):373–382. Review. Erratum in: *Radiographics* 1999;19(4):1092. PubMed PMID: 10194785.

12 Answer D.   Carney complex consists of multiple myxomas (including cardiac and extracardiac), endocrine neoplasm (pituitary adenoma), and skin hyperpigmentation. It is an autosomal dominant and is more common in females. The other syndromes do not include cardiac myxomas. In gorlin syndrome, patients have an increased risk for cardiac fibroma.

References: Ghadimi Mahani M, Lu JC, Rigsby CK, et al. MRI of pediatric cardiac masses. *AJR Am J Roentgenol* 2014;202(5):971–981. doi: 10.2214/AJR.13.10680. Review. PubMed PMID: 24758649.

Tao TY, Yahyavi-Firouz-Abadi N, Singh GK, et al. Pediatric cardiac tumors: clinical and imaging features. *Radiographics* 2014;34(4):1031–1046. doi: 10.1148/rg.344135163. PubMed PMID: 25019440.

13a Answer B. The contour abnormality is along the left heart border, which is consistent with a LV abnormality.

13b Answer A. The most common type of cardiac tumor in infants and children is a rhabdomyoma. Myxomas are most common in adults. Fibromas are the second most common cardiac tumor in children. Cardiac teratoma is rare in the pediatric population.

13c Answer C. This is a large tumor along the LV lateral wall with enhancement most consistent with a cardiac fibroma in this 3-year-old boy. Fibromas are derived from fibroblasts. Treatment is watchful waiting as this cannot be resected due to the large size and involvement of a large portion of the LV. Unlike rhabdomyomas, fibromas do not typically regress, so for this patient, cardiac transplantation may ultimately be required. Alcohol ablation is used for hypertrophic cardiomyopathy patients with left ventricular outflow tract obstruction.

References: Ghadimi Mahani M, Lu JC, Rigsby CK, et al. MRI of pediatric cardiac masses. *AJR Am J Roentgenol* 2014;202(5):971–981. doi: 10.2214/AJR.13.10680. Review. PubMed PMID: 24758649.

Tao TY, Yahyavi-Firouz-Abadi N, Singh GK, et al. Pediatric cardiac tumors: clinical and imaging features. *Radiographics* 2014;34(4):1031–1046. doi: 10.1148/rg.344135163. PubMed PMID: 25019440.

14 Answer C. Proton density-weighted (Image A) and triple inversion recovery images (Image B) show a dumbbell-shaped lesion in the interatrial septum sparing the fossa ovalis. This is classic for lipomatous hypertrophy of the interatrial septum. This lesion can show PET activity due to presence of metabolically active brown fat.

Reference: Kimura F, Matsuo Y, Nakajima T, et al. Myocardial fat at cardiac imaging: how can we differentiate pathologic from physiologic fatty infiltration? *Radiographics* 2010;30(6):1587–1602. doi: 10.1148/rg.306105519. PubMed PMID: 21071377.

15 Answer C. CT shows an infiltrative mass in the right atrium and ventricle with a pericardial effusion and a left lung nodule. This is most consistent with a cardiac angiosarcoma, the most common primary malignant tumor of the heart. It is more common in males and carries a poor prognosis with median survival rate of 6 months.

Reference: Araoz PA, Eklund HE, Welch TJ, et al. CT and MR imaging of primary cardiac malignancies. *Radiographics* 1999;19(6):1421–1434. Review. PubMed PMID: 10555666.

16 Answer B. This is a mass in the left atrium most consistent with a left atrial myxoma. It shows T2 prolongation with gradual post contrast enhancement. The treatment is surgery.

Reference: Araoz PA, Eklund HE, Welch TJ, et al. CT and MR imaging of primary cardiac malignancies. *Radiographics* 1999;19(6):1421–1434. Review. PubMed PMID: 10555666.

17 Answer D. This left atrial tumor is most consistent with left atrial thrombus given the lack of enhancement (Image B). Thrombus can have variable signal on T1W, T2W, and PDW images depending on the age of thrombus. The lack of enhancement is essentially diagnostic of thrombus as the other entities should all show enhancement.

Reference: Sparrow PJ, Kurian JB, Jones TR, et al. MR imaging of cardiac tumors. *Radiographics* 2005;25(5):1255–1276. Review. PubMed PMID: 16160110.

18a Answer C. The mass is located between the left and right coronary cusps. The noncoronary cusp is typically located at the interatrial septum. The right coronary cusp is located anteriorly (look for the sternum/right ventricular outflow tract). The left coronary cusp is adjacent to the left atrial appendage.

Reference: Bennett CJ, Maleszewski JJ, Araoz PA. CT and MR imaging of the aortic valve: radiologic-pathologic correlation. *Radiographics* 2012;32(5):1399–1420. doi: 10.1148/rg.325115727. PubMed PMID: 22977027.

18b Answer C. The image shows an aortic valvular mass most consistent with a papillary fibroelastomas given the lack of history of endocarditis. When it involves the aortic valve, it is more commonly seen on the aortic side, and when it involves the mitral valve, it is more commonly on the left atrial surface. It is much rarely seen in the cardiac chambers. These tumors can cause embolization/coronary occlusion. In symptomatic patients, surgical resection should be considered.

Reference: Mariscalco G, Bruno VD, Borsani P, et al. Papillary fibroelastoma: insight to a primary cardiac valve tumor. *J Card Surg* 2010;25(2):198–205. doi: 10.1111/j.1540-8191.2009.00993.x. Epub 2010 Feb 9. Review. PubMed PMID: 20149002.

19 Answer B. Cardiac rhabdomyomas are associated with tuberous sclerosis so one would look for renal angiomyolipomas. Treatment is usually watchful waiting since these lesions tend to regress. Surgery is given their intramyocardial distribution considered when there is flow obstruction. No chemotherapy is necessary. Cardiac rhabdomyomas can be diagnosed on prenatal ultrasound.

References: Ghadimi Mahani M, Lu JC, Rigsby CK, et al. MRI of pediatric cardiac masses. *AJR Am J Roentgenol* 2014;202(5):971–981. doi: 10.2214/AJR.13.10680. Review. PubMed PMID: 24758649.

Tao TY, Yahyavi-Firouz-Abadi N, Singh GK, et al. Pediatric cardiac tumors: clinical and imaging features. *Radiographics* 2014;34(4):1031–46. doi: 10.1148/rg.344135163. PubMed PMID: 25019440.

20 Answer D. Multiple fatty lesions are seen in the LV myocardium. The first image is T1W double inversion recovery (DIR) black blood imaging (Image A) showing myocardial areas of increased signal, which shows fat suppression (Image B). These fatty myocardial lesions can be seen in patients with tuberous sclerosis. These are not fatty changes from prior infarct.

Reference: Kimura F, Matsuo Y, Nakajima T, et al. Myocardial fat at cardiac imaging: how can we differentiate pathologic from physiologic fatty infiltration? *Radiographics* 2010;30(6):1587–1602. doi: 10.1148/rg.306105519. PubMed PMID: 21071377.

21 Answer B. Metastatic involvement of the heart is more common than primary cardiac tumors. The most common site of metastatic involvement is the pericardium. Tumor thrombus will usually show heterogeneous enhancement, while thrombus will show no enhancement. Metastatic tumors (excluding melanoma) tend to show low signal on T1W.

Reference: Sparrow PJ, Kurian JB, Jones TR, et al. MR imaging of cardiac tumors. *Radiographics* 2005;25(5):1255–1276. Review. PubMed PMID: 16160.

22 Answer B. Postcontrast images show a mass along the right atrium and ventricle with heterogeneous enhancement. This is a nonspecific finding and should be correlated with patient's history to narrow the differential. Metastatic involvement of the heart is more common than primary cardiac tumors. Therefore, the most helpful history would be prior lymphoma. Cardiac echinococcosis should show cystic lesions, which are not seen here. Uptake on PET is nonspecific and will not necessarily narrow the differential since this mass already shows enhancement on MRI. However, if PET also shows other areas of abnormal uptake that may be helpful if a primary is suggested. Endocarditis/abscess can show enhancement, but in this case, the appearance is more consistent with mass rather than abscess.

References: Buckley O, Madan R, Kwong R, et al. Cardiac masses, part 1: imaging strategies and technical considerations. *AJR Am J Roentgenol* 2011;197(5):W837–W841. doi: 10.2214/AJR.10.7260. Review. PubMed PMID: 22021530.

Jeudy J, Kirsch J, Tavora F, et al. From the radiologic pathology archives: cardiac lymphoma: radiologic-pathologic correlation. *Radiographics* 2012;32(5):1369–1380. doi: 10.1148/rg.325115126. PubMed PMID: 22977025.

O'Donnell DH, Abbara S, Chaithiraphan V, et al. Cardiac tumors: optimal cardiac MR sequences and spectrum of imaging appearances. *AJR Am J Roentgenol* 2009;193(2):377–387. doi: 10.2214/AJR.08.1895. Review. PubMed PMID: 19620434.

Sparrow PJ, Kurian JB, Jones TR, et al. MR imaging of cardiac tumors. *Radiographics* 2005;25(5):1255–1276. Review. PubMed PMID: 16160110.

23a Answer B. CT (Image A) shows a calcified lesion along the right atrial wall along the crista terminalis. Postcontrast MRI (Image B) shows a nonenhancing mass in the same location. This is most consistent with an old calcified right atrial thrombus. Most likely history in this case would be a patient with history of central line placement.

Typical history for a cardiac fibroma could be a 13-year-old with heart failure. For angiosarcoma, a 40-year-old with shortness of breath may be the best history. For a patient with hypertension and tachycardia, a cardiac paraganglioma may be possible due to the excessive production of catecholamines. If the images showed valvular vegetations, then a history of endocarditis could be likely. For asymptomatic patients, a benign pseudomass such as a prominent crista terminalis could be seen. For patients with history of echinococcus infection, there could be residuals such as calcified masses.

23b Answer G. CT shows a calcified lesion along the inferior lateral heart. The best answer here would be a patient with history of echinococcus infection as this is most consistent with hydatid cyst residuals. Please see prior discussion for discussion on other answer choices.

Reference: Kantarci M, Bayraktutan U, Karabulut N, et al. Alveolar echinococcosis: spectrum of findings at cross-sectional imaging. *Radiographics* 2012;32(7):2053–2070. doi: 10.1148/rg.327125708. Review. PubMed PMID: 23150858.

24a Answer B. Noncontrast CT (Image A) shows a mass anterior and to the left of the ascending aorta. Note the sternotomy wires. PET (Image B) shows no significant activity in this mass. Given the sternotomy wires, this may be a saphenous graft aneurysm, so the best next step is to evaluate for possible aneurysm with contrast-enhanced CTA. If there is a concern for a vascular pathology, biopsy should not be performed. Lack of PET activity makes this less likely to be a malignancy. This is not a lesion that can be left alone without further evaluation.

24b Answer A. Images show a saphenous vein graft aneurysm. These patients typically present with chest pain/angina. However, a significant number of cases are discovered incidentally (up to ⅓ of reported cases). There is no consensus on treatment depending on aneurysm size; however, some have advocated treating the aneurysm >1 cm. Currently, surgery is performed more often than percutaneous treatment (covered stent). SVG aneurysms most often occur in the RCA territory, likely due to larger number of SVGs to the RCA territory and possibly the larger caliber of the RCA grafts.

Reference: Ramirez FD, Hibbert B, Simard T, et al. Natural history and management of aortocoronary saphenous vein graft aneurysms: a systematic review of published cases. *Circulation* 2012;126(18):2248–2256. doi: 10.1161/CIRCULATIONAHA.112.101592. Review. PubMed PMID: 23109515.

25 Answer B. There is a low-attenuation lesion in the right atrium on the CT (Image A). The postcontrast MRI (Image B) shows no mass in the right atrium. This is most consistent with a pseudofilling defect in the right atrium from unopacified blood returning to the right atrium, most likely due to patient doing a Valsalva maneuver as she held her breath. This has been described as transient interruption of the contrast in PE studies. It is unlikely for a large mass in the right atrium to embolize without any symptoms. The mass is also unlikely to have equal enhancement to the blood pool and not show up on the any of the images on MRI.

Reference: Wittram C, Yoo AJ. Transient interruption of contrast on CT pulmonary angiography: proof of mechanism. *J Thorac Imaging* 2007;22(2):125–129. PubMed PMID: 17527114.

7 Valvular Disease

QUESTIONS

1. The Bernoulli equation is an example of the law of conservation of
   A. Mass
   B. Energy
   C. Momentum
   D. Charge

2. The aortic valve has a systolic measured area of 0.7 cm². How would you grade the severity of stenosis?
   A. Normal
   B. Mild
   C. Moderate
   D. Severe

3. Enlargement of which cardiac structure would be the most reliable sign of pulmonary valve stenosis?
   A. Right ventricle
   B. Main pulmonary trunk
   C. Main trunk and left pulmonary artery
   D. Right and left pulmonary arteries

4. Which of the following valvular abnormalities have the worst acute prognosis?
   A. Bicuspid aortic valve
   B. Drug-induced tricuspid valvulopathy
   C. Infarcted papillary muscle with rupture
   D. Multivalvular rheumatic fever

5. Which is the most common cause of mitral stenosis worldwide?
   A. Rheumatic heart disease
   B. Myxomatous degenerative disease
   C. Carcinoid syndrome
   D. Congenital mitral stenosis

6 What would be the primary contributor to this patient's mitral insufficiency?

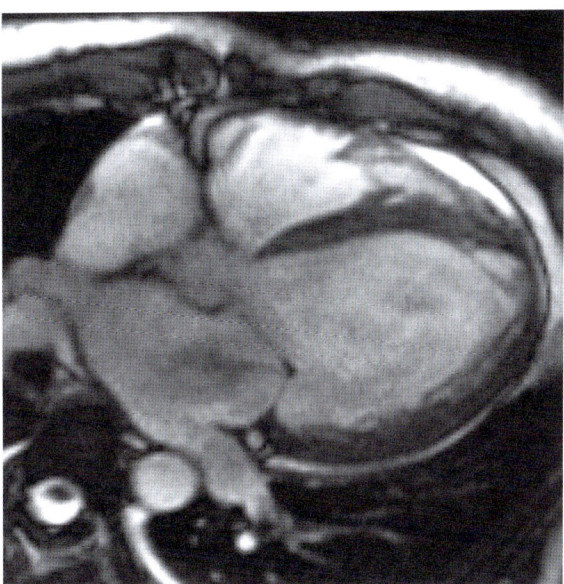

A. Mitral valve prolapse
B. Annular dilation
C. Congenital mitral stenosis
D. Infective endocarditis

7 Which is the most common cause of pulmonic stenosis?

A. Congenital stenosis
B. Rheumatic disease
C. Degenerative thickening
D. Carcinoid syndrome

8 Rheumatic disease involving the aortic valve is most commonly associated with

A. Aortic insufficiency
B. Isolated involvement
C. Bicuspid aortic valve
D. Aortic stenosis

9 The classic diagnostic criteria for mitral valve prolapse include displacement of the mitral leaflets of

A. >1 mm beyond the annulus into the left ventricle and leaflet thickening of >3 mm
B. >5 mm beyond the annulus into the left ventricle and leaflet thickening of >2 mm
C. >3 mm beyond the annulus into the left atrium and leaflet thickening of >1 mm
D. >2 mm beyond the annulus into the left atrium and leaflet thickening of >5 mm

10 Complications in infective endocarditis of the aortic valve include

A. Cardiac arrhythmias
B. Septic pulmonary emboli
C. Valvular stenosis
D. Rasmussen aneurysm

11 Patient presents with severe left atrial enlargement and new atrial fibrillation. Given the clinical history and imaging findings, what hemodynamic consequences can occur?

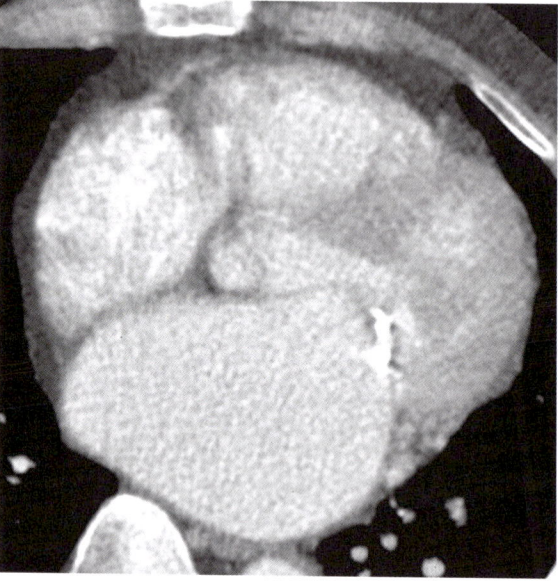

A. Elevated right atrial pressure
B. Blunting of hepatic vein waveforms
C. Blunting of pulmonary venous waveforms
D. Increased pulmonary arterial flow

12 After obtaining a preoperative contrast-enhanced CT, an abnormality was incidentally noted on the aortic valve (below). Patient has no history of endocarditis or septicemia.

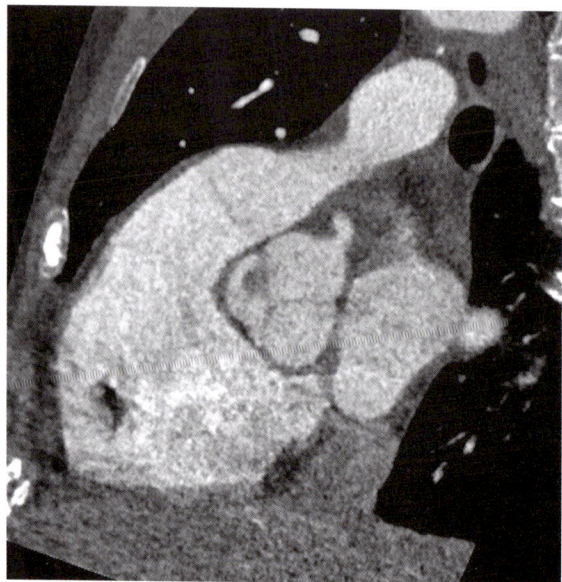

Given the clinical history and imaging findings, the most likely etiology would be
A. Fibroma
B. Metastasis
C. Rhabdomyosarcoma
D. Papillary fibroelastoma

13 A 59-year-old with chronic mitral insufficiency now presents with acute decompensation and pulmonary edema.

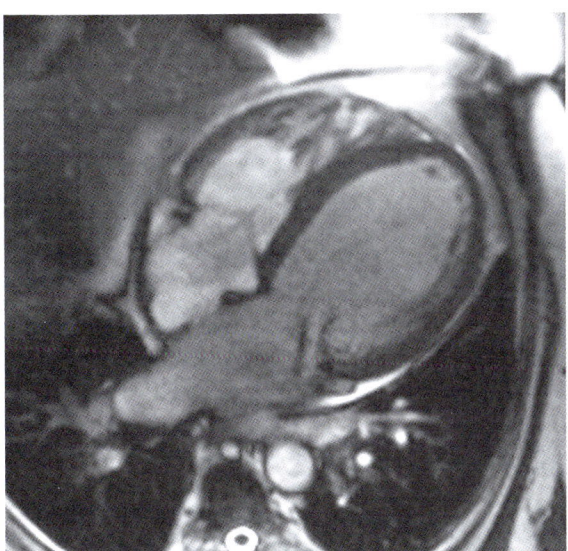

What is the most likely diagnosis?
A. Flail leaflet
B. Rheumatic mitral valve disease
C. Mitral stenosis
D. Mitral valve prolapse

14 What is the most likely diagnosis?

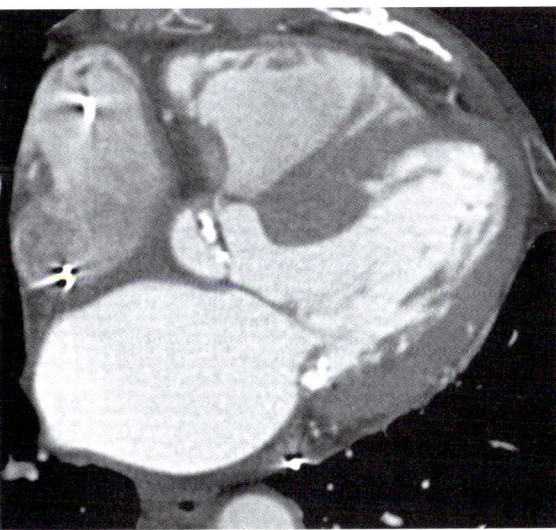

A. Flail leaflet
B. Rheumatic mitral valve disease
C. Mitral valve prolapse
D. Mitral regurgitation

15 A 36-year-old man with severe aortic calcification and valvular stenosis is referred for preoperative coronary CT angiography. Which of the following CT imaging findings are most likely to be observed?

  A. Asymmetric LV hypertrophy
  B. Normal aortic valve area
  C. Left atrial enlargement
  D. Bicuspid valve

16 Horizontal long-axis images from a cardiac MR demonstrating end-diastolic (left) and end-systolic (right) MR images of the mitral valve.

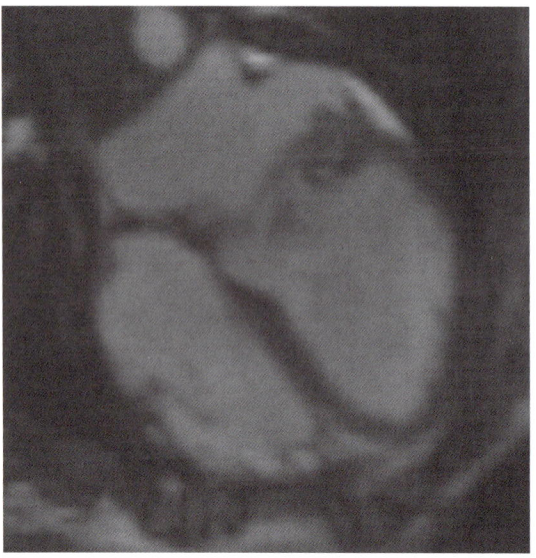 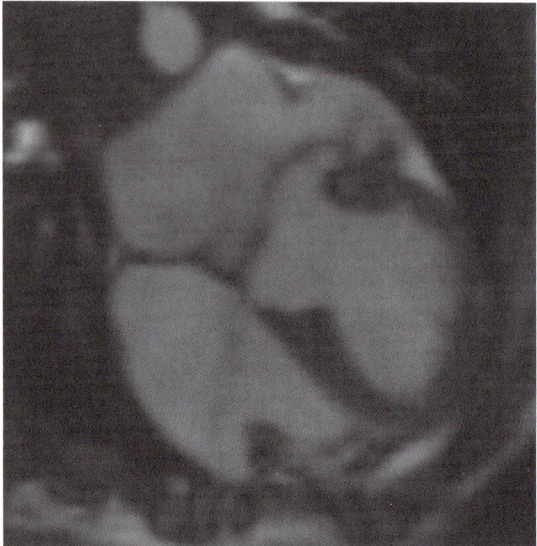

What is the most likely diagnosis?

  A. Flail leaflet
  B. Rheumatic mitral valve disease
  C. Mitral stenosis
  D. Mitral valve prolapse

17 An 86-year-old patient with severe aortic stenosis undergoes transcatheter aortic valve implantation. The postoperative course was largely uncomplicated; however, a new left bundle branch block is observed on telemetry. Which of the following is the most likely etiology?

  A. Cardiac sarcoidosis
  B. Complication of TAVI surgery
  C. Acute myocardial infarction
  D. Drug toxicity

18 What are the pathologic features that are associated with mitral stenosis?

  A. Commissural fusion with subvalvular shortening of chordae
  B. Myxomatous degeneration of the valve leaflets
  C. Calcific deposits in the annulus fibrosis
  D. Inflammatory vegetations with leaflet destruction

19 What hemodynamic effects can be seen with mitral stenosis?

  A. Increased left atrial pressure
  B. Decreased pulmonary capillary resistance
  C. Increased pulmonary venous flow
  D. Decreased left atrial volume

20 A clinician calls your office to consult about a cardiac MR for one of her patients. The patient is status post prosthetic mitral valve repair 8 months prior and is unsure whether this will be safe for cardiac MR. What would be your recommendation?

A. Cardiac MR imaging would not be safe to perform with any valve prosthesis.
B. Reviewing the make and model of the valve and date of surgery may be helpful in determining safety.
C. All metallic prosthetic valves are contraindicated, and all biologic valves are considered MR safe.
D. Valve prosthesis placed less than 12 months should not undergo imaging by MR.

21 Which is the most optimal cardiac imaging plane for evaluating the atrioventricular valves?

A. Vertical long axis
B. Short axis
C. Horizontal long axis
D. Coronal

22 A 33-year-old patient with a history of murmur undergoes a cardiac MRI. The MR depicts the following:

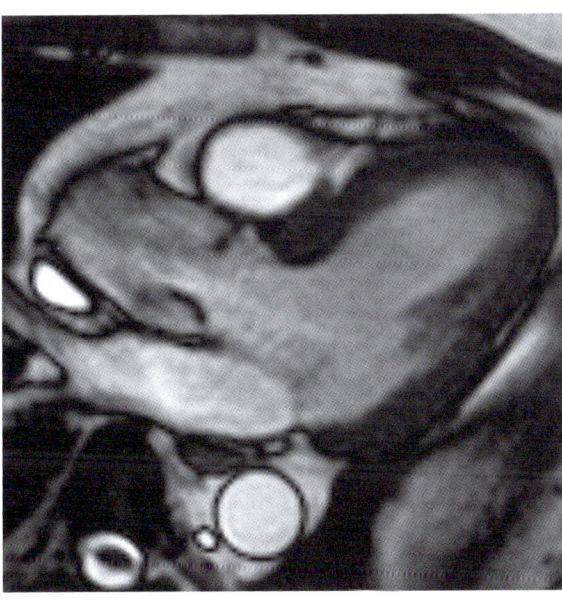
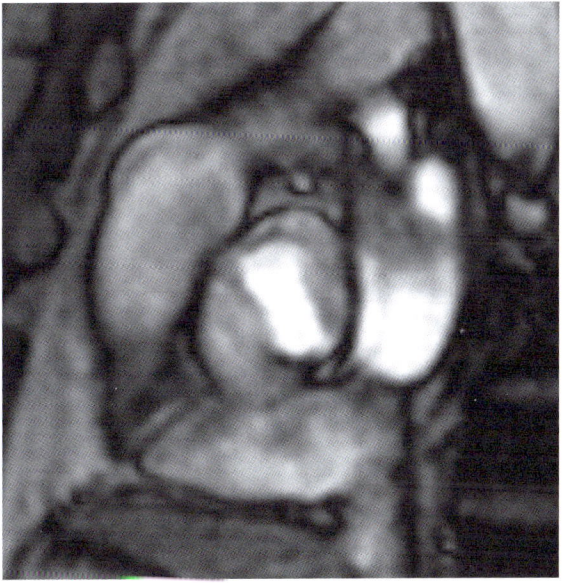

Which is the most appropriate diagnosis?

A. Critical aortic valve stenosis
B. Bioprosthetic aortic valve
C. Aortic valve endocarditis
D. Bicuspid aortic valve

23 Mitral valve prolapse may occur in association with which condition?

A. Shone syndrome
B. Carcinoid disease
C. Marfan syndrome
D. Rheumatic heart disease

24 Patient with fever and chest pain presents with the following imaging. What is the most likely diagnosis?

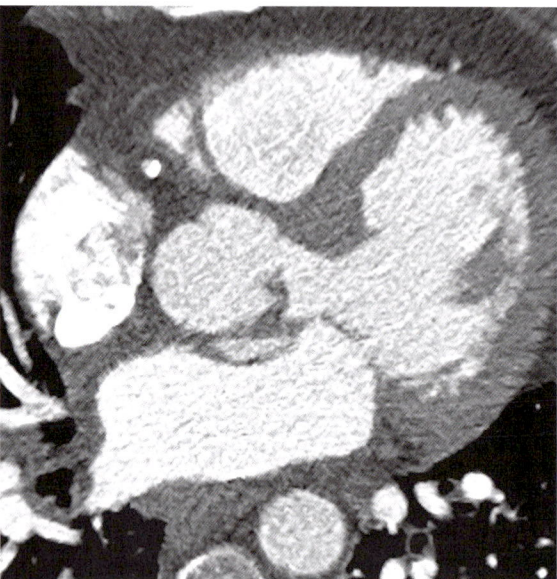

A. Paravalvular abscess
B. Aortic aneurysm
C. Aortic dissection
D. Pericardial effusion

25a A 34-year-old presents to the emergency department with atypical chest pain. Images from her CT are provided below.

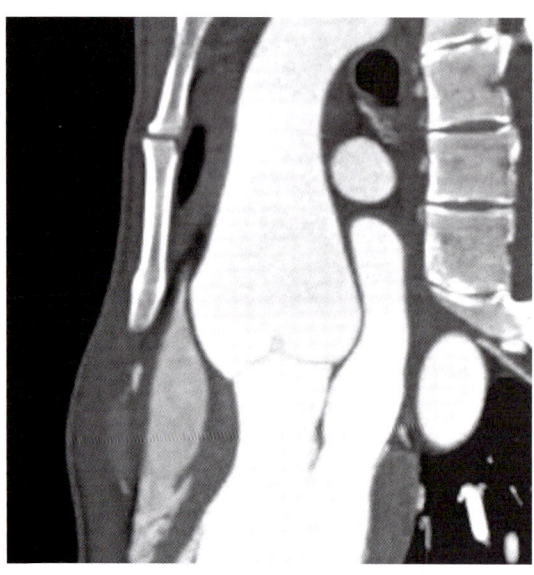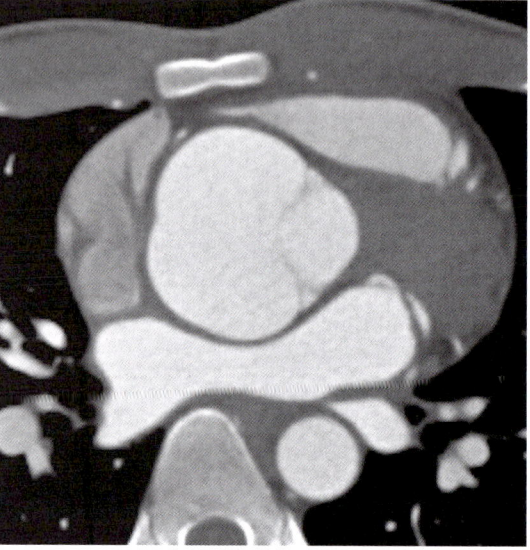

Which best describes the underlying pathology?
A. Acute aortic syndrome
B. Annuloaortic ectasia
C. Subvalvular aortic stenosis
D. Rheumatic heart disease

10 Answer A. The complications of infective endocarditis (IE) depend on the virulence of the organism and may include cusp perforation, chordal rupture, aneurysmal bulging of the valve, and perivalvular abscess formation. Uncommonly, this may result in a fistulous connection between major vessels and cardiac chambers or between chambers themselves resulting into congestive heart failure. Infection extending beyond valvular tissue may also result in disruption of the conduction system with electrocardiographic conduction abnormalities and arrhythmias.

Stenosis due to IE is uncommon. Septic pulmonary emboli and Rasmussen aneurysms are complications of right-sided cardiac valves.

Reference: Karchmer CM. Infectious endocarditis. In: Bonow RO, Braunwald E (eds.). *Braunwald's heart disease: a textbook of cardiovascular medicine*. Philadelphia, PA: Saunders, 2012:1540–1560.

11 Answer C. Contrast-enhanced CT demonstrates significant mitral valve calcification and marked left atrial enlargement consistent with mitral stenosis.

Severe mitral stenosis results in a significant increase in left atrial pressure. This pressure is reflected backward, causing blunting of pulmonary venous waveforms and an increase in pulmonary venous, capillary, and arterial pressures and resistance. Ultimately, pulmonary hypertension develops which then eventually leads to right ventricular hypertrophy and enlargement, tricuspid regurgitation, increased right atrial pressure, and the development of right-sided heart failure.

Reference: Otto CM, Bonow RO. Valvular heart disease. In: Bonow RO, Braunwald E (eds.). *Braunwald's heart disease: a textbook of cardiovascular medicine*. Philadelphia, PA: Saunders, 2012:1468–1539.

12 Answer D. MPR of cardiac-gated CT of the chest demonstrates a small well-circumscribed lesion on the aortic valve.

Papillary fibroelastomas are the third most common primary cardiac tumor in adults and the most common tumor of the cardiac valves. Papillary fibroelastomas can become quite large and occur on any valve surface or area of the endocardium. Histologically, they are composed of a core of myxoid connective tissue containing abundant mucopolysaccharide matrix and elastic fibers that is covered by a surface endothelium. Recurrences are rare, and valve-sparing surgery should be considered whenever possible, as regrowth of partially resected lesions does not always occur.

The remaining pathologies rarely involve the valves primarily.

Cardiac rhabdomyomas are the most frequently encountered primary cardiac tumor in infants and children. Cardiac rhabdomyoma arises more commonly in the ventricles, although up to 30% of cases can involve either atrium.

Patients with tuberous sclerosis have a 40% to 86% incidence of cardiac rhabdomyomas so it is an important association to screen for.

Fibromas of the heart are connective tissue tumors derived from fibroblasts and are very similar to soft tissue fibromas. About 90% of the reported cases occur in children before the age of 1 year, although fibromas can occur in any age group. Fibromas are associated with Gorlin syndrome in which patients develop odontogenic cysts, epidermal cysts, multiple nevi, and basal cell carcinomas of the skin.

Reference: Burke A, Jeudy J, Virmani R. Cardiac tumours: an update. *Heart* 2008;94(1):117–123.

13 Answer A. Balanced steady-state free precession (b-SSFP) cardiac MR demonstrates prolapse of the anterior mitral leaflet into the left atrium consistent with a flail leaflet. This is typically secondary to rupture of a component of the mitral valve tensor apparatus (chordae tendineae and papillary muscles).

Leaflet prolapse and elongated chordae are common in degenerative mitral valve disease. Superimposed chordal rupture may develop from chronic damage resulting in a flail segment and associated severe mitral insufficiency.

Reference: Otto CM, Bonow RO. Valvular heart disease. In: Bonow RO, Braunwald E (eds.). *Braunwald's heart disease: a textbook of cardiovascular medicine*. Philadelphia, PA: Saunders, 2012:1468-1539.

14 Answer B. CT of the chest demonstrated thickening and calcification of both mitral and aortic valve leaflets, most consistent with rheumatic heart disease.

Rheumatic fever is an immunologically mediated, multisystem inflammatory disorder that occurs after an episode of group A streptococcal pharyngitis. A rheumatic carditis occurs during the active phase of rheumatic fever and may progress over time to chronic rheumatic heart disease. Significant valve thickening and commissural fusion and thickening of the chordae tendineae are characteristic by histology.

The mitral valve is most commonly affected in 65% to 70% of cases and along with the aortic valve in another 25% of cases. Tricuspid valve involvement is infrequent, and the pulmonary valve is very rarely affected.

Reference: Schoen FJ, Mitchell RN. The heart. In: Kumar V, Abbas AK, Fausto N, et al. (eds.). *Robbins and Cotran pathologic basis of disease*. Saunders, 2009:529-588.

15 Answer D. The abnormal morphology of a bicuspid aortic valve (BAV) results in valvular dysfunction and hemodynamic derangements. Echocardiographic studies have shown that sclerosis of the aortic cusps begins as early as the second decade of life while calcification becomes prominent in most middle-aged patients. This early degeneration may be related to more aggressive inflammatory changes of the aortic valve, characterized by increased macrophage infiltration and neovascularization.

Chronic aortic stenosis leads to ventricular pressure overload and concentric left ventricular hypertrophy will increased wall thickness and normal LV chamber size.

With worsening AS, diastolic dysfunction with impaired relaxation and increased diastolic filling pressure may result. This can lead to left atrial dilatation; however, this is a late finding in the progression of the disease.

Reference: Losenno KL, Goodman RL, Chu MWA. Bicuspid aortic valve disease and ascending aortic aneurysms: gaps in knowledge. *Cardiol Res Pract* 2012;2012:16. PMCID: PMC3503270.

16 Answer D. Balanced steady-state free precession images in the horizontal long axis demonstrate thickening and redundancy of the mitral valve at end diastole (left). End-systolic images (right) show prolapse of the leaflets beyond the annular plane and into the left atrium, consistent with mitral valve prolapse.

Mitral valve prolapse (MVP) is defined as single or bileaflet prolapse at least 2 mm beyond the long-axis annular plane, with or without thickening of the valve leaflets. The prevalence of prolapse is estimated at 2% to 3% and is equally distributed between men and women. Uncommonly, MVP is associated with heritable disorders of connective tissue including Marfan syndrome.

Although the great majority of persons with MVP have no untoward effects, approximately 3% develop one of four serious complications: (1) infective endocarditis, (2) mitral insufficiency, (3) stroke or other systemic infarct, or (4) arrhythmias, both ventricular and atrial.

References: Hayek E, Gring CN, Griffin BP. Mitral valve prolapse. *Lancet* 2005;365(9458): 507-518.

Schoen FJ, Mitchell RN. The heart. In: Kumar V, Abbas AK, Fausto N, et al. (eds.). *Robbins and Cotran pathologic basis of disease*. Saunders, 2009:529-588.

17 **Answer B.** Transcatheter aortic valve implantation (TAVI) has become an established treatment option for patients with aortic stenosis at prohibitive risk to undergo conventional surgical aortic valve replacement. Among potential complications that may arise with TAVI surgery, new conduction abnormalities and arrhythmias frequently occur.

New left bundle branch block has been reported in 29 to 65% of patients after Medtronic CoreValve system and in 4% to 18% of patients receiving the balloon-expandable Edwards SAPIEN valve. In the PARTNER study, new-onset atrial fibrillation was present in 41% of patients acutely after TAVI and 9% within 30 days from the procedure.

Reference: van der Boon RMA, Houthuizen P, Nuis R-J, et al. Clinical Implications of conduction abnormalities and arrhythmias after transcatheter aortic valve implantation. *Curr Cardiol Rep* 2013;16(1):1–7.

18 **Answer A.** The most common cause of mitral stenosis is rheumatic heart disease. With acute rheumatic fever, focal inflammatory lesions are found in various tissues including the cardiac valves. The inflammation of the endocardium and the left-sided valves typically results in fibrinoid necrosis within the cusps or along the tendinous cords.

Microscopically, there is organization of the acute inflammation and subsequent diffuse fibrosis and neovascularization that obliterate the leaflet architecture. Subsequent leaflet thickening, commissural fusion and shortening, and thickening and fusion of the chordae tendineae occur, leading to the characteristic changes seen in mitral stenosis.

Myxomatous degeneration is the pathologic hallmark of mitral valve prolapse. Infective endocarditis leads to deposition of inflammatory vegetations and leaflet destruction. Calcification of the mitral valve annulus generally does not affect valvular function or otherwise become clinically important.

Reference: Schoen FJ, Mitchell RN. The heart. In: Kumar V, Abbas AK, Fausto N, et al. (eds.). *Robbins and Cotran pathologic basis of disease*. Saunders, 2009:529–588.

19 **Answer A.** The most useful descriptor of the severity of mitral valve obstruction is the mitral valve orifice area. In normal adults, the cross-sectional area of the mitral valve orifice (MVO) is 4 to 6 cm². An MVO of <1 cm² leads to high resistance across the stenotic mitral valve, thereby increasing LA volume and pressure. This elevated left atrial pressure, in turn, raises pulmonary venous and capillary pressures, resulting in exertional dyspnea.

The left ventricle is usually normal and may have normal systolic pressure and end-diastolic function. With increased severity of mitral stenosis, resultant passive backward transmission of the elevated left atrial pressure, and pulmonary arteriolar constriction, may develop leading to pulmonary hypertension. Right ventricular enlargement and even dilatation of the hepatic veins may be seen in the most severe and chronic forms of mitral stenosis but are not common findings.

Reference: Otto CM, Bonow RO. Valvular heart disease. In: Bonow RO, Braunwald E (eds.). *Braunwald's heart disease: a textbook of cardiovascular medicine*. Philadelphia, PA: Saunders, 2012:1468–1539.

20 **Answer B.** Investigative studies have demonstrated a lack of substantial magnetic field interactions and negligible heating in heart valve prostheses and annuloplasty rings evaluated during MR testing. These findings indicate that MR procedures may be conducted safely in individuals with these implants using MR systems with static magnetic fields of 1.5 T or less.

With respect to clinical MR procedures, there has never been a report of a patient incident or injury related to the presence of a heart valve prosthesis. An often quoted exception to this used to be the Starr-Edwards Pre-6000 series valves, but these too have now been deemed acceptable for MRI.

Theoretical concerns for patients with heart valves that have metal leaflets undergoing MR procedures on MR systems >1.5 T, although this has never been demonstrated or reported.

For an object that is weakly magnetic, it is typically necessary to wait a period of 6 to 8 weeks prior to performing an MR procedure. In this case, retentive or counterforces provided by tissue in growth, scarring, or granulation serve to prevent the object from presenting a risk or hazard to the patient in the MR environment. In this particular case, it would be fine to image the patient.

References: Edwards M-B, Taylor KM, Shellock FG. Prosthetic heart valves: evaluation of magnetic field interactions, heating, and artifacts at 1.5 T. *J Magn Reson Imaging* 2000;12(2):363–369.

Shellock FG. Magnetic resonance safety update 2002: implants and devices. *J Magn Reson Imaging* 2002;16(5):485–496.

21 **Answer C.** The horizontal long axis (4-chamber view) provides a view of both atria, atrioventricular valves, and both ventricles. The short axis may provide a supplemental view of the valves but remains limited since the leaflets move in and out of plane. Vertical long axis may provide depiction of one of the valves, depending upon which ventricle the plane passes through. Coronal projections are also suboptimal in visualizing of the valves.

Reference: Miller SW. *Cardiac imaging: the requisites.* Elsevier Health Sciences, 2009.

22 **Answer D.** Balanced steady-state free precession images in three-chamber view (left) and en face view through the valve (right) demonstrate thickening of the aortic valve with "fish-mouth" morphology consistent with a bicuspid aortic valve.

Bicuspid aortic valve (BAV) is the most frequent congenital cardiovascular malformation in humans with a prevalence of approximately 1%. Structural abnormalities of the aortic wall commonly accompany bicuspid valves even when the valve is hemodynamically normal, potentiating aortic dilation or aortic dissection. The other available choices typically present with additional clinical history and complaints.

Reference: Schoen FJ, Mitchell RN. The heart. In: Kumar V, Abbas AK, Fausto N, et al. (eds.). *Robbins and Cotran pathologic basis of disease*. Saunders, 2009:529–588.

23 **Answer C.** Mitral valve prolapse (MVP) is a variable clinical syndrome that results from diverse pathogenic mechanisms. MVP occurs as a primary condition that is not associated with other diseases and can be familial or nonfamilial. It can also be associated with heritable disorders of connective tissue including Marfan syndrome, which is usually caused by mutations in fibrillin-1 (FBN-1).

Carcinoid heart disease generally involves the endocardium and valves of the right heart and is the cardiac manifestation of the systemic associated with carcinoid tumors. These changes are restricted to the right side of the heart due to inactivation of both serotonin and bradykinin during passage through the lungs.

Shone syndrome classically presents with four cardiovascular defects: a supravalvular mitral membrane, valvular mitral stenosis due to a parachute mitral valve, subaortic stenosis (membranous or muscular), and aortic coarctation. Most presenting cases are incomplete with only two or three of these components present.

References: Otto CM, Bonow RO. Valvular heart disease. In: Bonow RO, Braunwald E (eds.). *Braunwald's heart disease: a textbook of cardiovascular medicine*. Philadelphia, PA: Saunders, 2012:1468–1539.

Schoen FJ, Mitchell RN. The heart. In: Kumar V, Abbas AK, Fausto N, et al. (eds.). *Robbins and Cotran pathologic basis of disease*. Saunders, 2009:529–588.

24 **Answer A.** The case demonstrates thickening of aortic valve leaflets and a paravalvular collection around the aortic root as a result of aortic valve endocarditis. Resulting complications include disruption of the conduction system with electrocardiographic conduction abnormalities and arrhythmias or purulent pericarditis.

Reference: Karchmer CM. Infectious endocarditis. In: Bonow RO, Braunwald E (eds.). *Braunwald's heart disease: a textbook of cardiovascular medicine*. Philadelphia, PA: Saunders, 2012:1540–1560.

25a Answer B. The image demonstrates dilatation of the aortic root with effacement of the sinotubular junction, consistent with annuloaortic ectasia. Annuloaortic ectasia (AE) is symmetric dilation of the aortic root and ascending aorta with effacement of the sinotubular junction. AE may cause aortic regurgitation, aortic dissection, and rupture. It is most often associated with Marfan syndrome, but it can also be seen in other conditions, such as Ehlers-Danlos syndrome, osteogenesis imperfecta, or homocystinuria, or be idiopathic. Ascending aortic aneurysm is also seen in syphilis, bicuspid aortic valve, aortitis, and postoperative patients.

Rheumatic heart disease causes thickening of the aortic valve and aortic stenosis. Subvalvular aortic stenosis is the second most common form of AS and refers to narrowing at the outlet of the left ventricle just below the aortic valve.

Reference: Litmanovich D, Bankier AA, Cantin L, et al. CT and MRI in diseases of the aorta. *AJR Am J Roentgenol* 2009;193(4):928–940.

25b Answer A. Loeys-Dietz syndrome (LDS) is an autosomal-dominant connective tissue disorder defined as those with mutations in transforming growth factor–β (TGF-β) receptor TGFBR1 (predominantly presenting with craniofacial features) and TGFBR2 (predominantly presenting with cutaneous features). LDS is characterized by the triad of arterial tortuosity and aneurysms, hypertelorism, and bifid uvula or cleft palate. Aortic root aneurysms are present in up to 98% of patients with LDS, with thoracic aortic dissection being the leading cause of death (67%), followed by abdominal aortic dissection (22%) and cerebral hemorrhage (7%).

Shone syndrome is a rare congenital heart disease comprising a series of four obstructive or potentially obstructive left-sided cardiac lesions: supravalvular mitral membrane, parachute mitral valve, subaortic stenosis (membranous or muscular), and coarctation of the aorta.

Heyde syndrome is a syndrome of aortic valve stenosis associated with gastrointestinal bleeding from colonic angiodysplasia.

Williams syndrome is a rare genetic disorder that affects a child's growth, physical appearance, and cognitive development. Cardiovascular defects include supravalvular aortic stenosis, pulmonary arterial stenosis, aortic coarctation, cardiomyopathy, tetralogy of Fallot, aortic valve defect (aortic stenosis or insufficiency), and mitral valve defect (mitral stenosis or mitral insufficiency).

References: Chu LC, Johnson PT, Dietz HC, et al. CT angiographic evaluation of genetic vascular disease: role in detection, staging, and management of complex vascular pathologic conditions. *AJR Am J Roentgenol* 2014;202(5):1120–1129.

Eronen M, Peippo M, Hiippala A, et al. Cardiovascular manifestations in 75 patients with Williams syndrome. *J Med Genet* 2002;39(8):554–558.

Islam S, Cevik C, Islam E, Attaya H, et al. Heyde's syndrome: a critical review of the literature. *J Heart Valve Dis* 2011;20(4):366–375.

Roche KJ, Genieser NB, Ambrosino MM, et al. MR findings in Shone's complex of left heart obstructive lesions. *Pediatr Radiol* 1998;28(11):841–845.

26 Answer C. Cardiac CT demonstrates marked enlargement of right-sided cardiac chambers with thickening and tethering of the anterior tricuspid leaflet, consistent with the diagnosis of carcinoid valvular disease. Notably, there is also deviation of the interventricular septum toward the left compatible with elevated right-sided pressures.

Cardiac involvement from carcinoid disease is a rare and unique manifestation typically inducing abnormalities of the right side of the heart. Valvular dysfunction in carcinoid heart disease is caused by proliferation of endocardial fibroblasts in response to chronic inflammation or induced by a number of circulating vasoactive mediators. Plaque deposition leads to thickening, retraction, and impaired leaflet motion. Compared to the right side of the heart, the left-sided valves are rarely affected because of the pulmonary metabolism and deactivation of the hormonal substances.

Eisenmenger syndrome is a complication of uncorrected large intracardiac left-to-right shunts. Long-standing shunts lead to increased pulmonary resistance leading to bidirectional shunting and then to right-to-left shunting. Rheumatic heart disease causes significant thickening of valve leaflets and valvular stenosis; however, superimposed insufficiency may result when leaflets remain fixed in an open position. Calcified deposits on the mitral valve annulus do not typically affect valvular function or otherwise become clinically important.

References: Grozinsky-Glasberg S, Grossman AB, Gross DJ. Carcinoid heart disease: from pathophysiology to treatment "something in the way it moves." *Neuroendocrinology* 2015.

Miles LF, Leong T, McCall P, Weinberg L. Carcinoid heart disease: correlation of echocardiographic and histopathological findings. *BMJ Case Reports* 2014;2014.

27. **Answer C.** The gradient across a valve can be estimated using the peak velocity and the Bernouli equation ($4*v^2$). With a peak velocity of >4.0 m/sec, the mean aortic gradient corresponds to a mean aortic valve gradient of >40 mm Hg. The peak gradient would be estimated at 64 mm Hg.

Reference: Nishimura RA, Otto CM, Bonow RO, et al.; ACC/AHA Task Force Members. 2014 AHA/ACC guideline for the management of patients with valvular heart disease: a report of the American College of Cardiology/American Heart Association Task Force on Practice Guidelines. *Circulation* 2014;129(23):e521–e643. doi: 10.1161/CIR.0000000000000031. Epub 2014 Mar 3. Erratum in: *Circulation* 2014;129(23):e651. PubMed PMID: 24589853.

28. **Answer D.** Current generation (2014/2015) of endovascular access sheath requires at least 6 mm diameter for the CoreValve system. The SAPIEN system ranges from 6 to 8 mm for the minimal diameter. Current sheath sizes range from 18 French to 22–24 French.

Reference: Achenbach S, Delgado V, Hausleiter J, et al. SCCT expert consensus document on computed tomography imaging before transcatheter aortic valve implantation (TAVI)/transcatheter aortic valve replacement (TAVR). *J Cardiovasc Comput Tomogr* 2012;6(6):366–380. doi: 10.1016/j.jcct.2012.11.002. Epub 2012 Nov 14. PubMed PMID: 23217460.

29. **Answer C.** Coronal MPR of a cardiac CT demonstrates a linear but incomplete web arising in the left ventricular outflow tract, below the level of the aortic valve.

Left ventricular outflow tract obstruction includes a spectrum of stenotic lesions that are generally categorized as subvalvular, valvular, or supravalvular. These obstructions to forward flow may present alone or in concert, as in the frequent association of a bicuspid aortic valve with coarctation of the aorta. All of these lesions impose increased afterload on the left ventricle and, if severe and untreated, result in hypertrophy and eventual dilatation and failure of the left ventricle.

Subaortic stenosis (SAS) may be focal, as in a discrete membrane, or more diffuse, resulting in a tunnel leading out of the left ventricle. Fibromuscular SAS is most frequently encountered (90%), but the tunnel-type lesions are associated with a greater degree of stenosis. Congenital valvular stenosis due to bicuspid aortic valve (BAV) occurs with an estimated incidence of 1% to 2%. BAV usually occurs in isolation but is associated with other abnormalities, the most common being coarctation of the aorta, patent ductus arteriosus, or ascending aortopathy. Supravalvular aortic stenosis (SVAS) is obstruction constriction occurring above the level of the aortic valve. SVAS is frequently associated with Williams syndrome. Aortic insufficiency results from malcoaptation of the aortic leaflets due to abnormalities of the aortic leaflets, their supporting structures (aortic root and annulus), or both.

Reference: Aboulhosn J, Child JS. Left ventricular outflow obstruction subaortic stenosis, bicuspid aortic valve, supravalvar aortic stenosis, and coarctation of the aorta. *Circulation* 2006;114(22):2412–2422.

8 Pericardial Disease

QUESTIONS

1. The patient presents with dyspnea and has cardiomegaly based on a radiograph (not shown). Which of the following cardiac findings shown on the four-chamber balanced steady-state image?

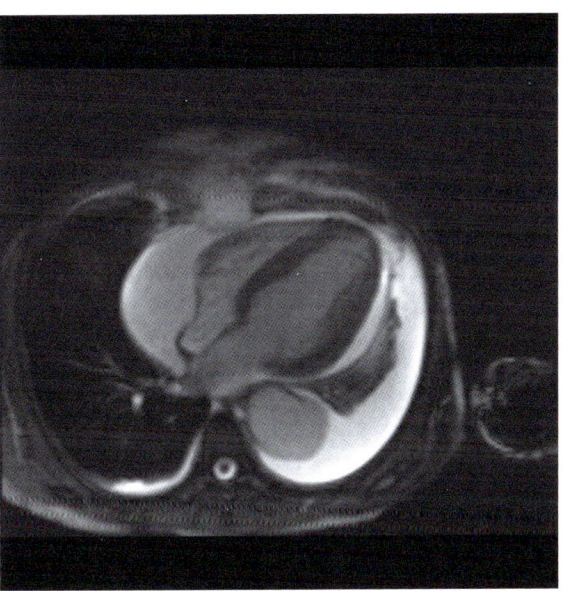

   A. Atrial septal defect
   B. Enlarged left ventricle
   C. Mitral valve prolapse
   D. Pericardial effusion
   E. Pericarditis

2. What contributes to MRI overestimating the pericardial thickness?
   A. Chemical shift artifact at the fat fluid interface
   B. Higher spatial resolution compared to CT
   C. Lack of motion of the pericardial layers
   D. Low temporal resolution

3 The pericardial abnormality is from what process?

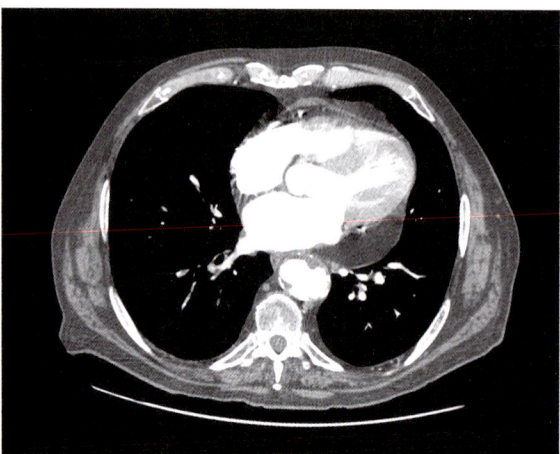

A. Constrictive pericarditis
B. Pericardial lipoma
C. Pericardial lymphoma
D. Pneumopericardium

4 The pericardial mass can be associated with which of the following?

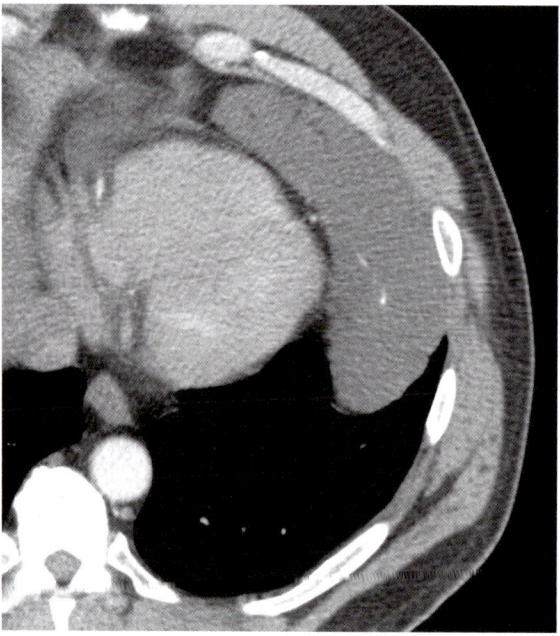

A. Calcifications
B. Serous pericardial effusion
C. Restrictive physiology
D. Systemic malignancy

5a The image shows?

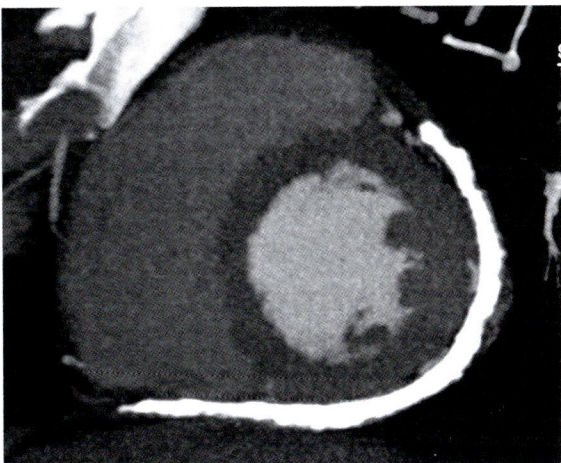

   A. Absent pericardium
   B. Calcific pericarditis
   C. Pericardial effusion
   D. Pericardial metastasis

5b Constrictive pericarditis can cause which of the following changes?

   A. Decreased right ventricular volume
   B. Decreased IVC caliber
   C. Normal-sized liver
   D. Rightward displaced interventricular septum

6 What radiographic finding shown here is most suggestive of a pericardial effusion?

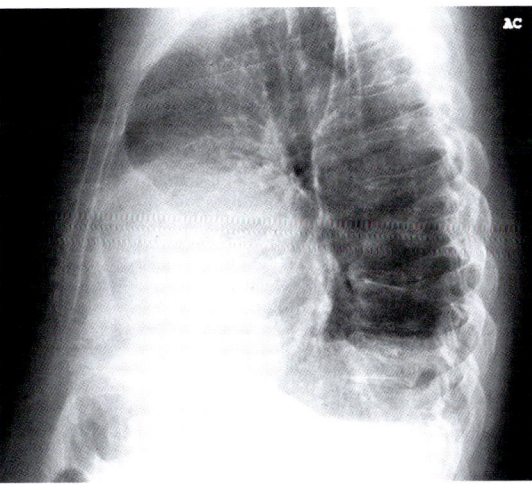
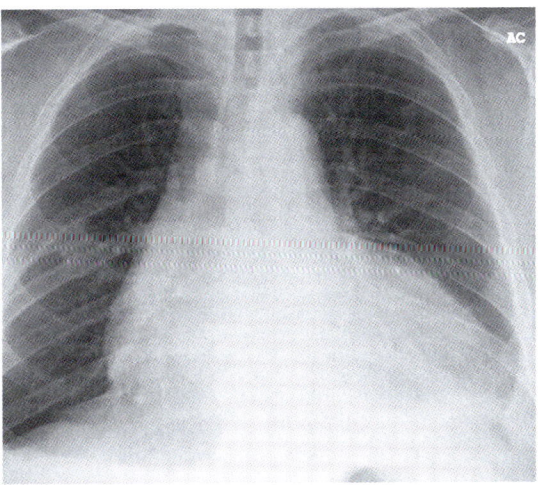

   A. Dilated heart
   B. Pericardial calcification
   C. Separation of the epicardial and pericardial fat
   D. Widening of the mediastinum

7 The mass is best characterized by which of the following?

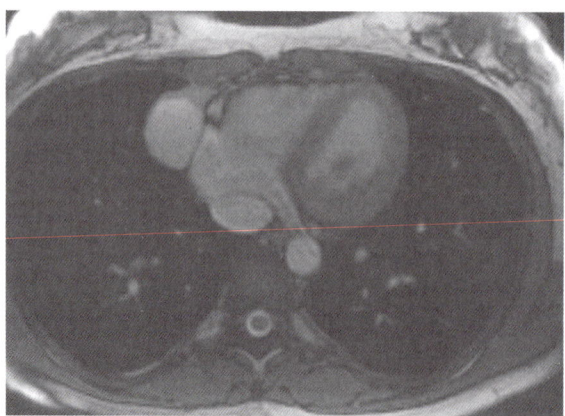

A. Compression of the cardiac chambers
B. Enhancement on postcontrast MR imaging
C. Intermediate signal on T1 images if it is simple
D. Most commonly located at the right cardiophrenic angle
E. Septations on T2 images

8 Which of the following is the most likely diagnosis?

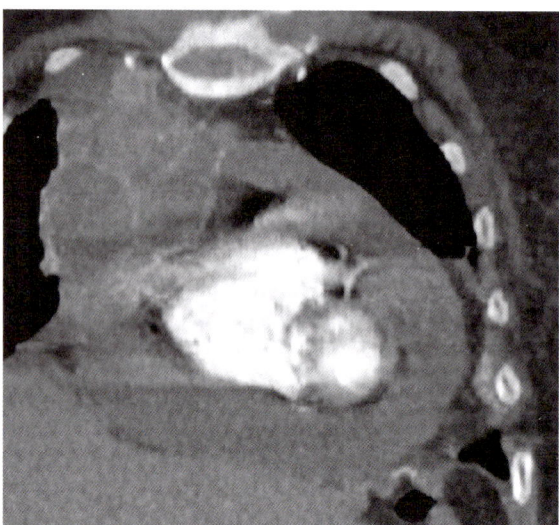

A. Calcific pericarditis
B. Constrictive pericarditis
C. Malignant pericardial effusion
D. Pericardial effusion
E. Pericardial lymphangioma

9   What is the most likely procedure done to result in this complication shown?

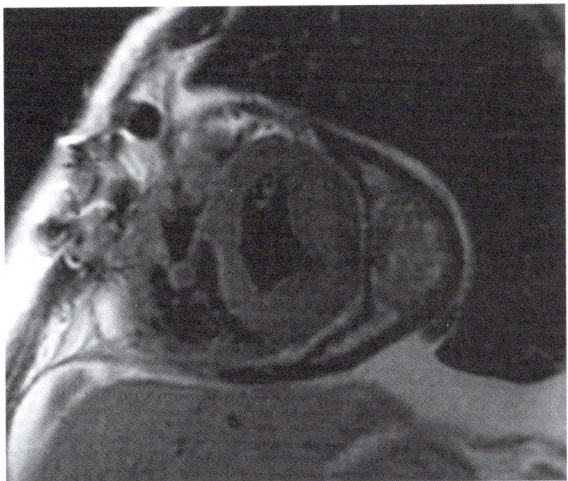

   A. Aneurysmectomy
   B. CABG
   C. Pericardectomy
   D. Radiation therapy

10 Which of the following is associated with the finding?

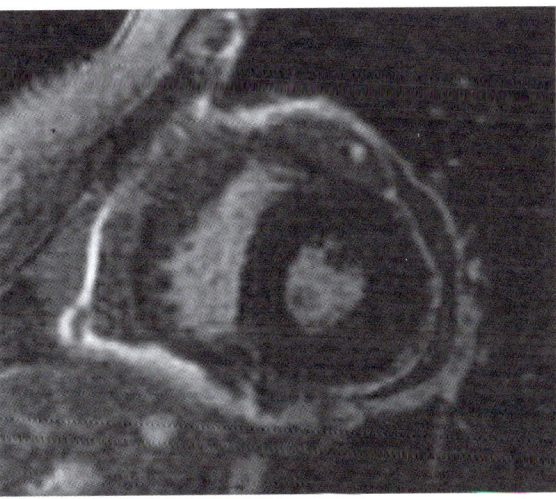

   A. Absent inflammation
   B. Mild disease
   C. Fatty proliferation
   D. Increased neovascularization

11 What best describes the principle of ventricular independence as it relates to septal bounce?
   A. Increased in volume of one ventricle causes a reduced volume in the opposite ventricle.
   B. The bounce is decreased during inspiration.
   C. A decrease in right ventricular pressure causes the shift toward the left ventricle.
   D. Increased venous return has no impact on ventricular interdependence.

12a What is the most likely diagnosis?

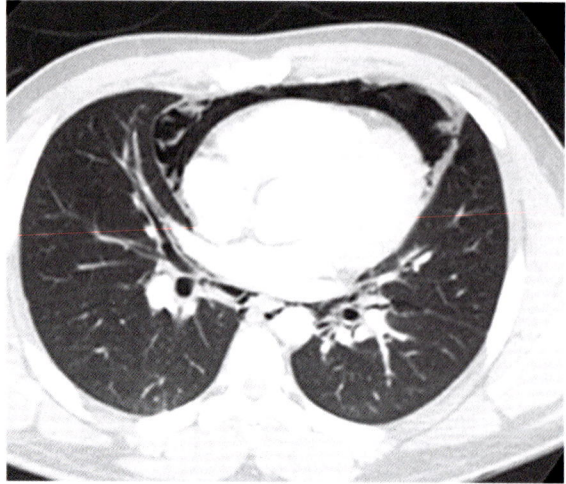

A. Atrioesophageal fistula
B. Fistula to the mediastinum
C. Pneumothorax
D. Pneumopericardium
E. Pneumoperitoneum

12b Which of the following characterizes the physiology of cardiac tamponade?

A. Bradycardia
B. Hypertension
C. Elevated jugular venous distension
D. Decrease in systolic blood pressure

13 A pericardial window can be performed to drain a pericardial effusion. Which of the following describes pericardial window procedure?

A. Removal of a small segment of the pericardium
B. Chylopericardium is a contraindication to a pericardial window.
C. It is performed when the pericardium is compliant.
D. A tube will remain in place when draining is <200 mL/24 h.

14 Restrictive and constrictive cardiac physiology share similar physiologic findings. Which of the following can occur in both entities?

A. Diastolic dysfunction
B. Thickened pericardium
C. Abnormal myocardium

15 The diagnosis of acute pericarditis involves the clinical criteria of chest pain, pericardial friction rub, pericardial effusion, and EKG changes. What EKG changes are most suggestive of acute pericarditis?

A. Upward concave ST elevation and PR segment depression
B. ST depression
C. Delta wave
D. Q waves

ANSWERS AND EXPLANATIONS

1 Answer D. The patient has a large pericardial effusion on the bright blood sequence. Normally, the pericardium is a thin sac composed of two layers enveloping the heart (an inner serous membrane and an outer fibrocollagenous layer). Normally, the pericardium contains 10 to 50 mL of an ultrafiltrate of plasma. If it contains a greater volume, it will cause a pericardial effusion.

References: Bogaert J, Francone M. Cardiovascular magnetic resonance in pericardial diseases. *J Cardiovasc Magn Reson* 2009;11:14.

Roberts WC, Spray TL. Pericardial heart disease: a study of its causes, consequences, and morphologic features. *Cardiovasc Clin* 1976;7:11-65.

2 Answer A. The pericardium normally measures up to 2 mm in systole and 1 mm in diastole; however, accurate measurement of the pericardium using MRI can be challenging. MRI has been shown to overestimate the pericardial thickness, which may be secondary to chemical shift artifact, spatial resolution limits, and motion of the pericardial layers.

References: Bogaert J, Francone M. Cardiovascular magnetic resonance in pericardial diseases. *J Cardiovasc Magn Reson* 2009;11:14.

Sechtem U, Tscholakoff D, Higgins CB. MRI of the abnormal pericardium. *AJR Am J Roentgenol* 1986;147:245-252.

3 Answer B. Primary pericardial tumors are uncommon. Pericardial lipomas have been reported to account for up to 10% of all primary pericardial neoplasms. The mass is of fat attenuation and is well encapsulated. Tumors are usually detected incidentally and are usually asymptomatic. In symptomatic patients, the tumor may lead to compression of the cardiac chambers.

References: Steger CM. Intrapericardial giant lipoma displacing the heart. *ISRN Cardiol* 2011;2011:4. Article ID 243637. http://dx.doi.org/10.5402/2011/243637

Stoian I, et al. Rare tumors of the heart-angiosarcoma, pericardial lipoma, leiomyosarcoma, three case reports. *J Med Life* 2010;3(2):178-182. Published online 2010 May 25.

4 Answer A. The mass is low in density, septated, and contains calcifications. These features are most characteristic of a pericardial lymphangioma. There are no areas of nodularity or enhancement in the mass, indicating it is not due to a primary cardiac malignancy or metastatic disease. Pericardial lymphangiomas are uncommon primary tumors that may extend into the mediastinum and may compress cardiac or adjacent mediastinal structures leading to respiratory distress or altered cardiac function.

References: Shaheen F, Lone N. A rare case of pericardial lymphangioma causing tamponade: routine and dynamic MR findings. *Eur J Radiol Extra* 2009;69(1):e9-e10.

Zakaria RH, et al. Imaging of pericardial lymphangioma. *Ann Pediatr Cardiol* 2011;4(1):65-67. doi: 10.4103/0974-2069.79628.

5a Answer B. The image shows the pericardium is thickened (measuring >4 mm) along the lateral and inferior wall of the heart and is densely calcified. These findings are compatible with calcific pericarditis. Calcific pericarditis can be secondary to prior inflammation, infection (tuberculosis), connective tissue disease, radiation therapy, or uremia. The finding of calcifications can be associated with constrictive physiology.

References: Macgregor JH, Chen JT, Chiles C, et al. The radiographic distinction between pericardial and myocardial calcifications. *AJR Am J Roentgenol* 1987;148(4):675-677.

Wang ZJ, Reddy GP, Gotway MB, et al. CT and MR imaging of pericardial disease. *Radiographics* 2003;23:S167-S180.

5b Answer A. Constrictive pericarditis can be associated with decrease in size of the right ventricle reduced right ventricular volume, dilation of the IVC and SVC, hepatomegaly, and ascites. The interventricular septum can be displaced toward the left ventricle or develop a sigmoid shape.

References: Higgins CB. Acquired heart disease. In: Higgins CB, Hricak H, Helms CA (eds.). *Magnetic resonance imaging of the body*. Philadelphia, PA: Lippincott-Raven, 1997:409-460.

Wang ZJ, Reddy GP, Gotway MB, et al. CT and MR imaging of pericardial disease. *Radiographics* 2003;23:S167-S180.

6 Answer C. The patient has a large pericardial effusion. Radiography is not sensitive for the diagnosis of a pericardial effusion large effusions can be identified using several radiographic findings. The effusion is best visualized on the lateral view and is outlined by the epicardial and pericardial fat ("oreo-cookie sign"). Other findings suggestive of a pericardial effusion include a dilated cardiac silhouette and widening of the subcarinal angle.

References: Chen JT, Putman CE, Hedlund LW, et al. Widening of the subcarinal angle by pericardial effusion. *AJR Am J Roentgenol* 1982;139(5):883-887.

Wang ZJ, Reddy GP, Gotway MB, et al. CT and MR imaging of pericardial disease. *Radiographics* 2003;23:S167-S180.

7 Answer D. The image shows a mass at the right cardiophrenic angle that is most compatible with a pericardial cyst. Pericardial cysts are most commonly located at the right cardiophrenic angle, have increased T2 signal, lack septations, and have no enhancement. Pericardial cysts are formed during development of the pericardial sac and while most common at the right cardiophrenic angle can be located in the anterior and posterior mediastinum. Less commonly, pericardial cysts can cause compression or become infected.

References: Patel J, Park C, Michaels J, et al. Pericardial cyst: case reports and a literature review. *Echocardiography* 2004;21:269-272.

White CS. MR evaluation of the pericardium. *Top Magn Reson Imaging* 1995;7:258-266.

8 Answer C. The image shows a large pericardial effusion with septations and nodular enhancement of the pericardium, compatible with a malignant pericardial effusion. Irregular and nodular pericardial thickening and enlarged mediastinal lymph nodes increase the specificity when diagnosing a malignant pericardial effusion. Fluid-based sampling and cytology are used to confirm the diagnosis of a malignant pericardial effusion.

References: Rienmüller R, Gröll R, Lipton MJ. CT and MR imaging of pericardial disease. *Radiol Clin North Am* 2004;42:587-601.

Sun JS, Park KJ, Kang DK. CT findings in patients with pericardial effusion: differentiation of malignant and benign disease. *AJR Am J Roentgenol* 2010;194(6):W489-W494.

9 Answer C. The patient has a thickened and enhancing pericardium and a hematoma indicating underlying constrictive pericarditis. The patient underwent a pericardiectomy. A pericardiectomy can be performed via either a median sternotomy or anterolateral thoracotomy. A pericardiectomy is performed as definitive treatment for constrictive pericarditis. During the procedure, the pericardium is removed to the greatest extent possible. However, despite the procedural success, hemodynamics may not return to their baseline state.

References: Maisch B, Seferovic PM, Ristic AD, et al. Guidelines on the diagnosis and management of pericardial diseases. *Eur Soc Cardiol* 2004;25(7):587-610.

Tiruvoipati R, Naid RD, Loubani M, et al. Surgical approach for pericardiectomy: a comparative study between median sternotomy and left anterolateral thoracotomy. *Cardiovasc Thorac Surg* 2003;2(3):322-326. doi: 10.1016/S1569-9293(03)00074-4.

10 Answer D. The patient has pericarditis with a thickened pericardium and late gadolinium enhancement. The presence of late gadolinium enhancement in pericarditis is associated with increased inflammation, neovascularization, proliferation of fibroblasts, and granulation tissue indicating ongoing inflammation. Patients without late gadolinium enhancement but a thickened pericardium are more likely to have mild or absent inflammation.

References: Srichai MB. CMR imaging in constrictive pericarditis: is seeing believing? *J Am Coll Cardiol Imaging* 2011;4(11):1192-1194. doi: 10.1016/j.jcmg.2011.09.009.

Young PM, Glockner JF, Williamson EE. MR imaging findings in 76 consecutive surgically proven cases of pericardial disease with CT and pathologic correlation. *Int J Cardiovasc Imaging* 2012;28(5):1099-1109. [E-pub ahead of print].

11 Answer A. The principle of ventricular interdependence defines how an increase in volume of one ventricle causes a decreased volume in the opposite ventricle. The septal bounce is characterized by movement of the interventricular septum initially toward the left ventricle and subsequently away from the left ventricle during early diastole. During early diastole, since right ventricular filling occurs before left ventricular filling, the increased right ventricular volume will shift the septum toward the left. This will reverse as the left ventricle subsequently fills increased venous return, which occurs during inspiration, will increase the septal bounce.

References: Giorgi B, Mollet NR, Dymarkowski S, et al. Clinically suspected constrictive pericarditis: MR imaging assessment of ventricular septal motion and configuration in patients and healthy subjects. *Radiology.* 2003;228:417-424.

Walker CM, Chung JH, Reddy GP. Septal bounce. *J Thorac Imaging* 2012;27(1):w1. doi: 10.1097/RTI.0b013e31823fdfbd.

12a Answer D. The patient has extensive pneumopericardium with air between the pericardium and right atrium and ventricle. Pneumopericardium can be secondary to trauma (blunt or penetrating), postoperative, infectious, or a fistula. If the air is extensive it can cause tamponade physiology.

References: Bejvan SM, Bejvan SM, Godwin JD. Pneumomediastinum: old signs and new signs. *AJR Am J Roentgenol* 1996;166(5):1041-1048.

Karoui M, Bucur PO. Images in clinical medicine. Pneumopericardium. *N Engl J Med* 2008;359(14):e16. doi: 10.1056/NEJMicm074422.

12b Answer C. Patients with cardiac tamponade physiology will have dyspnea, tachycardia, and elevated jugular venous pressure. Several other clinical finding complexes have also been reported which include:

> Beck triad—hypotension, elevated jugular venous pressure, and decreased heart sounds
> Pulsus paradoxus—decrease (by more than 12 mm Hg) in the systolic blood pressure during inspiration
> Kussmaul sign—increase in venous distension and pressure during inspiration

References: Roy CL, Minor MA, Brookhart MA, et al. Does this patient with a pericardial effusion have cardiac tamponade? *JAMA* 2007;297(16):9.

Yarlagadda C. Cardiac tamponade clinical presentation. *Medscape.* Available at: http://emedicine.medscape.com/article/152083-clinical#a0256

13 Answer A. A pericardial window is performed either for diagnosis or for therapy to drain pericardial fluid. The procedure is performed by placing a drain after a small amount of the pericardium has been removed, usually via a subxiphoid approach. Indications include symptomatic or asymptomatic simple pericardial effusions, chylous effusions, purulent effusions, delayed hemopericardium, or reaccumulating effusions. Concomitant surgery requiring a sternotomy and full pericardiectomy is a contraindication to a pericardial window.

References: Komanapalli C, Sukumar M. Thoracoscopic pericardial window. Available at: http://www.ctsnet.org/sections/clinicalresources/thoracic/expert_tech-32.html. Muller

Muller DK. Pericardial window. *Medscape*. Available at: http://emedicine.medscape.com/article/1829679-overview

14 Answer A. Constrictive pericarditis and restrictive cardiomyopathy may have overlapping clinical findings, which include normal to near-normal systolic function and diastolic dysfunction. Imaging will have a key role in the diagnosis allowing the clinician to distinguish between a thickened and enhancing pericardium in pericarditis and abnormal myocardium with late gadolinium enhancement in restrictive cardiomyopathy.

References: Chinnaiyan KM, Leff CB, Marsalese DL. Constrictive pericarditis versus restrictive cardiomyopathy: challenges in diagnosis and management. *Cardiol Rev* 2004;12(6):314–320.

Mookadam F, Jiamsripong P, Raslan SF, et al. Constrictive pericarditis and restrictive cardiomyopathy in the modern era. *Future Cardiol* 2011;7(4):471–483. doi: 10.2217/fca.11.18.

15 Answer A. EKG changes in pericarditis include upward, concave ST elevation and PR segment depression. The ST elevation reflects underlying epicardial inflammation and along with the PR depression occurs early in the disease process.

Over time, the ST and PR segments will return to normal and may lead to T-wave inversion, which can normalize.

Delta waves are associated with Wolff-Parkinson white syndrome, while Q waves are associated with prior myocardial infarction.

References: Ginzton LE, Laks MM. The differential diagnosis of acute pericarditis from the normal variant: new electrocardiographic criteria. *Circulation* 1982;65(5):1004–1009.

Khandaker MH, Espinosa RE, Nishimura RA, et al. Pericardial disease: diagnosis and management. *Mayo Clin Proc* 2010;85(6):572–593. doi: 10.4065/mcp.2010.0046.

16 Answer B. Hemopericardium is the accumulation of blood in the pericardial sac. Hemopericardium can be secondary to aneurysm rupture, trauma (blunt or penetrating), dissection, anticoagulation, or iatrogenic. It can lead to cardiac tamponade if the volume of blood accumulates rapidly leading to cardiovascular compromise.

References: Krejci CS, Blackmore CC, Nathens A. Hemopericardium an emergent finding in a case of blunt cardiac injury. *AJR Am J Roentgenol* 2000;175:250–250. Available at: http://www.ajronline.org/doi/full/10.2214/ajr.175.1.1750250

Levis JT, Delgado MC. Hemopericardium and cardiac tamponade in a patient with an elevated international normalized ratio. *West J Emerg Med* 2009;10(2):115–119.

17 Answer B. Cardiac metastases can involve the heart via hematogenous or lymphatic pathways and usually occur late in the disease process. Lymphatic pathways lead to pericardial involvement while pericardial pathways lead to cardiac involvement. Lung cancer (most common), breast cancer, lymphoma, and melanoma are the tumors that lead to cardiac metastasis and typically involve the pericardium.

References: Chiles C, Woddard PK, Gutierrez FR, et al. Metastatic involvement of the heart and pericardium: CT and MR imaging. *Radiographics* 2001;21(2):439–449.

Reynen K, Kockeritz U, Strasser RH. Metastases to the heart. *Ann Oncol* 2004;15(3):375–381. doi: 10.1093/annonc/mdh086.

18a Answer B. The image shows a mass in the free wall of the right ventricle with a pericardial effusion secondary to cardiac metastasis. The diagnosis can be confirmed via pericardiocentesis. The effusion can be treated with a pericardial window, radiation treatment, or infusion of a sclerotic agent.

References: Chiles C, Woddard PK, Gutierrez FR, et al. Metastatic involvement of the heart and pericardium: CT and MR imaging. *Radiographics* 2001;21(2):439-449.

Millaire A, Wurtz A, De Groote P, et al. Malignant pericardial effusions: usefulness of pericardioscopy. *Am Heart J* 1992;124:1030-1034.

18b Answer D. Malignant pericardial effusions can be diagnosed via pericardiocentesis. Cytology studies are positive in 80 to 90% of patients with malignant pericardial effusions. The finding of a malignant effusion can be associated with decreased survival.

References: Maher EA, Shepherd FA, Todd TJ. Pericardial sclerosis as the primary management of malignant pericardial effusion and cardiac tamponade. *J Thorac Cardiovasc Surg* 1996;112:637-643.

Meyers DG, Bouska DJ. Diagnostic usefulness of pericardial fluid cytology. *Chest* 1989;95:1142-1143.

19 Answer A. If the pericardial fluid accumulates rapidly, a volume of 100 can lead to pericardial pressure increasing by >30 mmHg. The sudden rise in pressure is secondary to decreased pericardial compliance. The reduced compliance results in a decreased ability of the pericardium to stretch and respond to the increased volume.

References: Holt JP, Rhode EA, Kines H. Pericardial and ventricular pressure. *Circ Res* 1960;8:1171-1181.

Shabetai R. Pericardial effusion: haemodynamic spectrum. *Heart* 2004;90(3):255-256. doi: 10.1136/hrt.2003.024810.

20 Answer B. Increased epicardial fat deposition (fat between the heart and visceral pericardium) has been suggested to contribute to coronary artery disease, increased coronary plaque burden, adverse cardiac events and atrial fibrillation.

Reference: Dey D, Nakazato R, Li D, et al. Epicardial and thoracic fat-noninvasive measurement and clinical implications. *Cardiovasc Diagn Ther* 2012;2(2):85-93. doi: 10.3798/j.issn.2223-3652.2012.04.03.

21 Answer A. CT is more accurate than MR to identify pericardial thickening and pericardial enhancement in patients with suspected pericarditis. MRI can better identify delayed pericardial enhancement, restricted movement of the pericardium and changes in waveforms in vessels.

Reference: Feng D, Glockner J, Kim K, et al. Cardiac magnetic resonance imaging pericardial late gadolinium enhancement and elevated inflammatory markers can predict the reversibility of constrictive pericarditis after antiinflammatory medical therapy: a pilot study. *Circulation* 2011;124(17):1830-1837. doi: 10.1161/circulationaha.111.026070.

22 Answer A. The normal pericardium will measure <4 mm on CT and will usually measure between 1 and 2 mm. A thickened pericardium can be suggestive of acute pericarditis; however, this should be confirmed with clinical findings and late gadolinium enhancement on MRI to confirm the diagnosis of acute pericarditis.

References: Ling LH, Oh JK, Breen JF, et al. Calcific constrictive pericarditis: is it still with us? *Ann Intern Med* 2000;132(6):444-450.

Maisch B, Seferovic PM, Ristic AD, et al. Guidelines on the diagnosis and management of pericardial diseases executive summary: The task force on the diagnosis and management of pericardial diseases of the European Society of Cardiology. *Eur Heart J* 2004;25(7):587-610.

23 Answer B. Epipericardial fat necrosis is a self-limited cause of acute chest pain. It is an uncommon cause of pain, and can be associated with mass adjacent to the pericardium on CT. The image will show infiltrated/necrotic fat. The mass may be mistaken for a diaphragmatic hernia, fat containing thymic tumor or sarcoma or a lipoma.

References: Fred HL. Pericardial fat necrosis: a review and update. *Texas Heart Inst J* 2010;37(1):82-84.

Van den Heuvel DAF, Van Es HW, Cirkel GA, et al. Images in thorax: acute chest pain caused by pericardial fat necrosis. *Thorax* 2010;65(2):188. doi: 10.1136/thx.2009.114637.

24 Answer D. The balanced steady state free precession image shows a septated pericardial mass. The septations indicate that the mass is not a simple pericardial cyst. Balanced steady state free precessions sequences have both fat and fluid weighing.

Reference: Bogaert J, Francone M. Pericardial disease: value of CT and MR imaging. *Radiology* 2013;267(2):340-356.

9 Congenital Heart Disease

QUESTIONS

1a A 48-year-old male with heart murmur. What is the most likely underlying condition based on the chest radiographs?

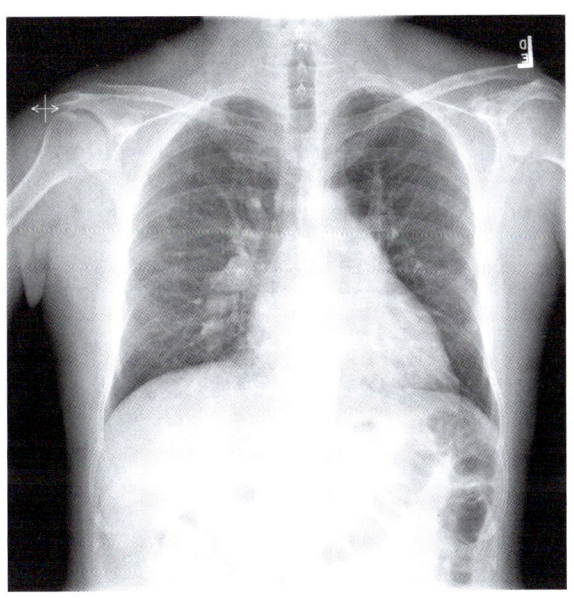
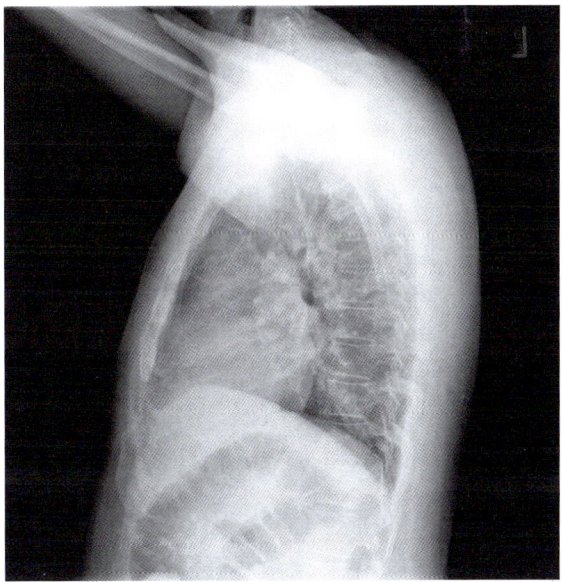

A. Aortic stenosis
B. Mitral stenosis
C. Atrial septal defect (ASD)
D. Normal
E. Ebstein anomaly

1b Which of the following is a contraindication to the procedure that was done?

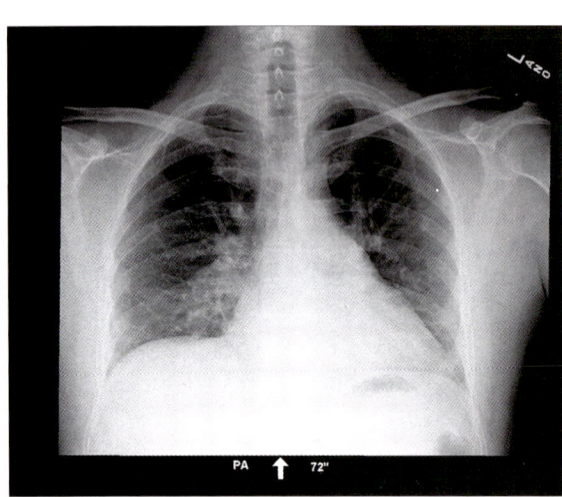
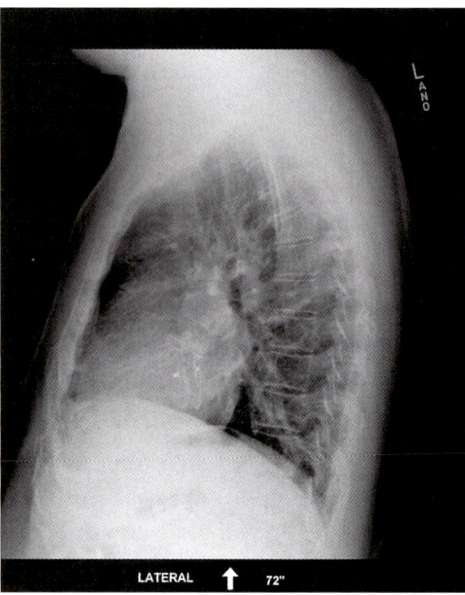

A. Qp/Qs > 2
B. Atrial fibrillation
C. Lack of adequate rims
D. Bilateral iliac artery thrombosis

1c Which of the following is a potential long-term complication of septal occluder device placement?

A. Atrial fibrillation
B. Heart block
C. Embolization/malpositioning
D. Erosion of the device

2 What is the treatment for this condition?

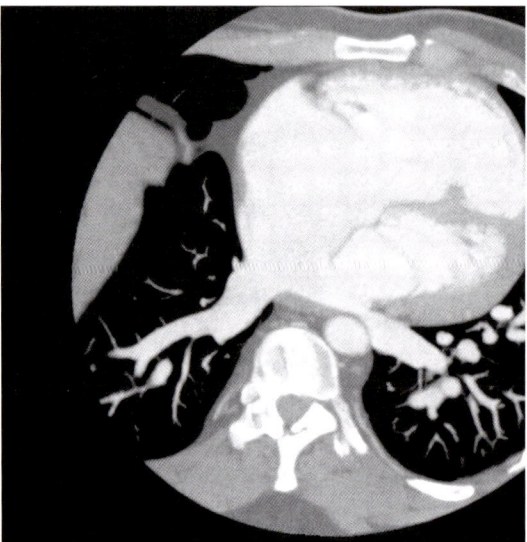

A. Medical
B. Surgical
C. Endovascular
D. None

3a This was an incidental finding on a gated CTA of an asymptomatic patient. What is the best next step?

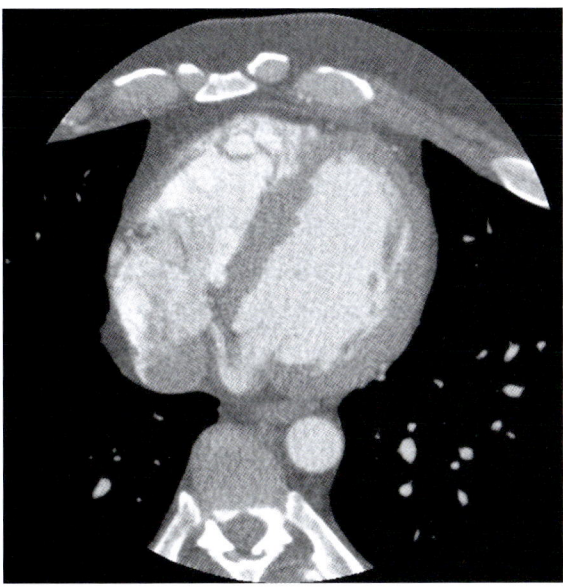
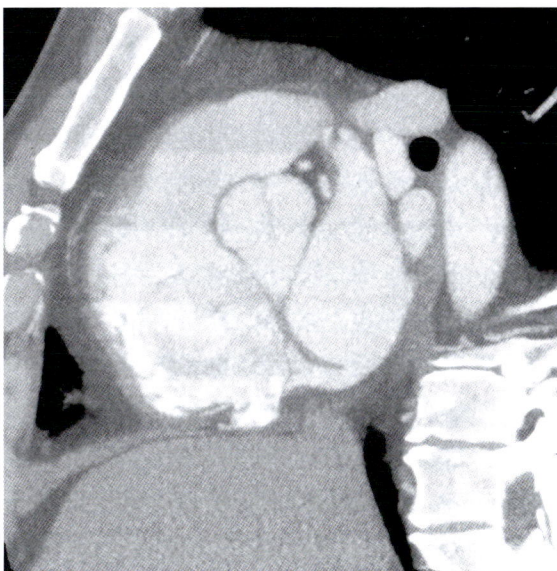

A. Surgical closure.
B. Catheter-based closure.
C. Leave it alone.

3b Unroofed coronary sinus is associated with which of the following vascular abnormalities?

A. Azygos continuation of the IVC
B. Coarctation of the aorta
C. Anomalous right pulmonary venous return
D. Left-sided SVC

4 How many types of atrial septal defects (ASD) are there?

A. There are two types of ASD.
B. There are three types of ASD.
C. There are four types of ASD.
D. There are five types of ASD.

5 What is a major difference between membranous versus muscular ventricular septal defects (VSD)?

A. Muscular VSD can undergo spontaneous closure.
B. Membranous VSD can undergo spontaneous closure.
C. Endocarditis prophylaxis is not required for muscular VSD.
D. Endocarditis prophylaxis is not required for membranous VSD.

6a A 61-year-old female presents with shortness of breath. What is the best next step?

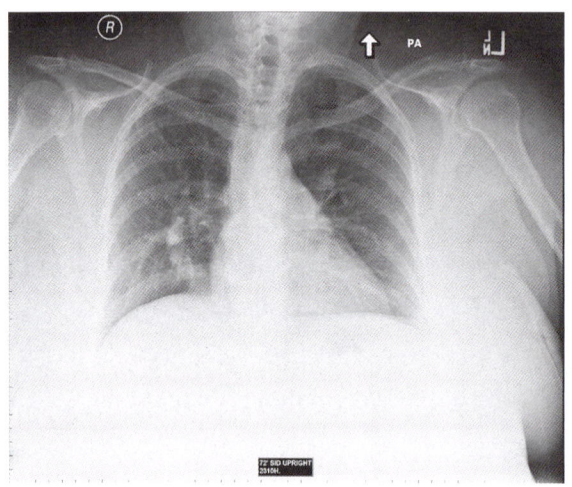
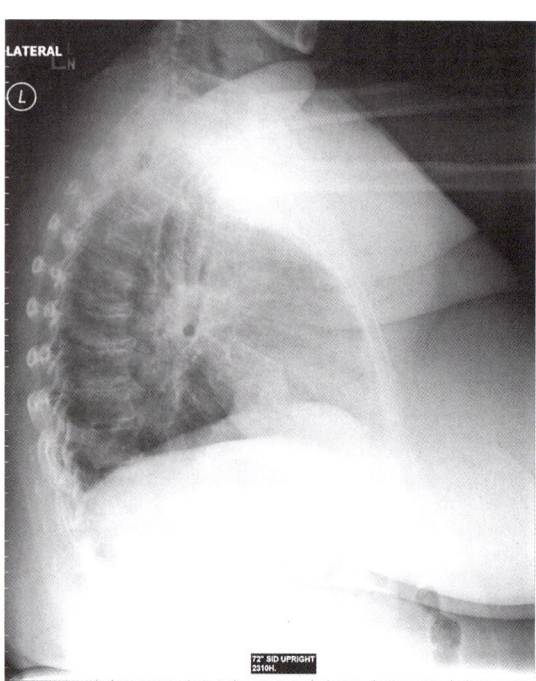

A. Biopsy
B. CT of the chest without contrast
C. CTA of the chest
D. VQ scan
E. No further imaging necessary

6b No atrial septal defect was seen in this patient. What type of shunt does the patient have?

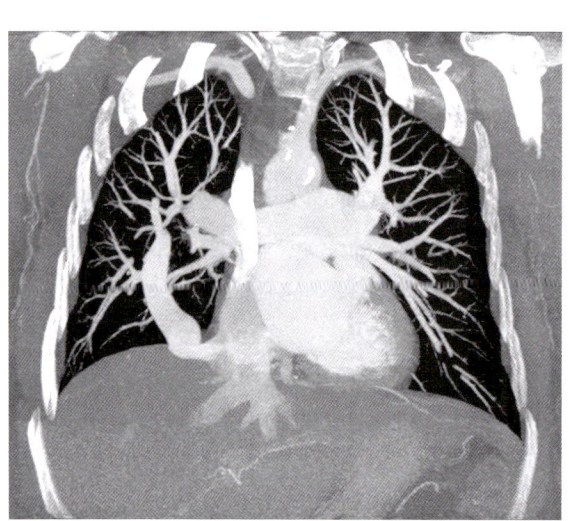
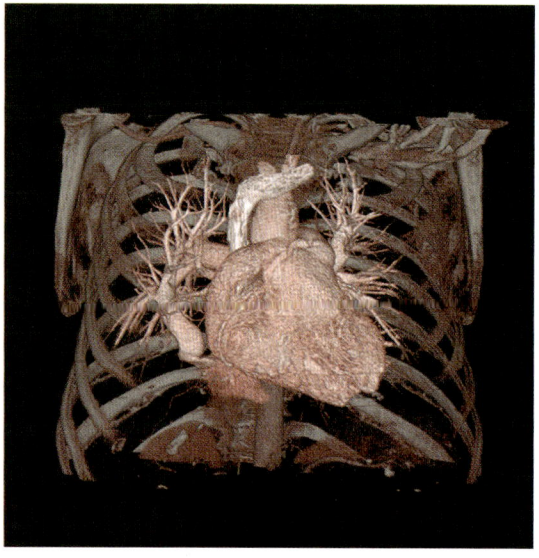

A. Left to right
B. Right to left
C. No shunt

7   A 51-year-old male presents with shortness of breath. What is the diagnosis?

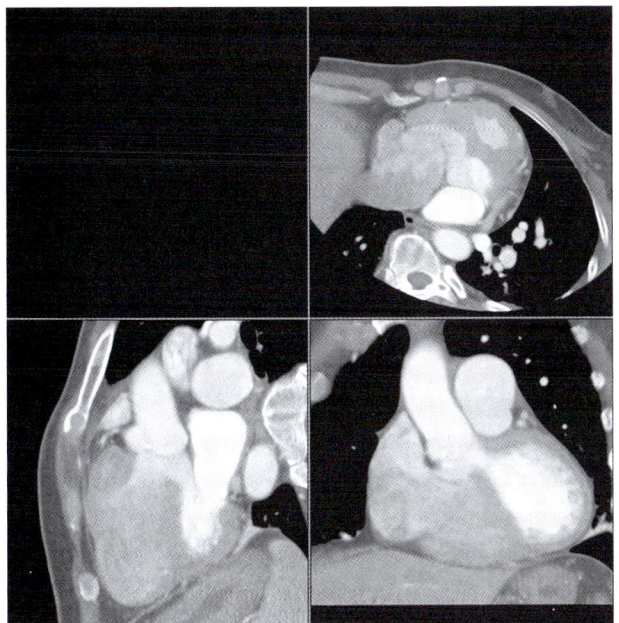
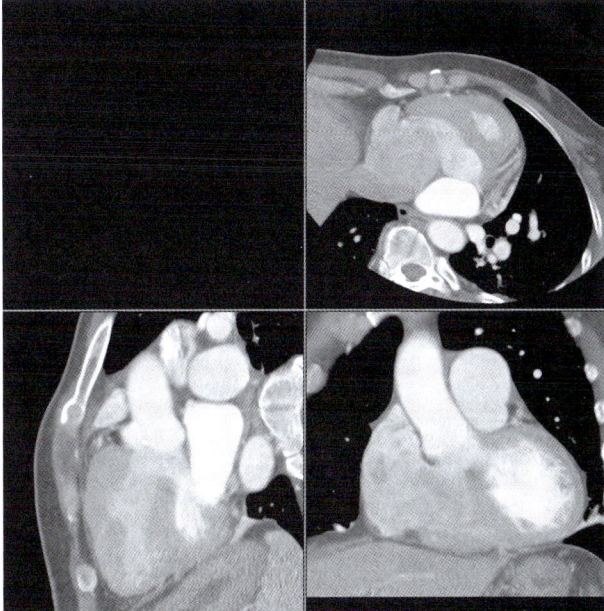
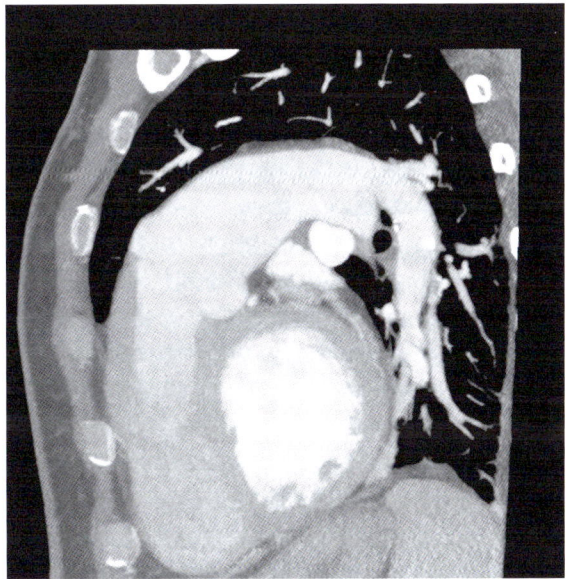

A. Muscular ventricular septal defect without Eisenmenger syndrome
B. Muscular ventricular septal defect with Eisenmenger syndrome
C. Membranous ventricular septal defect without Eisenmenger syndrome
D. Membranous ventricular septal defect with Eisenmenger syndrome

8a A 19-year-old female presents with chest pain. Where is the abnormality?

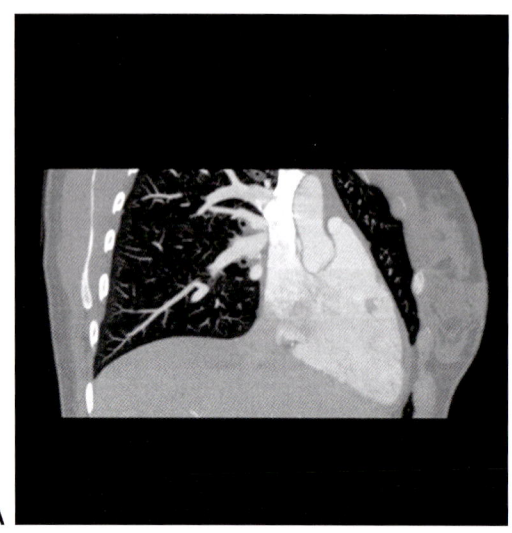
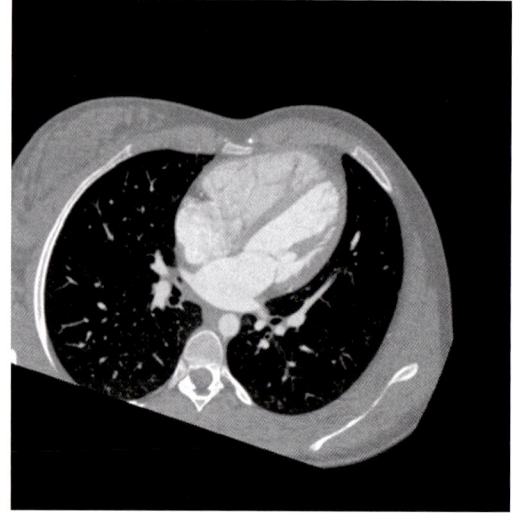

A. Left atrium
B. Aorta
C. Pulmonary vein
D. Left ventricle

8b A cardiac catheterization was subsequently performed. The Qp/Qs was determined to be 2.1. The Patient became symptomatic and developed atrial fibrillation. What is the best treatment?

A. Stent
B. Surgical repair
C. Medical treatment
D. Device closure

9a An 86-year-old female presents with shortness of breath. Where is the abnormality?

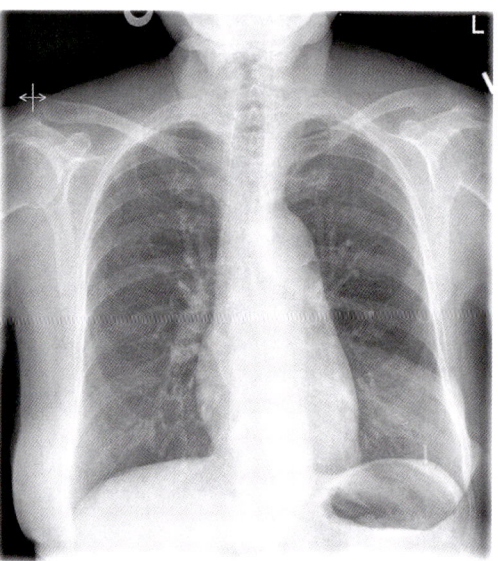

A. Aorta
B. Main pulmonary trunk
C. Left atrium
D. No abnormality

9b What type of shunt is this?

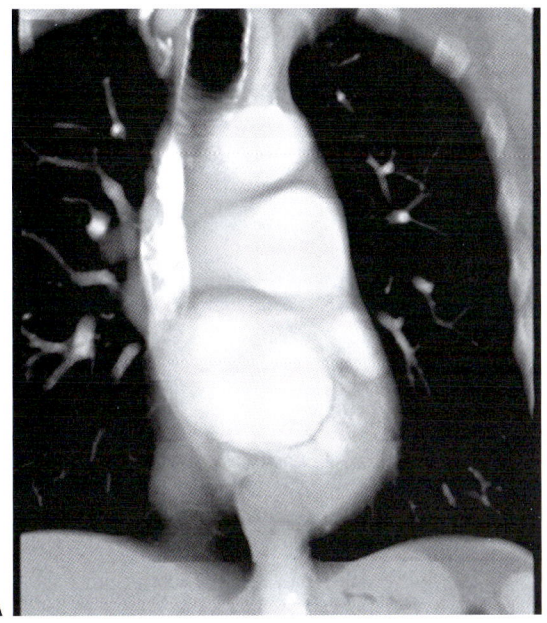
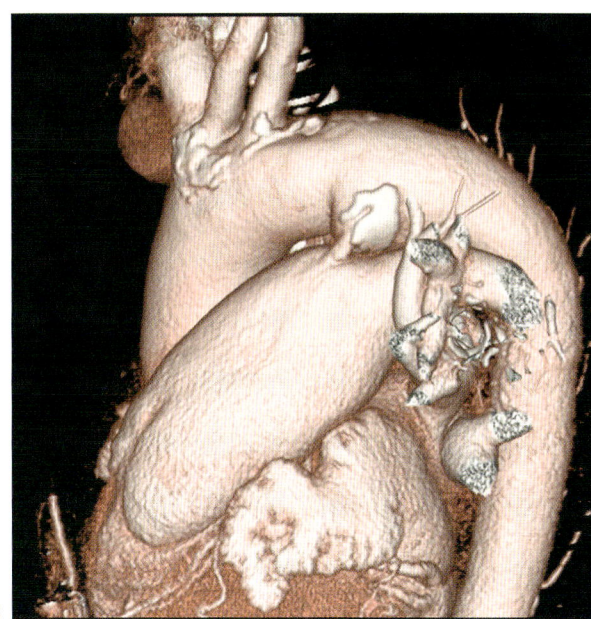

A. Left-to-left shunt
B. Right-to-left shunt
C. Left-to-right shunt
D. Right-to-right shunt
E. Mixed shunt

10a A 6-year-boy has a history of congenital heart disease. Which is true regarding these images?

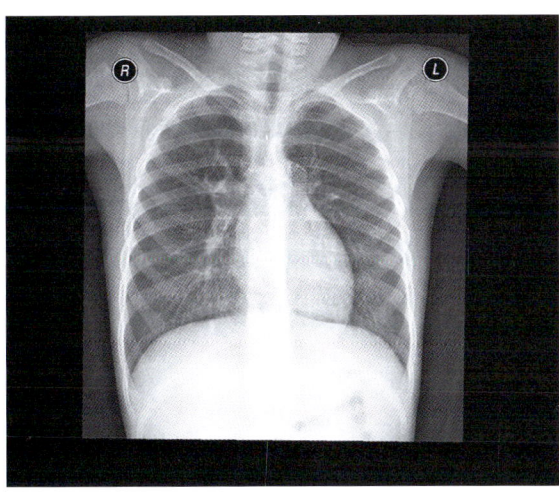
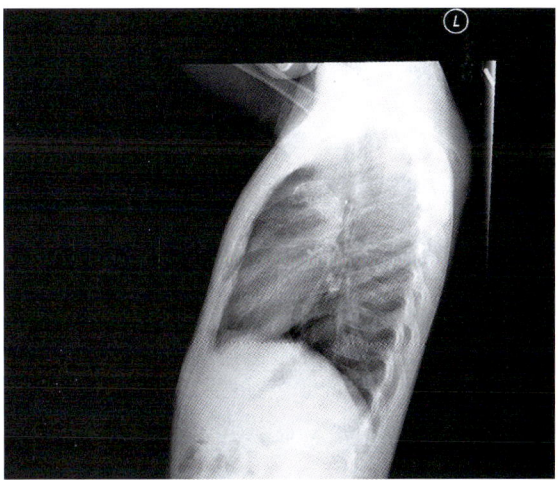

A. Aortic stent is in place.
B. Pulmonary artery stent is in place.
C. Pulmonary vein stent is in place.
D. Left SVC stent is in place.

10b What type of surgery did the patient have?

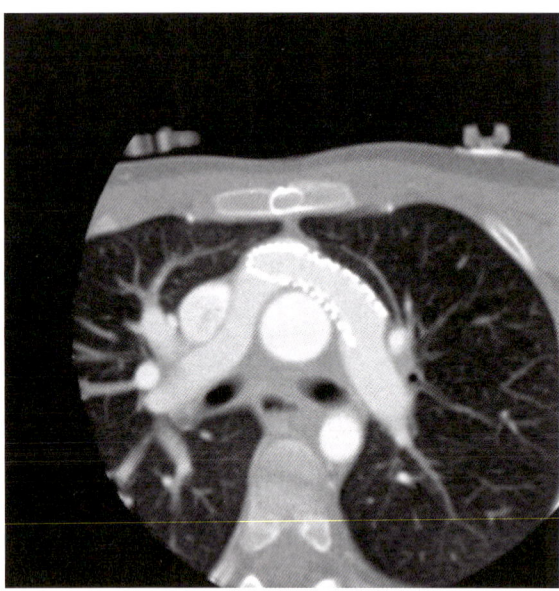
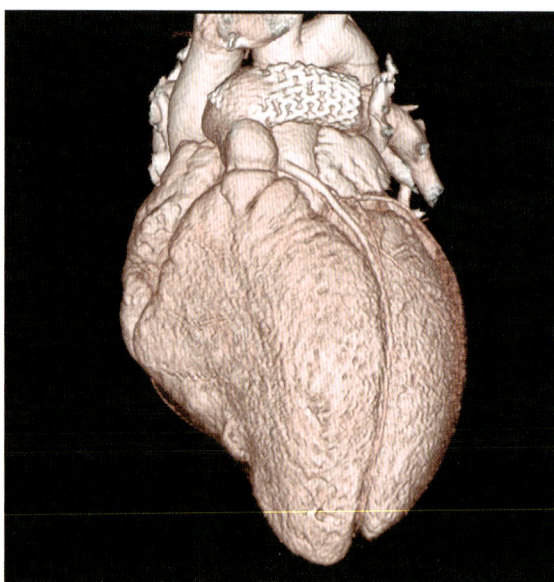

A. Arterial switch
B. Ross procedure
C. Mustard baffle
D. Fontan procedure

11a A 56-year-old female presents with shortness of breath. What is commonly associated with this condition?

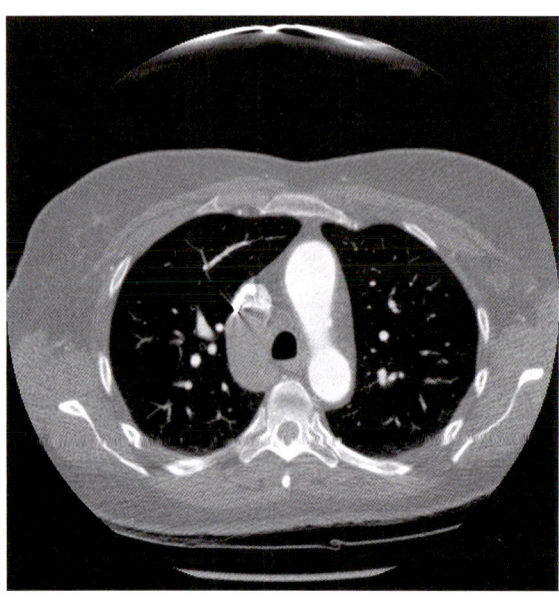
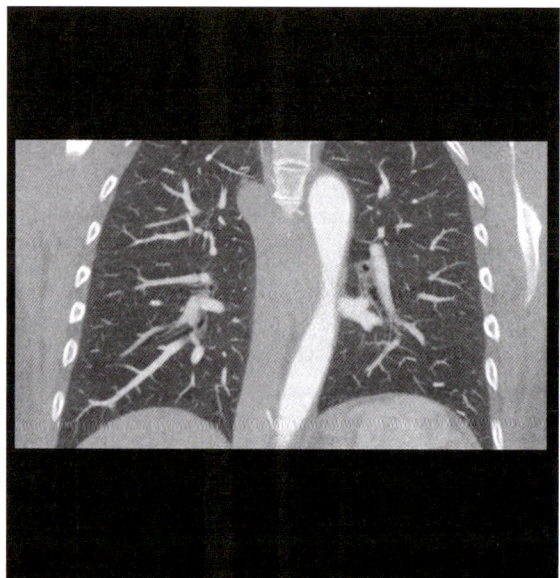

A. Polysplenia
B. Asplenia
C. Bicuspid aortic valve
D. Unicuspid aortic valve

11b This is the identical patient from 11a. What underlying condition does she have?

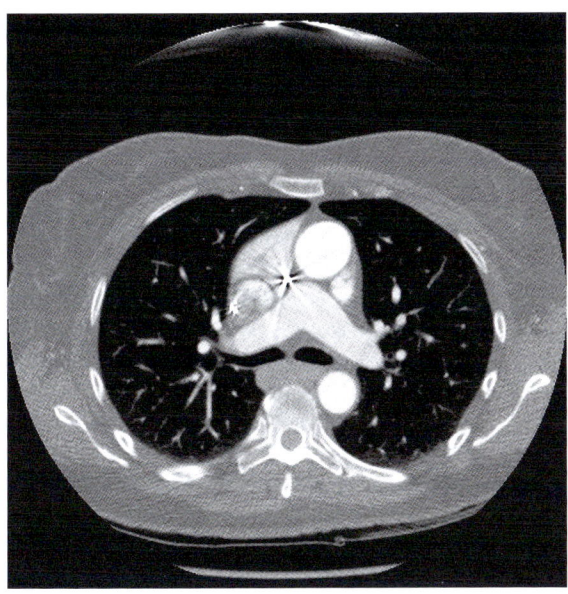
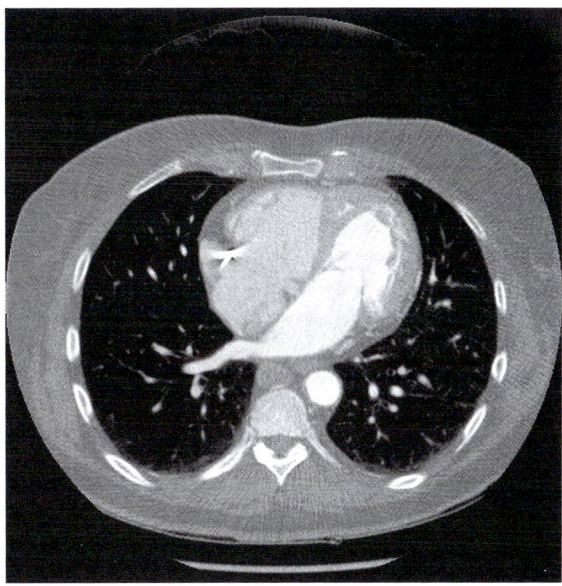

A. Dextrotransposition of the great arteries (D-TGA)
B. Levotransposition of the great arteries (L-TGA)
C. Truncus arteriosus
D. Normal anatomy

11c This patient also has this abnormality. What should be done?

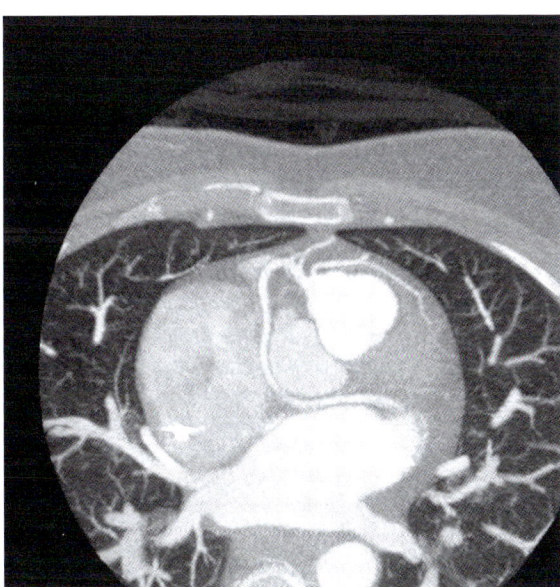

A. Surgical correction
B. No treatment
C. No contact sports
D. ICD placement

12 A 36-year-old female with congenital heart disease. What procedure did she have?

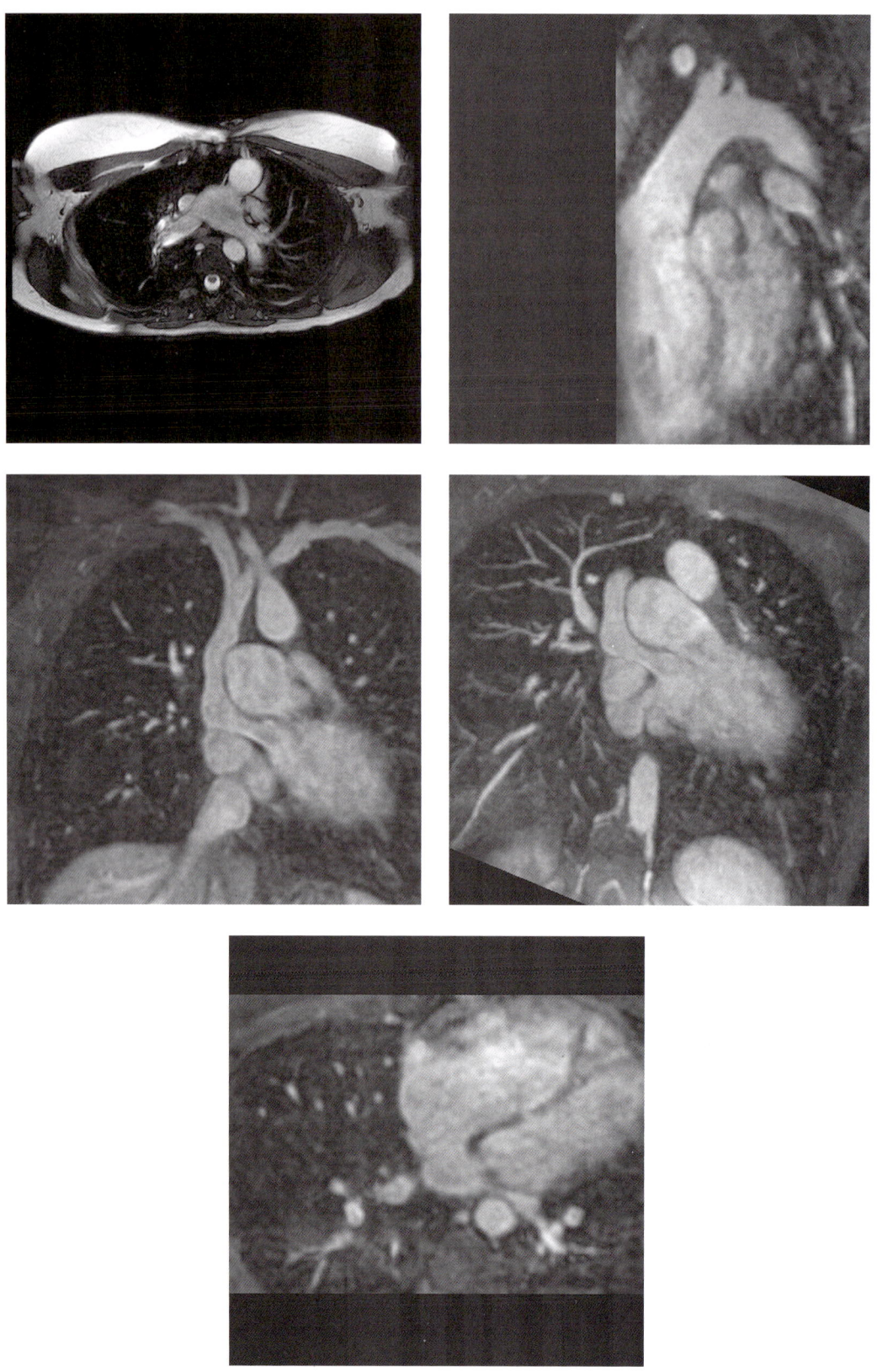

A. Tetralogy of Fallot repair
B. Mustard/Senning procedure
C. Jatene arterial switch
D. Rastelli procedure

13 In truncus arteriosus, that is the most common morphology of the truncal valve?
    A. Unicuspid
    B. Bicuspid
    C. Tricuspid
    D. Quadricuspid

14a What type of aortic abnormality is most associated with this condition?

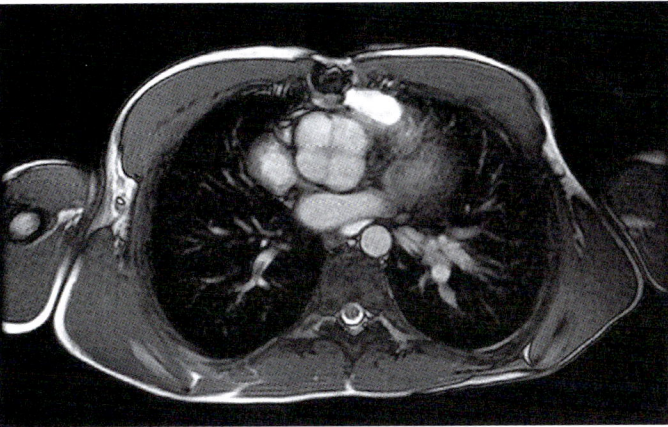

    A. Aortic insufficiency
    B. Aortic stenosis
    C. Aortic coarctation
    D. Aortic aneurysm

14b Which congenital heart disease is most associated with this abnormality?
    A. Tetralogy of Fallot
    B. Truncus arteriosus
    C. Dextrotransposition of the great vessels
    D. Levotransposition of the great vessels

15 This patient also has subaortic stenosis. What other abnormality should you also look for to exclude Shone complex/syndrome?

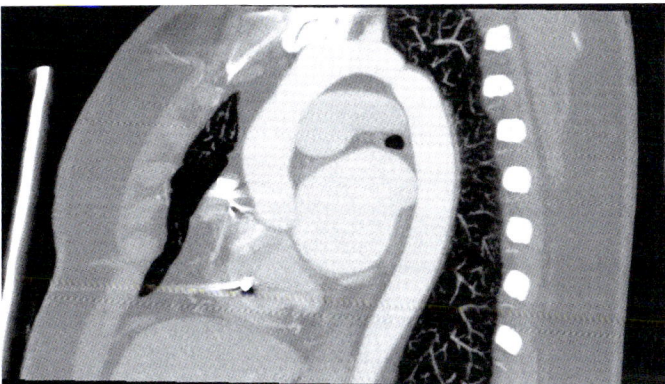

    A. Parachute mitral valve
    B. Bicuspid aortic valve
    C. Sex chromosomal abnormality (XO)
    D. Cor triatriatum

16 What valves are switched in Ross procedure?

　A. Mitral to tricuspid
　B. Aortic to pulmonic
　C. Pulmonic to aortic
　D. Mitral to pulmonic

17 A 12-year-old boy presents with chest pain. What is the best next step?

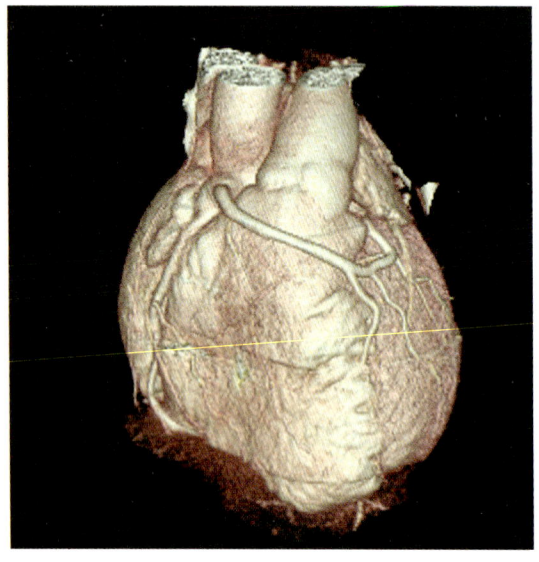
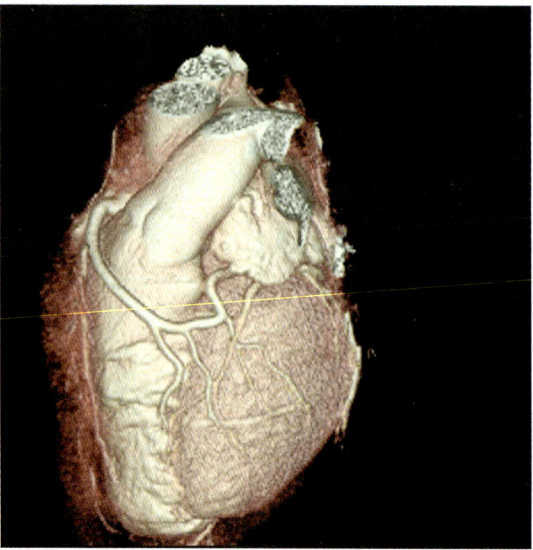

　A. Surgery given symptoms
　B. ICD to prevent sudden cardiac death
　C. No treatment is necessary.
　D. Follow-up CT in 1 year

18 Which one of the following is most associated with congenital heart disease?

　A. Situs solitus
　B. Situs inversus
　C. Situs ambiguous

19 What type of shunt is this?

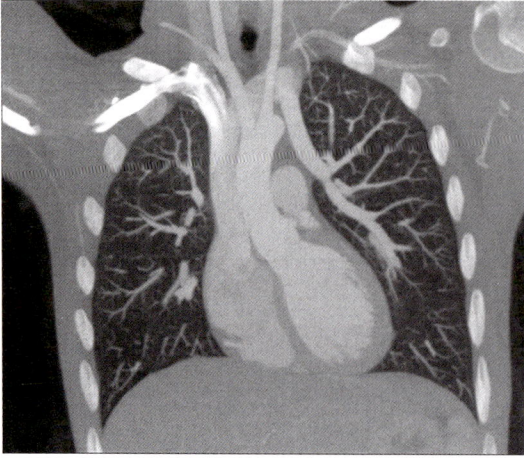

　A. Left to right
　B. Right to left
　C. Mixed

20 A 62-year-old male with arrhythmia. Where is the vein draining into?

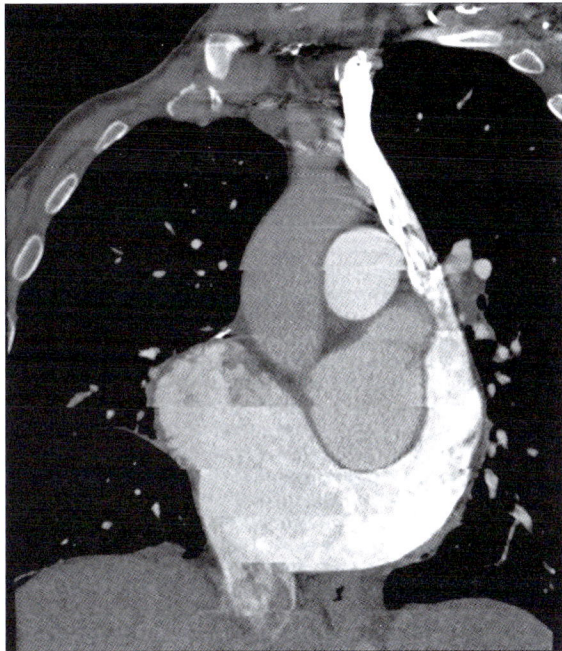

   A. Left atrium
   B. Left ventricle
   C. Coronary sinus
   D. IVC

21 Which commissures are fused?

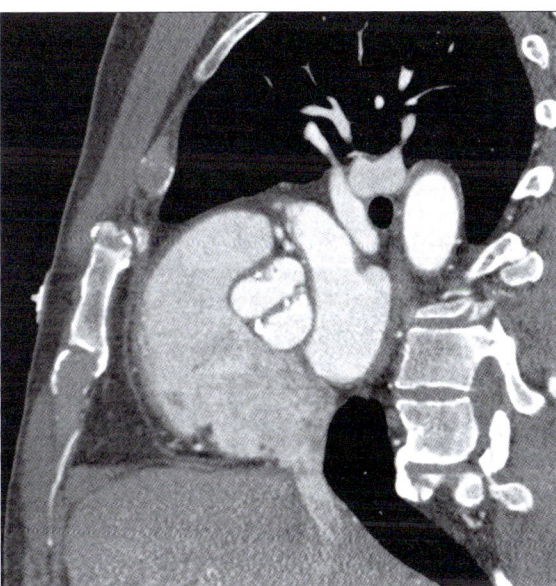

   A. Left and noncoronary sinus
   B. Noncoronary and right coronary sinus
   C. Right and left coronary sinus

22 Mitral valve clefts are associated with
   A. Primum atrial septal defect
   B. Secundum atrial septal defect
   C. Sinus venosus atrial septal defect
   D. Unroofed coronary sinus atrial septal defect

23 What tricuspid valvular abnormality is seen?

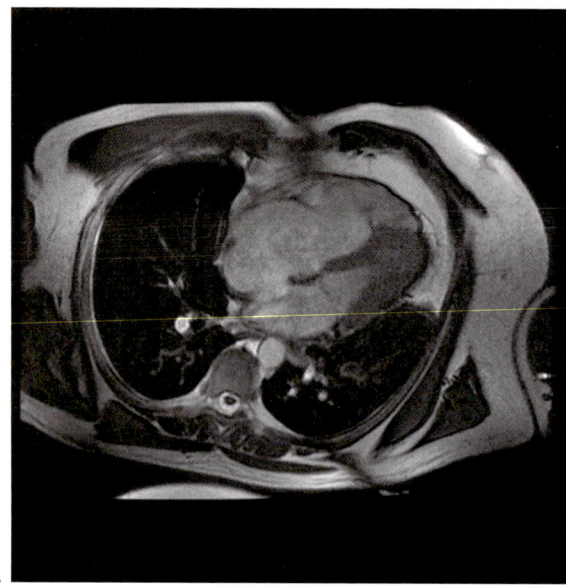

A

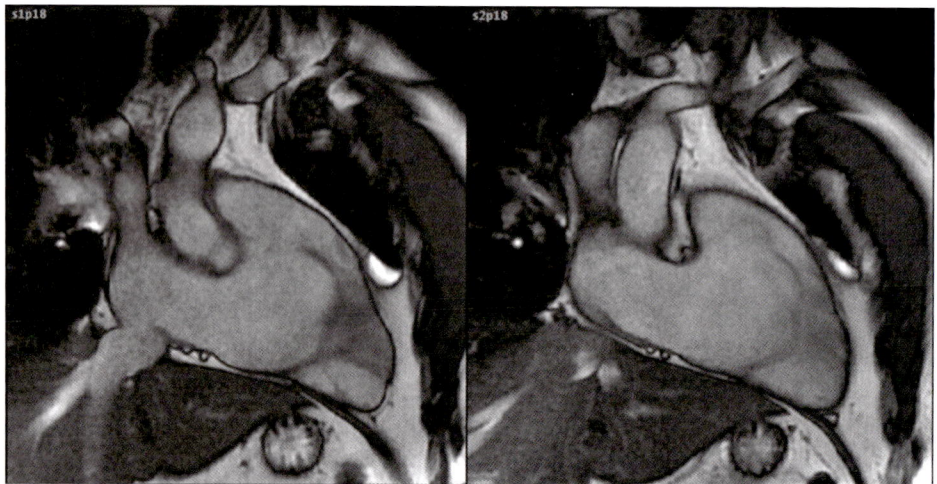

B

   A. Anteriorly displaced septal leaflets
   B. Sail-like anterior leaflet
   C. Fusion of the anterior and septal leaflets
   D. Hockey stick of the anterior leaflet

24 What is the relationship of the bronchi to the pulmonary arteries?

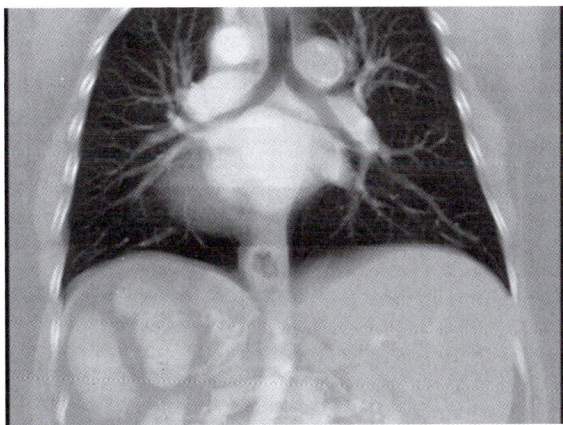

A. Right eparterial, left hyparterial
B. Right hyparterial, left eparterial
C. Right eparterial, left eparterial
D. Right hyparterial, left hyparterial

25a For each image below, select the most likely description of findings. Each option may be used once, more than once, or not at all.

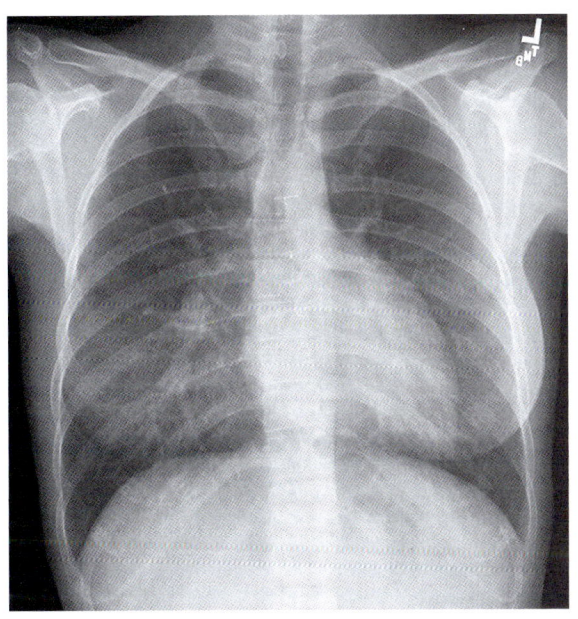
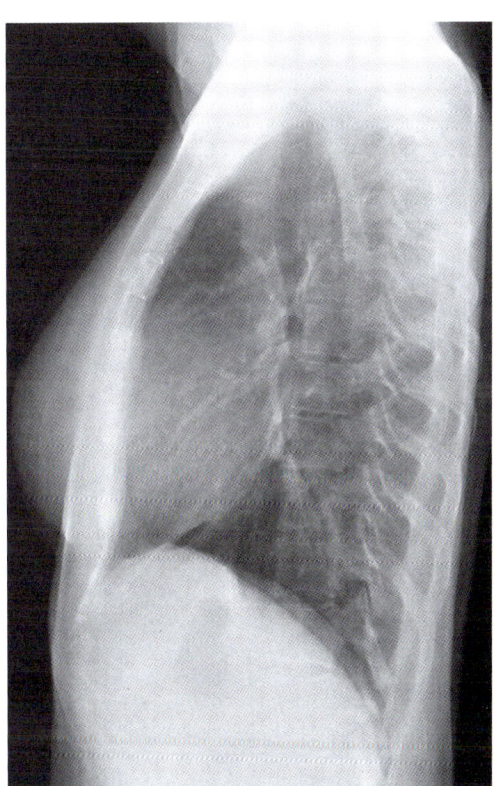

A. Egg-on-a-string sign
B. Boot-shaped heart
C. Boxed-shaped heart
D. Figure of three
E. Scimitar sign
F. Snowman sign

25b For each image below, select the most likely description of findings. Each option may be used once, more than once, or not at all.

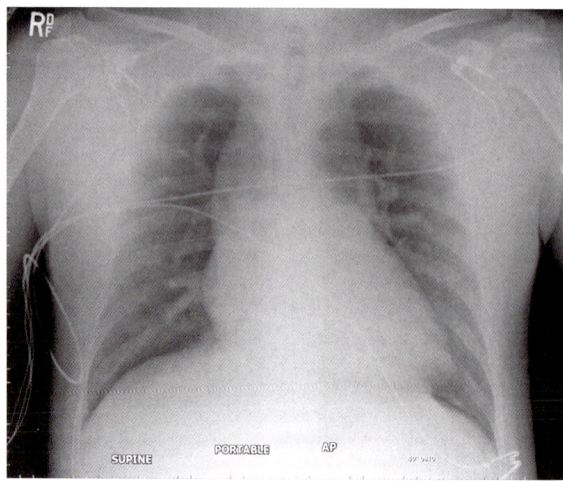

A. Egg-on-a-string sign
B. Boot-shaped heart
C. Box-shaped heart
D. Figure of three
E. Scimitar sign
F. Snowman sign

26 A 75-year-old male undergoes a Cardiac CTA. What is the best next step?

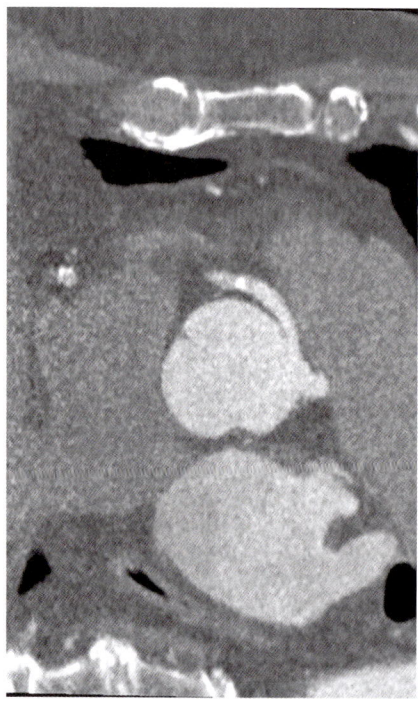

A. Surgical correction
B. ICD placement
C. No treatment
D. Stress test

27 Common complications after this procedure include baffle obstruction, baffle leak, arrhythmias, and which of the following?

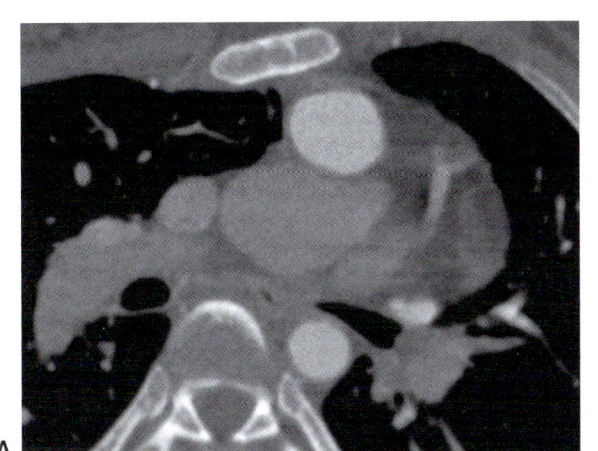
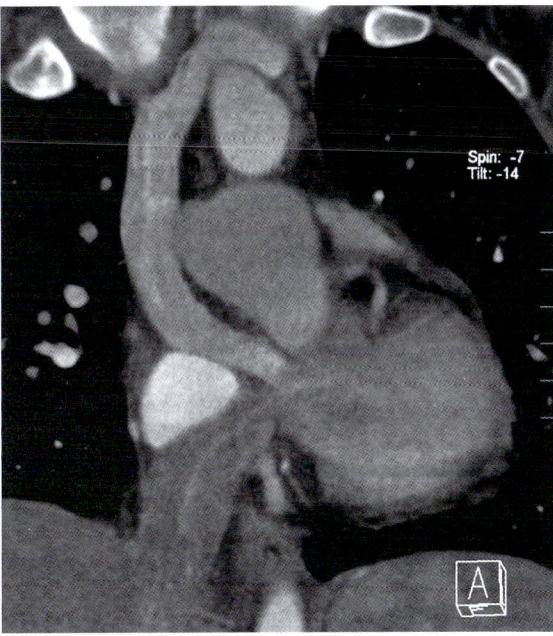
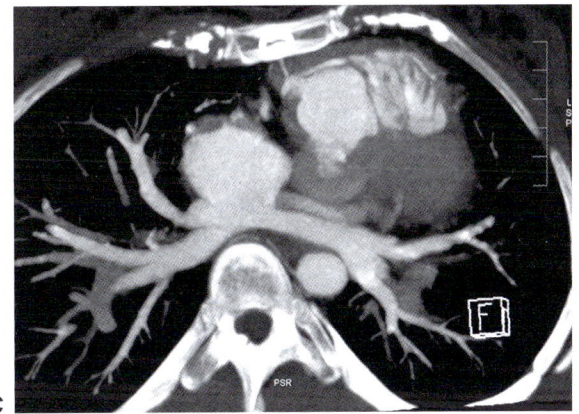

A. Left ventricular dysfunction
B. Right ventricular dysfunction
C. Mitral regurgitation
D. Mitral stenosis

28 What is the diagnosis?

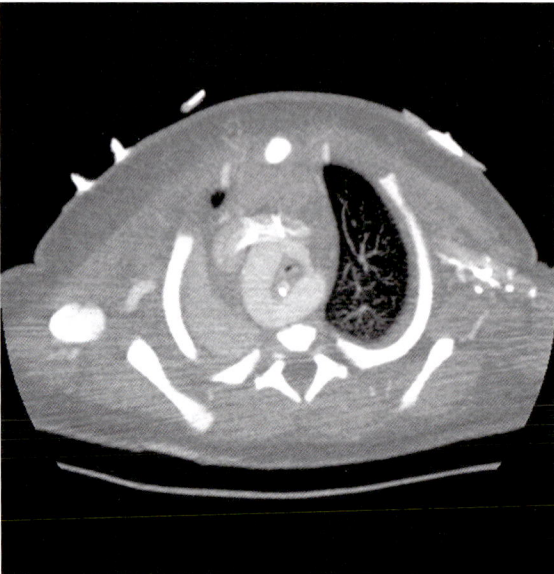

A. Right arch with aberrant left subclavian artery
B. Right arch with mirror image branching
C. Double aortic arch with dominant right arch
D. Double aortic arch with dominant left arch

29 Where is the most common location of rupture for this condition?

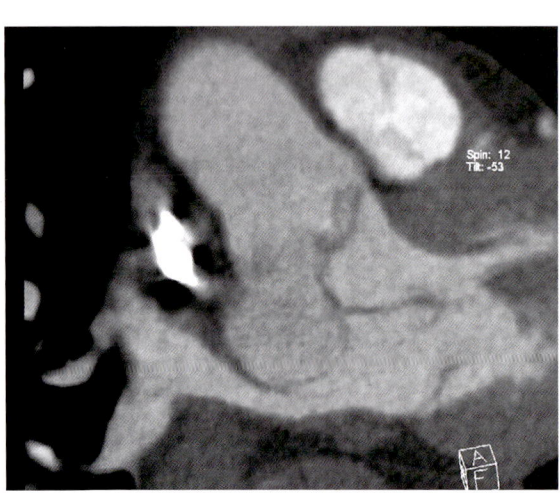 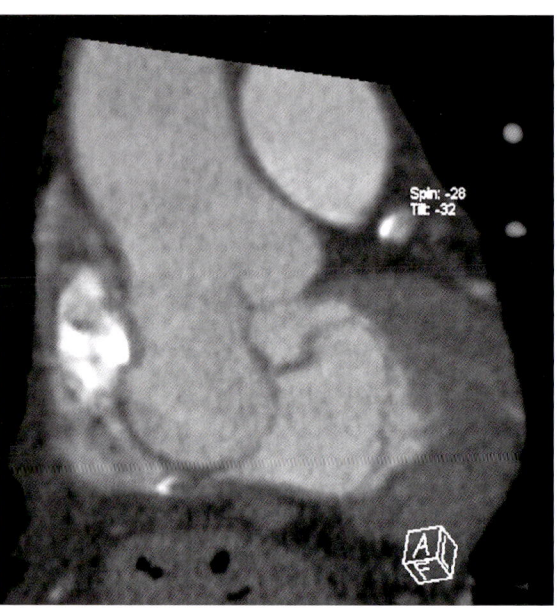

A. Right atrium
B. Right ventricle
C. Left atrium
D. Left ventricle

30 What is the best overall diagnosis?

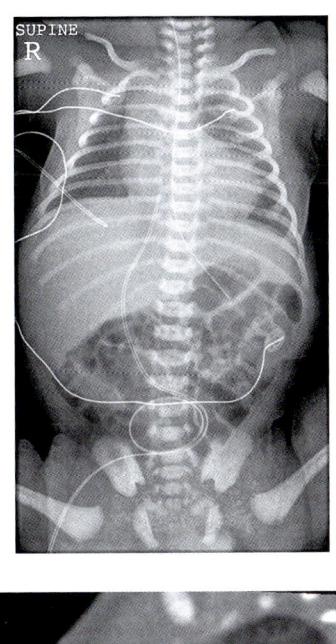
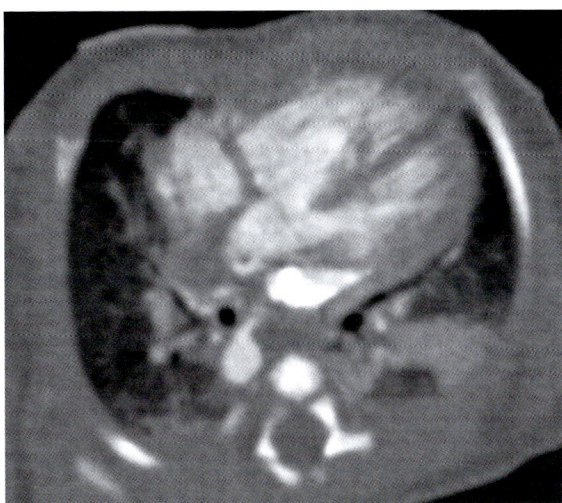
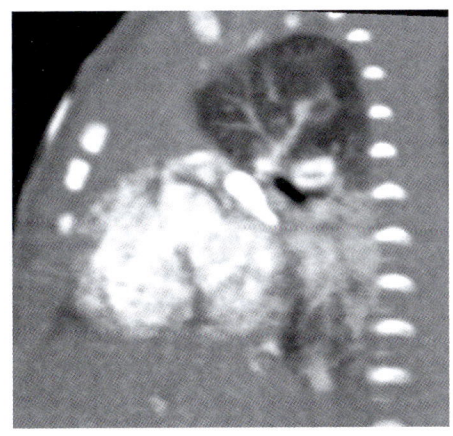
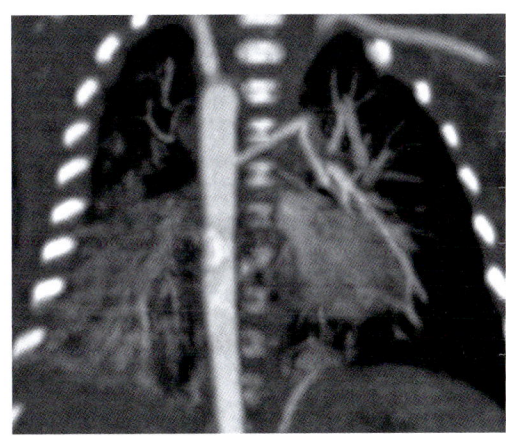
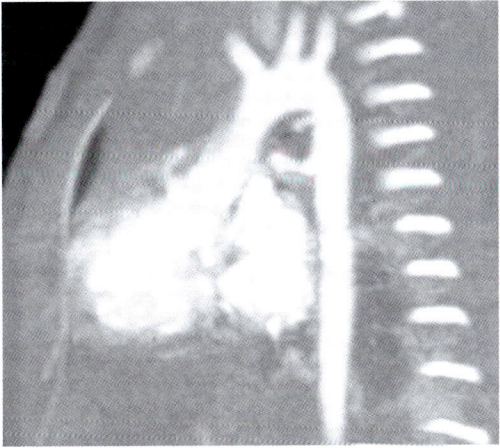

A. Tetralogy of Fallot (overriding aorta, ventricular septal defect, right ventricular hypertrophy, right ventricular outflow obstruction)
B. Pulmonary atresia with ventricular septal defect (PA-VSD), multiple aortopulmonary collateral arteries (MAPCAs)
C. Right arch with aberrant left subclavian artery, bronchial artery hypertrophy, ventricular septal defect
D. Right arch with mirror image branching, bronchial artery hypertrophy, ventricular septal defect

31 An 18-year-old male presents with chest pain. Which of the following is the best diagnosis?

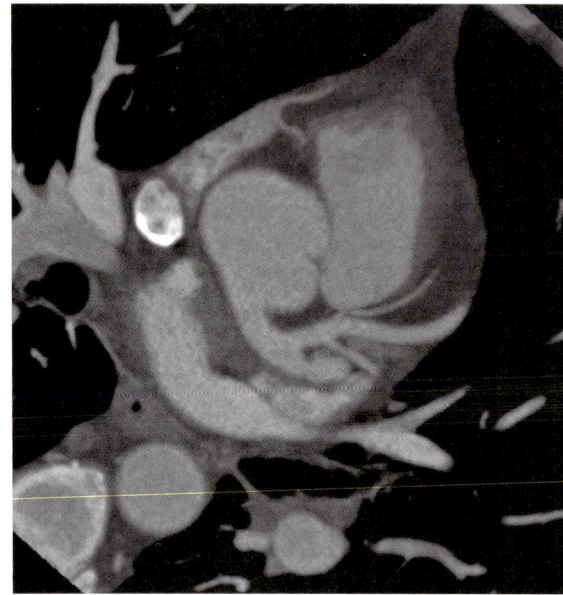
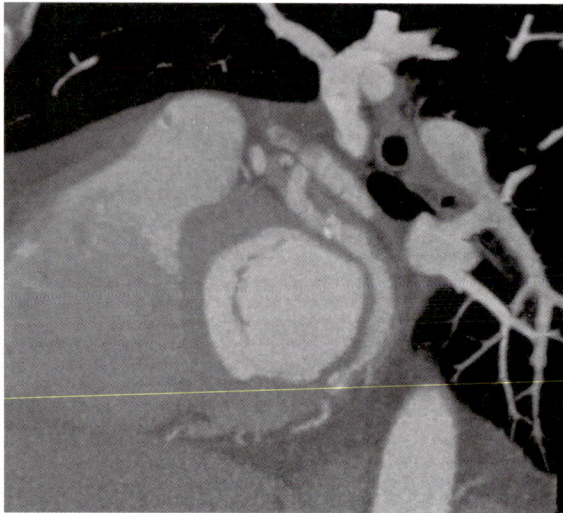
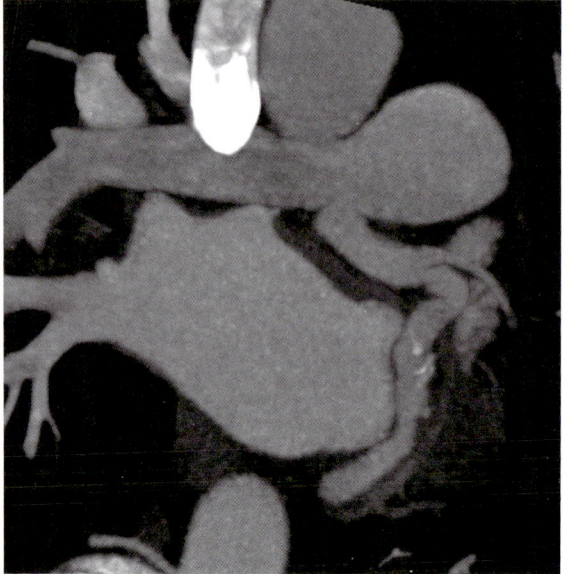

A. Normal coronary arteries post nitroglycerin
B. Premature atherosclerosis
C. Kawasaki disease
D. Coronary fistula

ANSWERS AND EXPLANATIONS

1a Answer C. Frontal and lateral chest radiographs demonstrate an enlarged pulmonary artery trunk and increased vascular flow. This is suggestive of underlying left to right shunting which can be caused by an atrial septal defect. Both aortic and mitral stenosis should not give an enlarged pulmonary artery trunk nor increased vascular flow. The findings are not normal given the enlarged pulmonary trunk and increased pulmonary flow. Ebstein anomaly would give a markedly enlarged right heart (e.g., boxed-shaped heart).

References: Baron MG, Book WM. Congenital heart disease in the adult: 2004. *Radiol Clin North Am* 2004;42(3):675–690, vii. Review.

Steiner RM, Gross GW, Flicker S, et al. Congenital heart disease in the adult patient: the value of plain film chest radiology. *J Thorac Imaging* 1995;10(1):1–25. Review.

1b Answer C. An Amplatzer septal occluder is now seen on the chest radiograph. Indications for percutaneous atrial septal defect (ASD) closure include hemodynamically significant ASD (such as Qp/Qs > 2) and paradoxical emboli. It is not indicated in patients with small secundum ASD of no hemodynamic significance. It is also not indicated in septum primum, sinus venosus, and unroofed coronary sinus type of ASDs. Atrial fibrillation is not a contraindication to ASD closure. Adequate rims are required for the placement of the Amplatzer device. Only venous access is needed to deploy the device.

References: Kazmouz S, Kenny D, Cao QL, et al. Transcatheter closure of secundum atrial septal defects. *J Invasive Cardiol* 2013;25(5):257–264. Review.

Lee EY, Siegel MJ, Chu CM, et al. Amplatzer atrial septal defect occluder for pediatric patients: radiographic appearance. *Radiology* 2004;233(2):471–476.

1c Answer D. Complications of ASD occlusion include atrial fibrillation, SVT, heart block, device malposition, embolization, and erosion. The most common immediate complication is device embolization and malpositioning. Atrial fibrillation and heart block also typically occur early. Cardiac erosion is a long-term complication that can be difficult to detect.

References: Crawford GB, Brindis RG, Krucoff MW, et al. Percutaneous atrial septal occluder devices and cardiac erosion: a review of the literature. *Catheter Cardiovasc Interv* 2012;80(2):157–167. doi: 10.1002/ccd.24347. Epub 2012 May 2. Review.

Lee T, Tsai IC, Fu YC, et al. MDCT evaluation after closure of atrial septal defect with an Amplatzer septal occluder. *AJR Am J Roentgenol* 2007;188(5):W431–W439. PubMed PMID: 17449739.

2 Answer B. This is an inferior type of sinus venosus atrial septal defect (ASD) associated with anomalous pulmonary venous return of the right inferior pulmonary vein. The treatment is surgical. While secundum ASD can potentially be treated endovascularly with closure devices, sinus venosus ASD cannot be treated endovascularly due to the lack of rims for the device to attach to.

Reference: Vyas HV, Greenberg SB, Krishnamurthy R. MR imaging and CT evaluation of congenital pulmonary vein abnormalities in neonates and infants. *Radiographics* 2012;32(1):87–98. doi: 10.1148/rg.321105764. PubMed PMID: 22236895.

3a Answer C. Images demonstrate unroofed coronary sinus (note the connection between the left and right atrium and the coronary sinus). In this case, the shunt appears small without evidence of left heart enlargement. Given the small shunt, no treatment is required. Surgical treatment would be considered if there is a significant shunt (Qp/Qs > 2). There is no role for catheter-based closure in unroofed coronary sinus.

3b **Answer D.** Unroofed coronary sinus is associated with left-sided SVC. Azygous continuation of the IVC is associated with polysplenia and many other congenital heart diseases. Coarctation is classically associated with bicuspid aortic valve. Anomalous right pulmonary venous return can be associated with sinus venosus atrial septal defects.

Reference: Shah SS, Teague SD, Lu JC, et al. Imaging of the coronary sinus: normal anatomy and congenital abnormalities. *Radiographics* 2012;32(4):991-1008. doi: 10.1148/rg.324105220. PubMed PMID: 22786990.

4 **Answer C.** There are 4 types of ASD: sinus venosus, ostium secundum, ostium primum, and unroofed coronary sinus.

Reference: Rojas CA, El-Sherief A, Medina HM, et al. Embryology and developmental defects of the interatrial septum. *AJR Am J Roentgenol* 2010;195(5):1100-1104. doi: 10.2214/AJR.10.4277. Review. PubMed PMID: 20966313.

5 **Answer A.** Muscular VSD can undergo spontaneous closure while membranous VSD will not close spontaneously. Endocarditis prophylaxis is necessary for both muscular and membranous VSDs.

Reference: Minette MS, Sahn DJ. Ventricular septal defects. *Circulation* 2006;114(20):2190-2197. Review. Erratum in: *Circulation* 2007;115(7):e205.

6a **Answer C.** PA and lateral chest radiographs show an abnormal vertical linear opacity along the right lower lung. On the lateral view, it appears to course inferiorly toward the IVC region. This is consistent with the "scimitar sign," which is suggestive of anomalous pulmonary venous return (scimitar vein). The differential also includes anomalous single pulmonary vein, which would drain normally into the left atrium. These conditions have different treatments (surgical for scimitar, no treatment for anomalous single pulmonary vein). The best next step would be to define the anatomy with a CTA chest. Biopsy would not be helpful and may even be dangerous. CT without IV contrast would not define the vascular anatomy well. VQ scan would not clarify what the tubular structure is. No further imaging would also not be helpful given we need to further define the abnormality.

References: Ferguson EC, Krishnamurthy R, Oldham SA. Classic imaging signs of congenital cardiovascular abnormalities. *Radiographics* 2007;27(5):1323-1334. Review. PubMed PMID: 17848694.

Nazarian J, Kanne JP, Rajiah P. Scimitar sign. *J Thorac Imaging* 2013;28(4):W61.

6b **Answer A.** A scimitar vein is draining into the IVC. This is a type of anomalous pulmonary venous return and a left to right shunt (remember that the pulmonary veins carry oxygenated blood so it is part of the left circulation).

In classic scimitar syndrome, there is anomalous right pulmonary vein, hypoplasia of the right lung along with pulmonary artery hypoplasia, dextrocardia, and systemic arterial supply to the lungs. These features are not always present on all patients. Atrial septal defect (ASD) is not part of the syndrome but can sometimes occur concurrently. If patient is symptomatic due to significant shunting, surgical correction to redirect the vein into the left atrium can be performed.

References: Ferguson EC, Krishnamurthy R, Oldham SA. Classic imaging signs of congenital cardiovascular abnormalities. *Radiographics* 2007;27(5):1323-1334. Review. PubMed PMID: 17848694.

Nazarian J, Kanne JP, Rajiah P. Scimitar sign. *J Thorac Imaging* 2013;28(4):W61.

7 **Answer D.** Images show a membranous VSD with evidence of both left to right and right to left shunting (note the mixing of the contrast material at the site of ventricular septal defect). This is consistent with Eisenmenger syndrome with suprasystemic right heart pressures causing right to left shunting. Note the marked right ventricular hypertrophy from the pulmonary hypertension due to long-standing shunt. Muscular ventricular septal defects are located along the muscular septum, which is not shown here.

Reference: Peña E, Dennie C, Veinot J, et al. Pulmonary hypertension: how the radiologist can help. *Radiographics* 2012;32(1):9-32. doi: 10.1148/rg.321105232. PubMed PMID: 22236891.

8a Answer C. Image A shows anomalous pulmonary venous return with right superior pulmonary vein (RSPV) returning to SVC. Note the right heart appears enlarged (Image B). Left atrium and ventricle appear normal. Visualized ascending aorta also appears normal.

Reference: Kafka H, Mohiaddin RH. Cardiac MRI and pulmonary MR angiography of sinus venosus defect and partial anomalous pulmonary venous connection in cause of right undiagnosed ventricular enlargement. *AJR Am J Roentgenol* 2009;192(1):259-266. doi: 10.2214/AJR.07.3430. PubMed PMID: 19098208.

8b Answer B. The images show anomalous pulmonary venous return with the right superior pulmonary vein (RSPV) entering to the SVC. There is significant shunting as evidenced by Qp/Qs of 2.1 and right heart enlargement. In addition, the presence of atrial fibrillation suggests significant volume overloading and chamber remodeling. The best treatment therefore is surgery. Note there is an association between right partial anomalous pulmonary venous return and sinus venosus atrial septal defects. Device closure is not feasible since the anomalous vein needs to be redirected to the left atrium. Medical treatment is not advisable given the significant shunting (Qp/Qs > 1.5) and development of atrial fibrillation. Stenting would not fix this problem.

References: Dillman JR, Yarram SG, Hernandez RJ. Imaging of pulmonary venous developmental anomalies. *AJR Am J Roentgenol* 2009;192(5):1272-1285. doi: 10.2214/AJR.08.1526. Review. PubMed PMID: 19380552.

Kafka H, Mohiaddin RH. Cardiac MRI and pulmonary MR angiography of sinus venosus defect and partial anomalous pulmonary venous connection in cause of right undiagnosed ventricular enlargement. *AJR Am J Roentgenol* 2009;192(1):259-266. doi: 10.2214/AJR.07.3430. PubMed PMID: 19098208.

9a Answer B. Frontal CXR shows an enlarged pulmonary trunk. The left mediastinal contour is composed of, starting superiorly, the left subclavian artery, left arch, main pulmonary trunk, left atrial appendage (if enlarged), and left ventricle. In this case, the contour below the arch is enlarged suggesting enlarged pulmonary trunk. Aortic enlargement can occur throughout its course so can involve the ascending aorta, arch, or descending aorta. Left atrial enlargement can be seen with enlarged left atrial appendage contour, or in extreme left atrial enlargement, a double contour is seen along the right heart border (double density sign). There can also be splaying of the carina.

Reference: Ferguson EC, Krishnamurthy R, Oldham SA. Classic imaging signs of congenital cardiovascular abnormalities. *Radiographics* 2007;27(5):1323-1334. Review. PubMed PMID: 17848694.

9b Answer C. Coronal reformat shows enlarged PA contour (Image A). 3D volume rendered images show a PDA (image B). Patent ductus arteriosus is a type of left to right shunt. However, it does not involve the right heart since the connection is between the aorta and pulmonary artery (so the right heart will not be enlarged). It is associated with rubella infection during pregnancy. It can lead to Eisenmenger syndrome in long-standing shunts.

References: Goitein O, Fuhrman CR, Lacomis JM. Incidental finding on MDCT of patent ductus arteriosus: use of CT and MRI to assess clinical importance. *AJR Am J Roentgenol* 2005;184(6):1924-1931. PubMed PMID: 15908555.

Morgan-Hughes GJ, Marshall AJ, Roobottom C. Morphologic assessment of patent ductus arteriosus in adults using retrospectively ECG-gated multidetector CT. *AJR Am J Roentgenol* 2003;181(3): 749-754. PubMed PMID: 12933475.

Schneider DJ, Moore JW. Patent ductus arteriosus. *Circulation* 2006;114(17):1873-1882.

10a Answer B. Frontal and lateral chest radiographs show a narrowed mediastinum with a left pulmonary artery stent. The stent is positioned anteriorly on the lateral view. Coarctation stents would be more superior and posterior in location along the course of the aorta. Pulmonary vein stents would be near the left atrium at a inferior and posterior position. Left SVC stent would be vertical in nature.

10b Answer A. The pulmonary artery draping over the aorta is a pathognomonic appearance of an arterial switch used to correct underlying dextrotransposition of the great arteries (d-TGA). In this case, the patient had the arterial switch with subsequent left pulmonary stenosis. This was treated with a stent.

In a Ross procedure, the native pulmonary valve is switched to the aortic position and a prosthetic pulmonic valve is put in place. Mustard baffle is used to treat dextrotransposition of the great arteries; the systemic and pulmonary venous returns are redirected via baffles to correct for the great vessel switch. In the Fontan procedure, the systemic venous return is connected into the pulmonary arteries directly, bypassing the heart; this is typically used in patients with single ventricular physiology.

Reference: Spevak PJ, Johnson PT, Fishman EK. Surgically corrected congenital heart disease: utility of 64-MDCT. *AJR Am J Roentgenol* 2008;191(3):854-861. doi: 10.2214/AJR.07.2889. Review. PubMed PMID: 18716119.

11a Answer A. The images show enlarged azygos vein seen in interrupted IVC with azygos continuation. This condition is associated with polysplenia. Bicuspid aortic valve is associated with coarctation but also aortic aneurysm from bicuspid aortopathy. Unicuspid aortic valve is associated with aortic stenosis.

Reference: Applegate KE, Goske MJ, Pierce G, et al. Situs revisited: imaging of the heterotaxy syndrome. *Radiographics* 1999;19(4):837-852; discussion 853-854. Review. PubMed PMID: 10464794.

11b Answer B. The Images show transposition of the vessels with the aorta arising anterior to the pulmonary artery. This is a levo-type of transposition of the great arteries (l-TGA) with ventricular inversion (morphologic RV on the left side, morphologic LV on the right side). With the ventricles switched in position, there is a transposition of the great arteries. However, the flow circuit is normal with the systemic blood going into the pulmonary artery and oxygenated pulmonary venous blood to the aorta. The systemic ventricle on the left is a morphologic right ventricle containing the tricuspid valve. This can cause problems later as the morphologic RV can fail and the tricuspid valve can be leaky. There is also a higher rate of arrhythmia from the systemic RV. As a result, these patients can sometimes present at a young age with already an ICD and valvular replacement.

Reference: Cohen MD, Johnson T, Ramrakhiani S. MRI of surgical repair of transposition of the great vessels. *AJR Am J Roentgenol* 2010;194(1):250-260. doi: 10.2214/AJR.09.3045. Review. PubMed PMID: 20028930.

11c Answer B. A retroaortic left circumflex artery is seen. This is a benign coronary anomaly and no surgery is necessary. There is no need for activity restriction or ICD placement.

References: Kim SY, Seo JB, Do KH, et al. Coronary artery anomalies: classification and ECG-gated multi-detector row CT findings with angiographic correlation. *Radiographics* 2006;26(2):317-333; discussion 333-334. Review. PubMed PMID: 16549600.

Shriki JE, Shinbane JS, Rashid MA, et al. Identifying, characterizing, and classifying congenital anomalies of the coronary arteries. *Radiographics*. 2012;32(2):453-468. doi: 10.1148/rg.322115097. Review. PubMed PMID: 22411942.

12 Answer B. There is d-TGA with Mustard/Senning baffle. The great vessels are switched so the procedure switches the inflow to redirect systemic blood to the left ventricle and the pulmonary venous return to the right atrium. Tetralogy repair involves closing the VSD and alleviating the right ventricular outflow tract obstruction. Arterial switch typically show a characteristic draping of the pulmonary artery over the aorta. Rastelli procedure would involve a right ventricular outflow conduit.

References: Cohen MD, Johnson T, Ramrakhiani S. MRI of surgical repair of transposition of the great vessels. *AJR Am J Roentgenol* 2010;194(1):250-260. doi: 10.2214/AJR.09.3045. Review. PubMed PMID: 20028930.

Lu JC, Dorfman AL, Attili AK, et al. Evaluation with cardiovascular MR imaging of baffles and conduits used in palliation or repair of congenital heart disease. *Radiographics* 2012;32(3):E107-E127. doi: 10.1148/rg.323115096. PubMed PMID: 22582368.

13 Answer C. A truncal valve is most often tricuspid, followed by quadricuspid and bicuspid. There is often a ventricular septal defect. Collette and Edwards described 4 types of truncus arteriosus.

Reference: Kimura-Hayama ET, Meléndez G, Mendizábal AL, et al. Uncommon congenital and acquired aortic diseases: role of multidetector CT angiography. *Radiographics* 2010;30(1):79-98. doi: 10.1148/rg.301095061. PubMed PMID: 20083587.

14a Answer A. A quadricuspid aortic valve is most associated with aortic insufficiency. It can also be seen with truncus arteriosus. There is no reported association with aortic stenosis, aortic coarctation, or aortic aneurysm.

14b Answer B. A quadricuspid aortic valve is most often seen with truncus arteriosus.

Reference: Bennett CJ, Maleszewski JJ, Araoz PA. CT and MR imaging of the aortic valve: radiologic-pathologic correlation. *Radiographics* 2012;32(5):1399-1420. doi: 10.1148/rg.325115727. PubMed PMID: 22977027.

15 Answer A. Shone syndrome/complex has four components—supravalvular mitral membrane (SVMM), parachute mitral valve, subaortic stenosis (membranous or muscular), and coarctation of the aorta. Bicuspid aortic valve, coarctation, and sex chromosomal abnormality are associated with Turner syndrome.

Reference: Bittencourt MS, Hulten E, Givertz MM, et al. Multimodality imaging of an adult with Shone complex. *J Cardiovasc Comput Tomogr* 2013;7(1):62-65. doi: 10.1016/j.jcct.2012.10.009. Epub 2012 Dec 1. PubMed PMID: 23347816.

16 Answer C. In a Ross procedure, the pulmonic valve is switched to the aortic position and a prosthetic valve is placed in the pulmonic position.

Reference: Lakoma A, Tuite D, Sheehan J, et al. Measurement of pulmonary circulation parameters using time-resolved MR angiography in patients after Ross procedure. *AJR Am J Roentgenol* 2010;194(4):912-919. doi: 10.2214/AJR.09.2897. PubMed PMID: 20308491.

17 Answer C. This is a prepulmonic course of the left coronary arising from the right sinus of Valsalva. No surgery is indicated given this is not prone to sudden death or compression. ICD is also not indicated for primary prevention. Follow-up CTA is not necessary given; this anatomy will not change.

Reference: Shriki JE, Shinbane JS, Rashid MA, et al. Identifying, characterizing, and classifying congenital anomalies of the coronary arteries. *Radiographics* 2012;32(2):453-468. doi: 10.1148/rg.322115097. Review. PubMed PMID: 22411942.

18 Answer C. Situs ambiguous is most associated with congenital heart disease. Situs solitus is normal anatomy and the least associated with congenital heart disease.

Reference: Applegate KE, Goske MJ, Pierce G, et al. Situs revisited: imaging of the heterotaxy syndrome. *Radiographics* 1999;19(4):837-852; discussion 853-854. Review. PubMed PMID: 10464794.

19 Answer A. Partial anomalous venous return is seen with the left superior pulmonary vein returning to the left brachiocephalic vein. This is a left to right shunt (pulmonary veins carry oxygenated blood). This can be incidental with treatment not considered unless there is evidence for a significant shunt (Qp/Qs > 1.5).

Reference: Wang ZJ, Reddy GP, Gotway MB, et al. Cardiovascular shunts: MR imaging evaluation. *Radiographics* 2003;23:S181-S194. Review. PubMed PMID: 14557511.

20 Answer C. Reformatted oblique image shows a left-sided SVC returning to the coronary sinus. This is a benign anatomical variant that requires no treatment. In rare cases, the left-sided SVC can drain into the left atrium and be associated with unroofed coronary sinus, a type of atrial septal defect.

Reference: Martinez-Jimenez S, Heyneman LE, McAdams HP, et al. Nonsurgical extracardiac vascular shunts in the thorax: clinical and imaging characteristics. *Radiographics* 2010;30(5):e41. doi: 10.1148/rg.e41. Epub 2010 Jul 9. PubMed PMID: 20622190.

21 Answer C. Bicuspid aortic valve is seen with fusion of the right and left coronary cusps. One can identify the sinuses by the following. The noncoronary sinus typically straddles the interatrial septum. The right sinus is anterior, so look for the sternum while left sinus is adjacent to the left atrial appendage.

Reference: Bennett CJ, Maleszewski JJ, Araoz PA. CT and MR imaging of the aortic valve: radiologic-pathologic correlation. *Radiographics* 2012;32(5):1399-1420. doi: 10.1148/rg.325115727. PubMed PMID: 22977027.

22 Answer A. Mitral valve clefts are seen with primum atrial septal defects (ASD). The ASD is a result of endocardial cushion defects, which result in a atrioventricular canal defect including a septum primum defect. Endocardial cushion defects and mitral valve clefts are associated with Down syndrome (trisomy 21). The other types of ASDs are not associated with mitral valvular abnormalities. A secundum ASD can often be seen in patients with Ebstein anomaly. Sinus venosus ASDs are often seen with right-sided partial anomalous venous return. An unroofed coronary sinus is associated with left-sided SVC.

Reference: Morris MF, Maleszewski JJ, Suri RM, et al. CT and MR imaging of the mitral valve: radiologic-pathologic correlation. *Radiographics* 2010;30(6):1603-1620. doi: 10.1148/rg.306105518. Review. PubMed PMID: 21071378.

23 Answer B. Cardiac MRI in horizontal (Image A) and vertical long-axis (Image B) views show abnormal location of the septal tricuspid leaflet, which is apically displaced (not anteriorly). There is also "atrialization" of the right ventricle due to the abnormal morphology of the tricuspid leaflet. The anterior leaflet is redundant and sail-like. This is consistent with an Ebstein anomaly. Note that Ebstein anomaly has a high association with secundum ASD. There is also an association with maternal lithium and benzodiazepine use.

There is no fusion of the anterior and septal leaflets. The hockey stick appearance of the anterior leaflet is seen in mitral stenosis.

Reference: Attenhofer Jost CH, Connolly HM, Dearani JA, et al. Ebstein's anomaly. *Circulation* 2007;115(2):277-285. Review. PubMed PMID: 7228014.

24 Answer B. Coronal reformat of a CT chest shows situs inversus. Note the left-sided liver and right-sided spleen. There is also azygos continuation in this patient (the large azygos vein on the left above the left bronchus). Right bronchus is now hyparterial while left bronchus is now eparterial. Normal relationship is right eparterial and left hyparterial. Bilateral right-sidedness (asplenia) is both hyparterial. Bilateral left-sidedness (polysplenia) is both hyparterial.

References: Applegate KE, Goske MJ, Pierce G, et al. Situs revisited: imaging of the heterotaxy syndrome. *Radiographics* 1999;19(4):837-852; discussion 853-854. Review. PubMed PMID: 10464794.

Lapierre C, Déry J, Guérin R, et al. Segmental approach to imaging of congenital heart disease. *Radiographics* 2010;30(2):397–411. doi: 10.1148/rg.302095112. Review. PubMed PMID: 20228325.

25a **Answer A.** Frontal and lateral chest radiograph shows a narrow mediastinum. The aortic and pulmonic contours are not well seen. This is classically associated with "egg-on-a-string" appearance seen with dextrotransposition of the great arteries. A boot-shaped heart is classically seen in tetralogy of Fallot. A box-shaped heart is seen with Ebstein anomaly. A figure of three is seen with coarctation. The scimitar sign is seen with partial anomalous pulmonary venous return. Finally, the snowman sign is seen with total anomalous pulmonary venous return (TAPVR).

Reference: Ferguson EC, Krishnamurthy R, Oldham SA. Classic imaging signs of congenital cardiovascular abnormalities. *Radiographics* 2007;27(5):1323–1334. Review. PubMed PMID: 17848694.

25b **Answer F.** Frontal chest radiograph shows a wide mediastinum with "snowman sign." This patient has total anomalous pulmonary venous return type I (supracardiac) in which all the pulmonary venous return is via the enlarged left vertical vein. The SVC contour is also enlarged due to the increased pulmonary venous return (both upper systemic and pulmonary venous return all run through the SVC). Note this condition is incompatible with life unless there is also another shunt that allows the mixed blood to enter the left (systemic) circulation (such as an atrial septal defect).

Reference: Ferguson EC, Krishnamurthy R, Oldham SA. Classic imaging signs of congenital cardiovascular abnormalities. *Radiographics* 2007;27(5):1323–1334. Review. PubMed PMID: 17848694.

26 **Answer D.** An anomalous RCA from the left sinus of Valsalva is seen. The RCA takes an interarterial course between the pulmonary artery and aortic root. This has been classically described as a "malignant" course. Treatment is considered surgical due to the theory that the vessel can be compressed between the pulmonary artery and aorta and cause ischemia. However, current treatment of this coronary anomaly is more nuanced. In a young patient with syncope/symptoms, this would certainly be a surgical lesion; however, in an older patient who have survived this incidental "malignant" course for 75 years, one could wonder if there is still a risk of sudden death. In this case, a stress test to see if there is any inducible ischemia from this anomaly is the best choice. ICD would not be indicated for primary prevention.

References: Angelini P. Coronary artery anomalies: an entity in search of an identity. *Circulation* 2007;115(10):1296–1305. Review. PubMed PMID: 17353457.

Shriki JE, Shinbane JS, Rashid MA, et al. Identifying, characterizing, and classifying congenital anomalies of the coronary arteries. *Radiographics* 2012;32(2):453–468. doi: 10.1148/rg.322115097. Review. PubMed PMID: 22411942.

27 **Answer B.** Axial image shows the aorta to be directly anterior to the pulmonary artery (Image A). This is typically seen with dextrotransposition of the great arteries (d-TGA). The coronal image (Image B) shows the intra-atrial baffle with the SVC baffle directing the upper venous return to the left atrium. Lower extremity venous return from IVC is also redirected to the left atrium. The axial MIP image (Image C) shows the pulmonary veins baffled to the right atrium, which is connected to the systemic right ventricle. Complications of the baffle repair include baffle obstruction, baffle leak, arrhythmias, and right ventricular dysfunction. The morphologic right ventricle is not made for systemic pressures and will tend to fail. There is no reported increased pathology of the mitral valve. There is increased tricuspid insufficiency due to the systemic pressures.

Reference: Lu JC, Dorfman AL, Attili AK, et al. Evaluation with cardiovascular MR imaging of baffles and conduits used in palliation or repair of congenital heart disease. *Radiographics* 2012;32(3):E107–E127. doi: 10.1148/rg.323115096. PubMed PMID: 22582368.

28 **Answer C.** Axial maximal intensity projection (MIP) image shows a double arch with a dominant right arch. A right arch with aberrant left subclavian artery can have a similar appearance but would not have the connecting vessel on the left. A right arch with mirror image branching would not have the posterior vessel to the trachea and esophagus. In a double aortic arch with a dominant left arch, the caliber of the left arch would be larger.

References: Kimura-Hayama ET, Meléndez G, Mendizábal AL, et al. Uncommon congenital and acquired aortic diseases: role of multidetector CT angiography. *Radiographics* 2010;30(1):79-98. doi: 10.1148/rg.301095061. PubMed PMID: 20083587.

Ramos-Duran L, Nance JW Jr, Schoepf UJ, et al. Developmental aortic arch anomalies in infants and children assessed with CT angiography. *AJR Am J Roentgenol* 2012;198(5):W466-W474. doi: 10.2214/AJR.11.6982. Review. PubMed PMID: 22528928.

29 **Answer B.** Images show a sinus of Valsalva (SOV) aneurysm involving the noncoronary cusp. SOV aneurysms most often occur in the right and noncoronary cusps. They are associated with aortic regurgitation and supracristal ventricular septal defects. They tend to rupture into the right ventricular outflow tract (RVOT), followed by the right atrium and rarely in the left atrium or ventricle.

Reference: Bricker AO, Avutu B, Mohammed TL, et al. Valsalva sinus aneurysms: findings at CT and MR imaging. *Radiographics* 2010;30(1):99-110. doi: 10.1148/rg.301095719. PubMed PMID: 20083588.

30 **Answer B.** Multiple images demonstrate a baby with complex congenital heart disease. There is a right arch with mirror image branching, VSD, overriding aorta, and multiple aortopulmonary collateral arteries (MAPCAs). This is most consistent with pulmonary atresia with ventricular septal defect (PA-VSD). This condition has been previously called as pseudotruncus and classified as type IV of truncus arteriosus. However, this condition is now considered its own entity and can have similar abnormalities as tetralogy of Fallot (TOF) except with pulmonary atresia and MAPCAS. TOF has the following four features: overriding aorta, ventricular septal defect, right ventricular hypertrophy, and right ventricular outflow obstruction.

References: Boechat MI, Ratib O, Williams PL, et al. Cardiac MR imaging and MR angiography for assessment of complex tetralogy of Fallot and pulmonary atresia. *Radiographics* 2005;25(6): 1535-1546. Review. PubMed PMID: 16284133.

Rajeshkannan R, Moorthy S, Sreekumar KP, et al. Role of 64-MDCT in evaluation of pulmonary atresia with ventricular septal defect. *AJR Am J Roentgenol* 2010;194(1):110-118. doi: 10.2214/AJR.09.2802. Review. PubMed PMID: 20028912.

31 **Answer C.** Multiple oblique reformatted MIP images show dilated coronary arteries with calcification. In a young patient, this is most consistent with history of Kawasaki disease. While the coronary arteries can dilate post nitroglycerin administration, this degree of diffuse ectasia should not be seen along the evidence for atherosclerosis. Premature atherosclerosis would typically not involve 18-year-old patients. Coronary fistula is within the differential for dilated coronary arteries, but there is no evidence for abnormal connections on the images provided.

Reference: Díaz-Zamudio M, Bacilio-Pérez U, Herrera-Zarza MC, et al. Coronary artery aneurysms and ectasia: role of coronary CT angiography. *Radiographics* 2009;29(7):1939-1954. doi: 10.1148/rg.297095048. Review. PubMed PMID: 19926755.

10 Acquired Disease of the Thoracic Aorta and Great Vessels

QUESTIONS

1. What is the most common cause of an ascending thoracic aortic aneurysm?
   A. Atherosclerosis
   B. Aortitis
   C. Marfan syndrome
   D. Aortic stenosis

2a. What is the most likely cause of this finding?

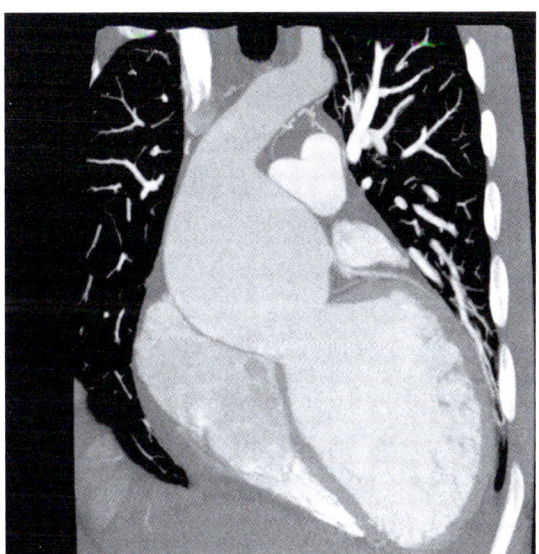

   A. Atherosclerosis
   B. Marfan syndrome
   C. Bicuspid aortopathy
   D. Hypertension

2b. In patients with Marfan syndrome, what associated valvular abnormality can be seen?
   A. Tricuspid stenosis
   B. Tricuspid valve prolapse
   C. Mitral stenosis
   D. Mitral valve prolapse

3 Which of the following characteristics favor traumatic pseudoaneurysm versus ductus diverticulum?

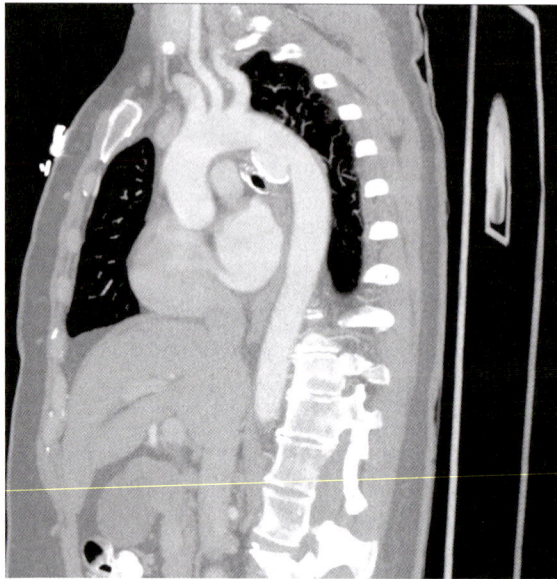

A. Aortic wall outer continuity
B. Smooth margins
C. Location at aortic isthmus
D. Intimal flap
E. Calcification

4 A 57-year-old female presents with chest pain. These images were obtained 4 months apart. What is the most likely cause of this aneurysm?

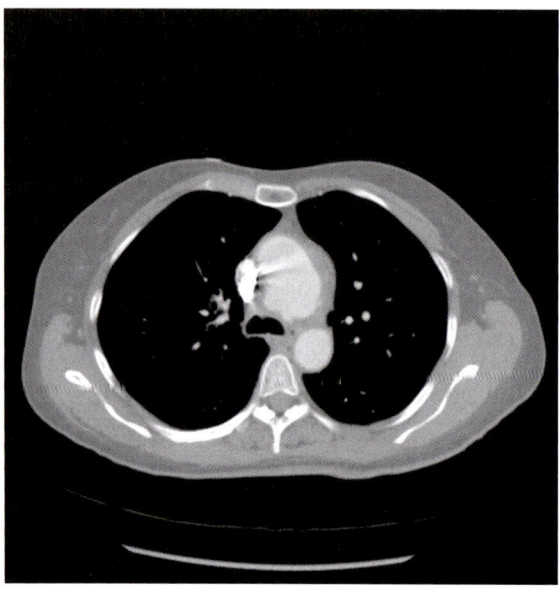
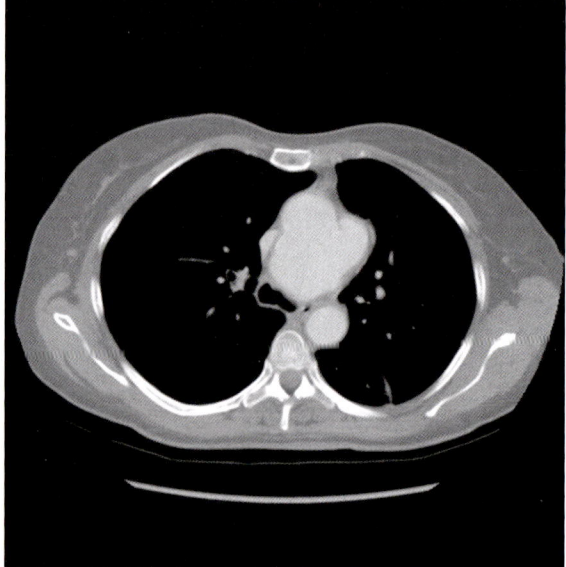

A. Atherosclerotic
B. Takayasu aortitis
C. Posttraumatic
D. Mycotic

5a A 61-year-old male presents with abdominal pain. What is the best next step?

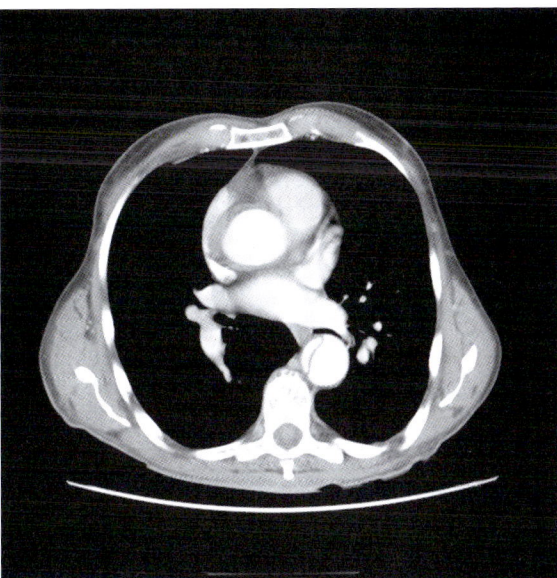

A. Medical treatment
B. Gated CTA chest
C. Immediate surgery
D. Endovascular treatment

5b A gated CTA is then obtained. What other type of imaging would be most helpful to determine the diagnosis?

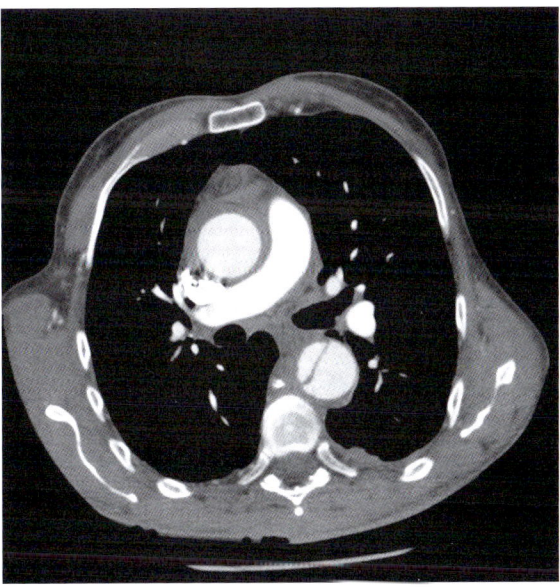

A. Left anterior oblique reformat of the thoracic aorta
B. Another cardiac phase in the gated CTA
C. Noncontrast images
D. Delayed images

5c This is the patient re-imaged a few hours later. What is the best next step in the management of this patient?

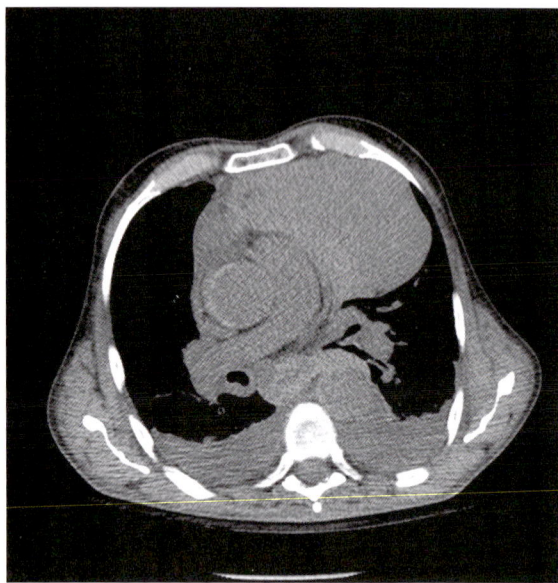
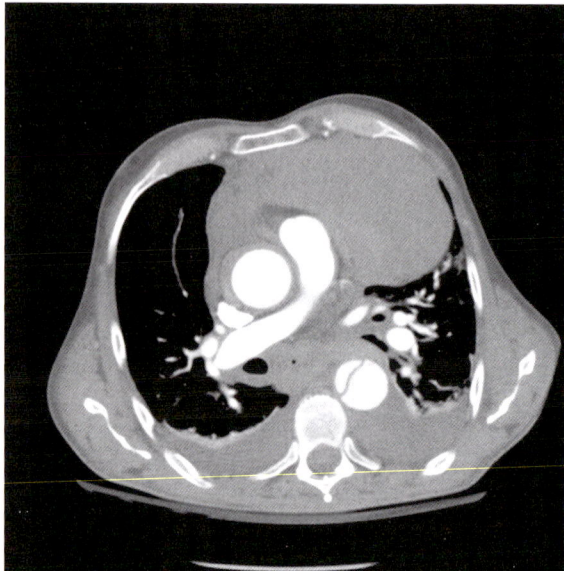

A. Medical management
B. Immediate surgery
C. Endovascular
D. Additional imaging

6 Annuloaortic ectasia is most commonly associated with Marfan syndrome. What other condition can also produce similar findings?

A. Syphilis
B. Bicuspid aortic valve
C. Takayasu arteritis
D. Ehlers-Danlos syndrome

7 In aortic dissection, what is the most diseased portion of the aorta?

A. Intima
B. Media
C. Adventitia
D. Vasa vasorum

8 Dissection at the aortic arch is considered what type of dissection using the Stanford classification?

A. Type A
B. Type B
C. Type C

9 What is the most common risk factor for aortic dissection?

A. Hypertension
B. Cystic medial degeneration
C. Marfan syndrome
D. Aortic aneurysm

10 What complication is being shown?

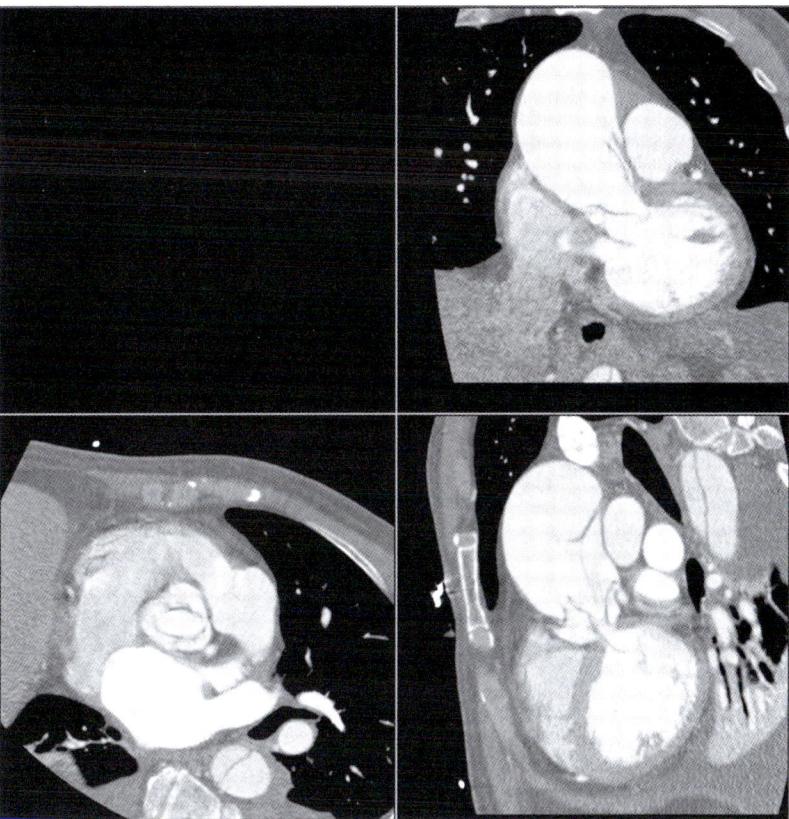

A. Aortic regurgitation
B. Aortic stenosis
C. Aortic valve endocarditis
D. Aortic rupture

11a In this condition, which layer of the aortic wall is intact?

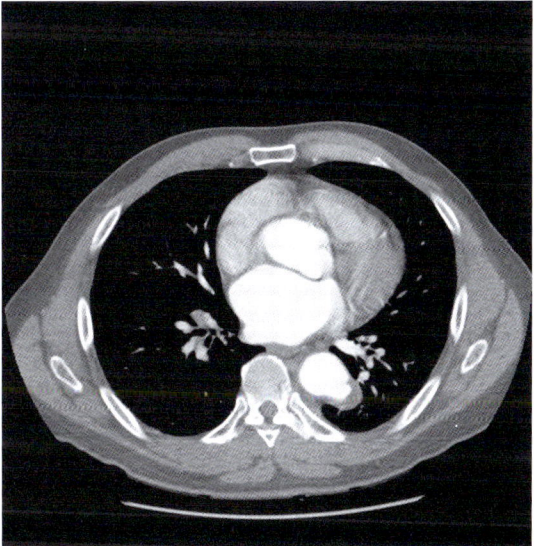

A. Intima
B. Media
C. Adventitia

11b The patient remains asymptomatic, what is the next step?
   A. Medical therapy
   B. Surgery
   C. Endovascular stenting

12 What is the most likely underlying condition that the 56-year-old male patient has?

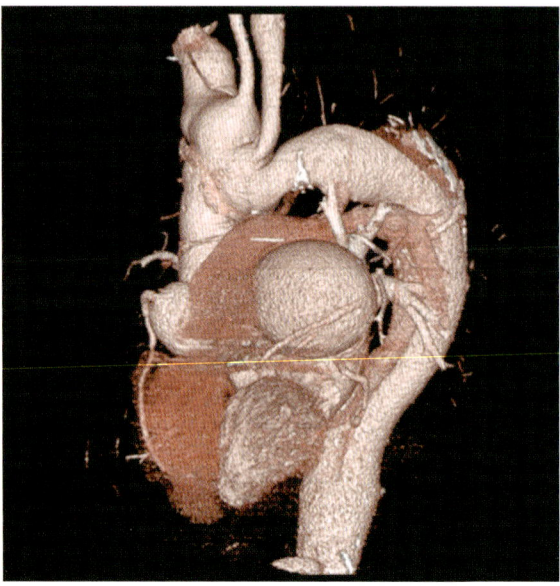

   A. Premature atherosclerosis
   B. Marfan syndrome
   C. Takayasu arteritis
   D. Prior syphilis infection

13 A 62-year-old male presents with leg pain. What is the best next step?

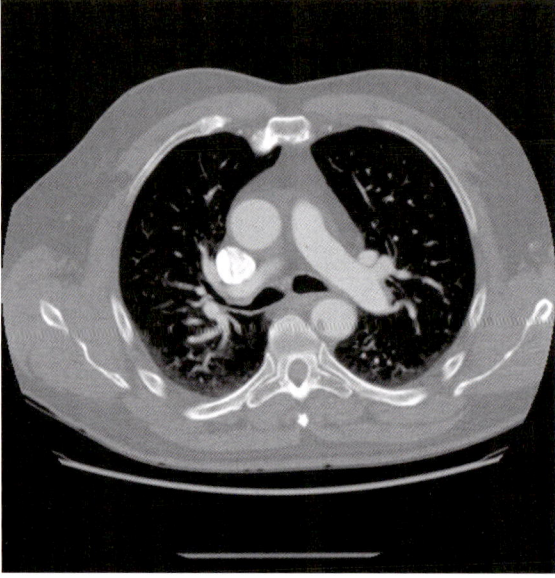

   A. Endovascular thrombectomy
   B. Surgical thrombectomy
   C. Medical treatment

14a What sign is suggested on this chest radiograph?

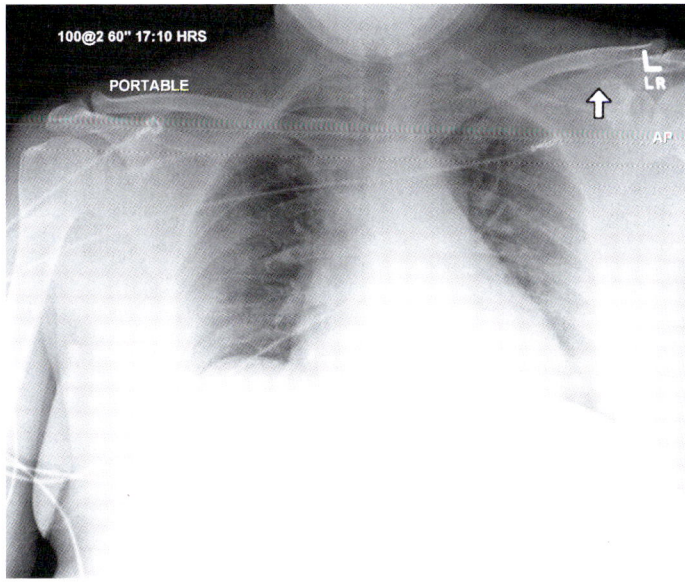

A. Snowman sign
B. Westermark sign
C. Golden S sign
D. Scimitar sign

14b What measurements can be obtained on these images to best assess for severity of pulmonary embolism?

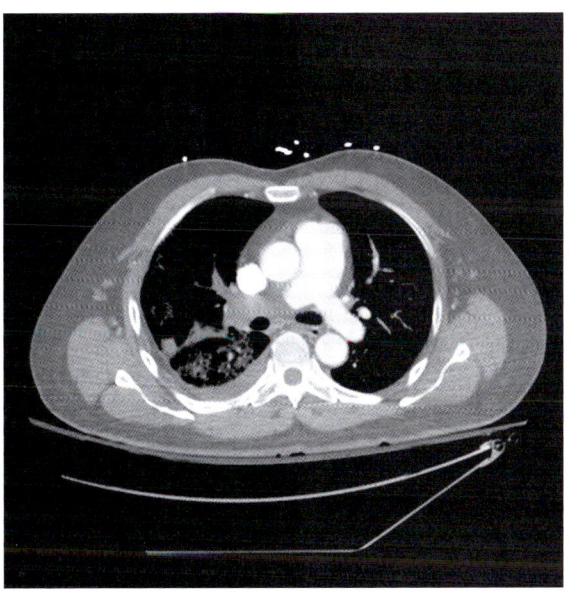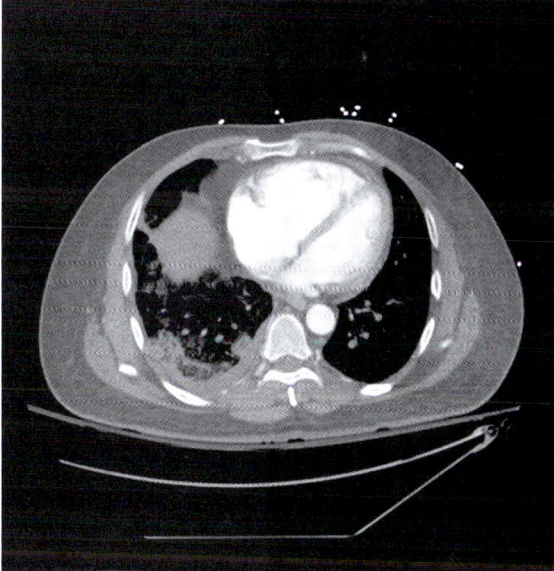

A. Right ventricle to left ventricle short-axis ratio
B. Left ventricle to right ventricle short-axis ratio
C. Interventricular septal wall thickness
D. Right ventricular wall thickness

15a A 28-year-old male presents with shortness of breath. What is the most likely cause of these findings?

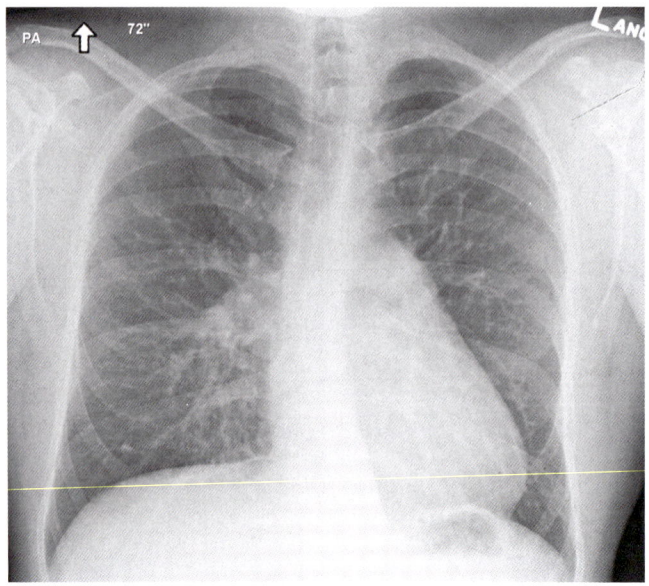

A. Pulmonary edema due to right heart failure
B. Pulmonary edema due to mitral regurgitation
C. Pulmonary hypertension due to left to right shunting
D. Pulmonary hypertension due to idiopathic cause

15b How is this complication best treated?

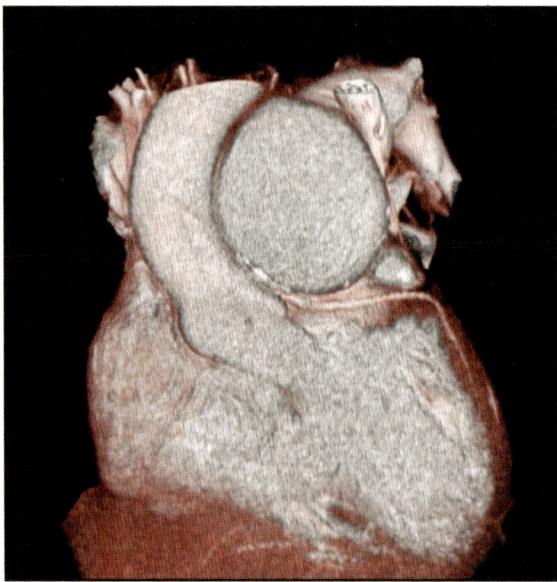

A. Observation
B. Stent
C. Medical

16 What type of arteriovenous malformation is this?

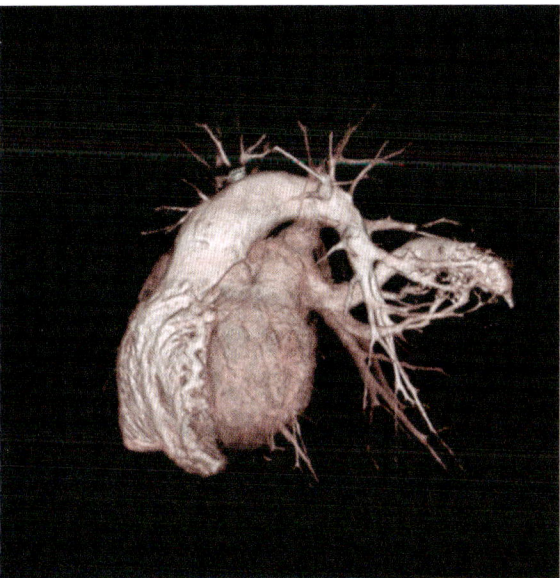

   A. Simple malformation
   B. Intermediate malformation
   C. Complex malformation

17 What type of shunt is pulmonary AVM?
   A. Right to left
   B. Left to right
   C. Right to right
   D. Left to left

18 Multiple pulmonary AVMs are associated with which of the following condition?
   A. Hereditary hemorrhagic telangiectasia (HHT)
   B. Von Hippel-Lindau
   C. Tuberous sclerosis
   D. Marfan syndrome

19 Traditionally, what has been the feeding vessel size cutoff for treatment of pulmonary AVMs?
   A. 1 mm
   B. 2 mm
   C. 3 mm
   D. 4 mm

20 What is the most common pulmonary vein anatomical variant?
   A. Common right pulmonary trunk
   B. Common left pulmonary trunk
   C. Separate trunk of right middle pulmonary vein
   D. Separate trunk of lingular pulmonary vein

21 What treatment is now considered the first-line therapy for this condition?

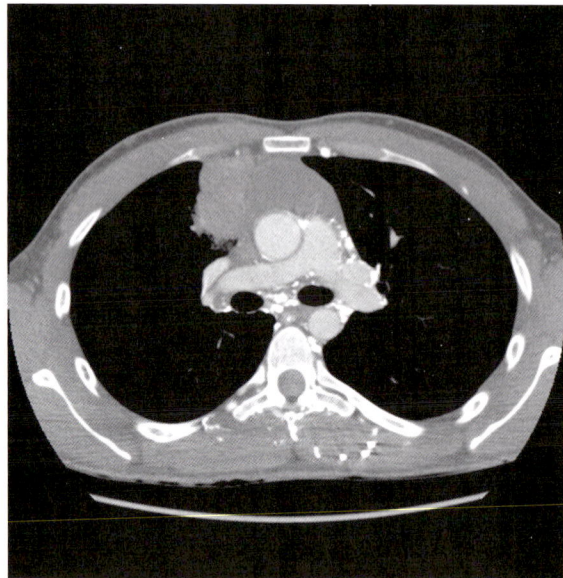

A. Surgery
B. Radiation
C. Chemotherapy
D. Stenting

22 A 33-year-old male is status post pulmonary vein ablation. What complication has occurred?

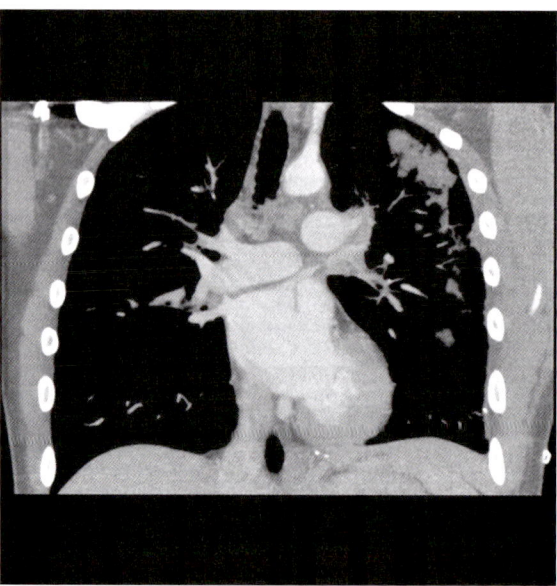

A. Esophagoatrial fistula
B. Pulmonary artery thrombosis
C. Pulmonary vein stenosis
D. Traumatic atrial septal defect

23 The differentials for this imaging finding include Takayasu arteritis and which of the following?

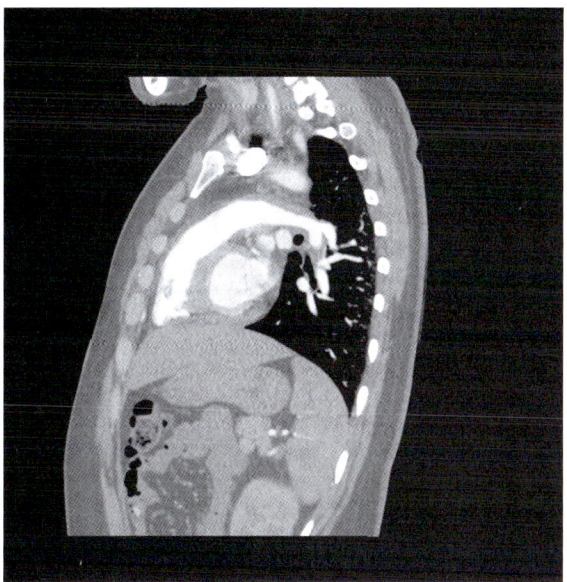
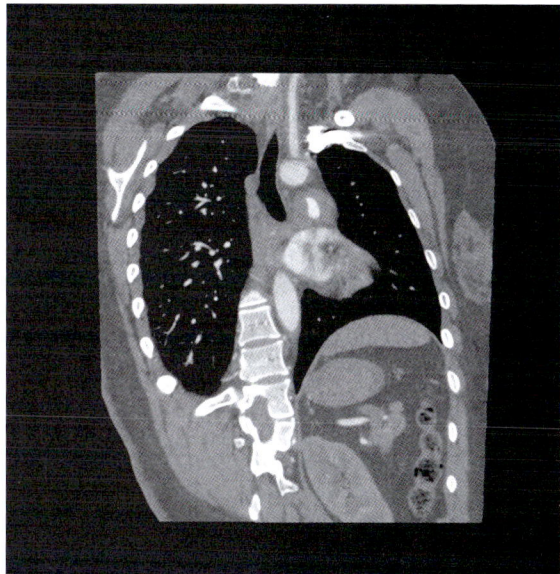
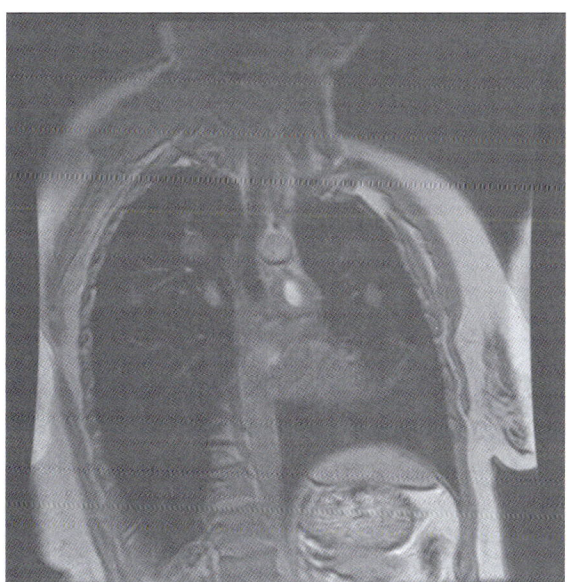
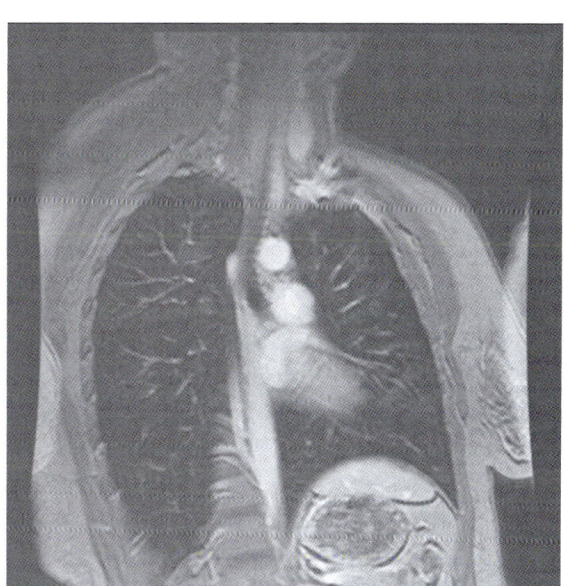

A. Polyarteritis nodosa
B. Kawasaki disease
C. Wegener granulomatosis
D. Giant cell arteritis

24 In adults with Marfan syndrome, what is the typical size of aorta that would meet surgical indication?
A. 4.0 cm
B. 5.0 cm
C. 6.0 cm
D. 7.0 cm

25 What is the next best step for this patient?

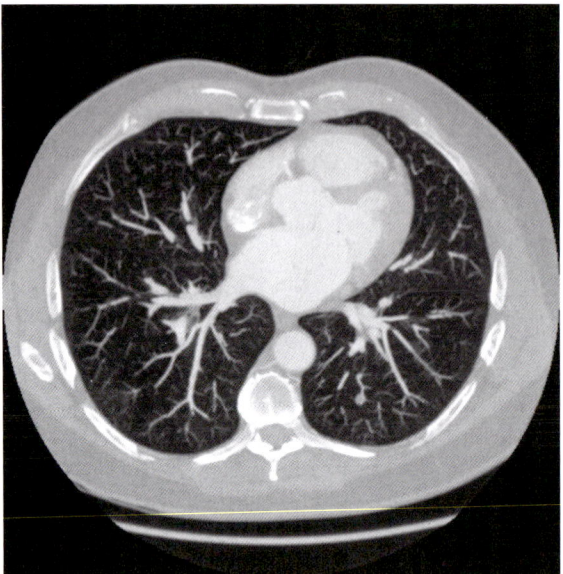

A. Refer for embolization
B. Refer for biopsy
C. Close observation
D. Look at thin axial images

26 What is the most likely cause of the arch abnormality?

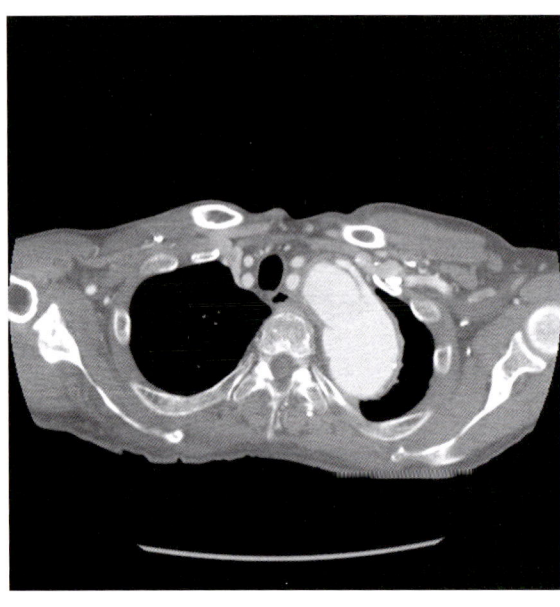 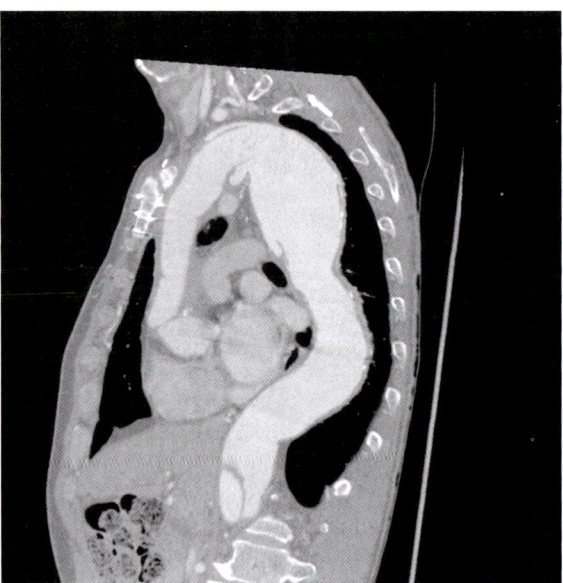

A. Residual dissection flap
B. Elephant trunk type repair
C. Limited intimal tear
D. Graft infection

27 Which of the following findings help identify the true lumen versus the false lumen on CTA?
    A. Larger luminal diameter
    B. Beak sign
    C. Lumen being wrapped by another lumen
    D. Inner wall calcification
    E. Cobweb sign

28 Which type of dissection is more common?
    A. Stanford type A
    B. Stanford type B
    C. Stanford type C
    D. Equal in prevalence

ANSWERS AND EXPLANATIONS

1 Answer A. Most common cause of aortic aneurysm is atherosclerosis and accounts for approximately 70% of cases. The other answer choices are all less common causes of ascending thoracic aortic aneurysm.

Reference: Agarwal PP, Chughtai A, Matzinger FR, et al. Multidetector CT of thoracic aortic aneurysms. *Radiographics* 2009;29(2):537-552. doi: 10.1148/rg.292075080. Review. PubMed PMID: 19325064.

2a Answer B. Coronal reformatted image shows annuloaortic ectasia (effacement of the sinotubular junction with dilated aortic root). Some have described this as a "pear-shaped/tulip bulb" appearance of the aorta. While atherosclerosis is the most common cause of aortic aneurysm, there does not appear to be atherosclerosis in this young patient. Bicuspid aortopathy can also cause aneurysm but does not typically give this classic appearance of annuloaortic ectasia. The appearance of aortic aneurysm caused by hypertension will also typically not involve annuloaortic ectasia.

References: Agarwal PP, Chughtai A, Matzinger FR, et al. Multidetector CT of thoracic aortic aneurysms. *Radiographics* 2009;29(2):537-552. doi: 10.1148/rg.292075080. Review. PubMed PMID: 19325064.

Ha HI, Seo JB, Lee SH, et al. Imaging of Marfan syndrome: multisystemic manifestations. *Radiographics* 2007;27(4):989-1004. Review. PubMed PMID: 17620463.

2b Answer D. Mitral valve prolapse can be seen with Marfan syndrome. The other valvular abnormalities listed are not associated with Marfan syndrome.

References: Agarwal PP, Chughtai A, Matzinger FR, et al. Multidetector CT of thoracic aortic aneurysms. *Radiographics* 2009;29(2):537-552. doi: 10.1148/rg.292075080. Review. PubMed PMID: 19325064.

Ha HI, Seo JB, Lee SH, et al. Imaging of Marfan syndrome: multisystemic manifestations. *Radiographics* 2007;27(4):989-1004. Review. PubMed PMID: 17620463.

3 Answer D. Classic ductus diverticulum features include smooth margins and gently sloping shoulders. It should form obtuse angles with the preserved aortic wall. There should not be an intimal flap; that would favor traumatic pseudoaneurysm. They can both be located at the aortic isthmus so that will not be a differentiating feature. Calcification can also occur in both chronic pseudoaneurysm and ductus diverticulum.

Reference: Steenburg SD, Ravenel JG, Ikonomidis JS, et al. Acute traumatic aortic injury: imaging evaluation and management. *Radiology* 2008;248(3):748-762. doi: 10.1148/radiol.2483071416. Review. PubMed PMID: 18710974.

4 Answer D. The rapid progression of the aneurysm is most consistent with mycotic aneurysm. Atherosclerosis would not be this rapid in course. Saccular type of aneurysm seen here is also more common in mycotic aneurysms. Takayasu arteritis typically causes narrowing but can also cause aneurysm; in this case, it could be in the differential but is considered a less likely cause. Posttraumatic aneurysm is also possible, but the rapid enlargement and irregular borders are more consistent with mycotic than posttraumatic aneurysm.

References: Agarwal PP, Chughtai A, Matzinger FR, et al. Multidetector CT of thoracic aortic aneurysms. *Radiographics* 2009;29(2):537-552. doi: 10.1148/rg.292075080. Review. PubMed PMID: 19325064.

Macedo TA, Stanson AW, Oderich GS, et al. Infected aortic aneurysms: imaging findings. *Radiology* 2004;231(1):250-257. Erratum in: *Radiology* 2006;238(3):1078. PubMed PMID: 15068950.

5a Answer B. Single-axial image shows a type B dissection in the descending thoracic aorta. There is suggestion of wall thickening at the aortic root, but this may be due to motion artifacts. The best next step would be a gated CTA chest to assess the aortic root better. Medical treatment would be fine if this were only an isolated descending thoracic dissection. Immediate surgery would be indicated if a type A dissection is confirmed (difficult to be certain given this may be motion artifacts on a nongated image). Endovascular treatment is not indicated given that there is no evidence for aneurysm and there is no role for endovascular treatment in type A dissections.

5b Answer C. Gated CTA confirms wall thickening/fluid surrounding the ascending aorta. This is concerning for a type A dissection/intramural hematoma. Blood can be confirmed with a noncontrast sequence, which should show high attenuating fluid in the aortic wall. Left anterior oblique reformat can visualize the aorta in its entirety but would not be helpful to determine the attenuation value of the wall. Another phase in the cardiac cycle will also not help determine if there is blood. Delay images can potentially be helpful by showing the wall better with less luminal contrast but will not be as good as the noncontrast images.

5c Answer B. The noncontrast image confirms high density surrounding the ascending aorta, which makes this a type A dissection equivalent with intramural hematoma versus retrograde extension of the dissection down the ascending thoracic aorta. The best next step is immediate surgery.

References: Karmy-Jones R, Aldea G, Boyle EM Jr. The continuing evolution in the management of thoracic aortic dissection. *Chest* 2000;117(5):1221-1223. PubMed PMID: 10807801.

Mészáros I, Mórocz J, Szlávi J, et al. Epidemiology and clinicopathology of aortic dissection. *Chest* 2000;117(5):1271-1278. PubMed PMID: 10807810.

6 Answer D. Annuloaortic ectasia is classically associated with Marfan syndrome. Other causes include Ehlers-Danlos syndrome, homocystinuria, and osteogenesis imperfecta. It can also be idiopathic without underlying genetic abnormality. Syphilitic aneurysm does not often involve the aortic root. Bicuspid aortopathy does not typically dilate the sinotubular junction. Takayasu arteritis tends to narrow the aorta.

Reference: Agarwal PP, Chughtai A, Matzinger FR, et al. Multidetector CT of thoracic aortic aneurysms. *Radiographics* 2009;29(2):537-552. doi: 10.1148/rg.292075080. Review. PubMed PMID: 19325064.

7 Answer B. Aortic dissection is defined by the disruption of the aortic intima with blood dissecting into the media of the aortic wall. The most diseased portion is therefore the media, which is disrupted. The intima can be mostly intact with an entry tear. If the adventitia is disrupted, there would be aortic rupture. The vasa vasorum is involved in intramural hematoma.

Reference: McMahon MA, Squirrell CA. Multidetector CT of aortic dissection: a pictorial review. *Radiographics* 2010;30(2):445-460. doi: 10.1148/rg.302095104. Review. PubMed PMID: 20228328.

8 Answer B. Dissection at the arch is considered a type B Stanford dissection. Type A involves the ascending aorta. Type B is any other type of dissection that does not involve the ascending aorta. There is no Stanford type C dissection.

Reference: McMahon MA, Squirrell CA. Multidetector CT of aortic dissection: a pictorial review. *Radiographics* 2010;30(2):445-460. doi: 10.1148/rg.302095104. Review. PubMed PMID: 20228328.

9 Answer A. Hypertension is the most common risk factor for aortic dissection, occurring in a majority of patients with dissection. All of the other answer choices are less common risk factors for dissection.

Reference: McMahon MA, Squirrell CA. Multidetector CT of aortic dissection: a pictorial review. *Radiographics* 2010;30(2):445-460. doi: 10.1148/rg.302095104. Review. PubMed PMID: 20228328.

10 Answer A. Reformatted images at the aortic root show type A dissection with the dissection flaps prolapsing into the aortic root during diastole causing aortic regurgitation.

Reference: McMahon MA, Squirrell CA. Multidetector CT of aortic dissection: a pictorial review. *Radiographics* 2010;30(2):445–460. doi: 10.1148/rg.302095104. Review. PubMed PMID: 20228328.

11a Answer C. An outpouching is seen in the descending thoracic aorta, which is consistent with a penetrating aortic ulcer (PAU). In a penetrating aortic ulcer, there is disruption of the inner layer (intima) by the penetrating ulcer with subsequent bleed in the medial layer. In this case, there is focal dilation of the aorta at the site of PAU. The adventitial/outer layer is intact or else there would be aortic rupture.

Reference: Castañer E, Andreu M, Gallardo X, et al. CT in nontraumatic acute thoracic aortic disease: typical and atypical features and complications. *Radiographics* 2003;23:S93-S110. Review. PubMed PMID: 14557505.

11b Answer A. Penetrating aortic ulcers typically occur in the descending aorta and is considered a type B aortic dissection equivalent. The most appropriate treatment in an asymptomatic patient is medical therapy (control blood pressure). It is only in patients who have aortic rupture/hemodynamic instability that surgery is considered. Endovascular treatment can be performed particularly given the high risk of surgical repair. Indications for treatment include symptomatic patients or if there is rapid enlargement of the ulcerating aneurysm.

Reference: Castañer E, Andreu M, Gallardo X, et al. CT in nontraumatic acute thoracic aortic disease: typical and atypical features and complications. *Radiographics* 2003;23:S93-S110. Review. PubMed PMID: 14557505.

12 Answer B. This is a patient with Marfan syndrome who had a Bentall composite aortic root replacement that developed large coronary button aneurysms. Note the dissection in the descending thoracic aorta. Due to the underlying aortic wall abnormality in Marfan patients, the reimplanted contrary buttons can be prone to aneurysm formation. While Takayasu and prior syphilis infection can give rise to aneurysms, they are not associated with coronary button aneurysms.

References: Bruschi G, Cannata A, Botta L, et al. Giant true aneurysm of the right coronary artery button long after aortic root replacement. *Eur J Cardiothorac Surg* 2013;43(5):e139-e140. doi: 10.1093/ejcts/ezt057. Epub 2013 Feb 20. PubMed PMID: 23425675.

Prescott-Focht JA, Martinez-Jimenez S, Hurwitz LM, et al. Ascending thoracic aorta: postoperative imaging evaluation. *Radiographics* 2013;33(1):73-85. doi: 10.1148/rg.331125090. Review. PubMed PMID: 23322828.

13 Answer C. Axial image shows a luminal thrombus in the descending thoracic aorta. There is no current role for aggressive management such as surgical or endovascular thrombectomy. Instead, patients are managed medically with anticoagulation.

Reference: Ferrari E, Vidal R, Chevallier T et al. Atherosclerosis of the thoracic aorta and aortic debris as a marker of poor prognosis: benefit of oral anticoagulants. *J Am Coll Cardiol* 1999;33(5):1317-1322. PubMed PMID: 10193733.

14a Answer B. Frontal chest radiograph shows right lung oligemia which is consistent with Westermark sign. Snowman sign is seen with total anomalous venous return. Golden S sign is seen with a hilar mass and upper lobe collapse. Scimitar sign is seen with anomalous pulmonary venous return.

Reference: Han D, Lee KS, Franquet T, et al. Thrombotic and nonthrombotic pulmonary arterial embolism: spectrum of imaging findings. *Radiographics* 2003;23(6):1521-1539. Review. PubMed PMID: 14615562.

14b Answer A. Right ventricle to left ventricle short-axis ratio is the best measurement to obtain for assessment of right heart strain and the severity of the pulmonary embolism. A ratio of >1 is indicative of RV strain, while >1.5 indicates a severe episode of PE. Interventricular septal wall thickness and right ventricular wall thickness have not been reported to correlate with acute pulmonary embolism outcomes.

Reference: Ghaye B, Ghuysen A, Bruyere PJ, et al. Can CT pulmonary angiography allow assessment of severity and prognosis in patients presenting with pulmonary embolism? What the radiologist needs to know. *Radiographics* 2006;26(1):23–39; discussion 39–40. Review. PubMed PMID: 16418240.

15a Answer C. Frontal chest radiograph shows enlarged pulmonary artery contour along with increased flow suggesting of underlying left to right shunt. This is therefore most consistent with pulmonary hypertension with underlying atrial or ventricular septal defect.

Reference: Peña E, Dennie C, Veinot J, et al. Pulmonary hypertension: how the radiologist can help. *Radiographics* 2012;32(1):9–32. doi: 10.1148/rg.321105232. PubMed PMID: 22236891.

15b Answer B. Volume-rendered image shows markedly enlarged pulmonary artery compressing the origin/proximal left coronary artery. This can be treated with surgery or stenting, but given the high mortality of pulmonary hypertension patients for surgery, stenting is now an accepted treatment.

References: Caldera AE, Cruz-Gonzalez I, Bezerra HG, et al. Endovascular therapy for left main compression syndrome. Case report and literature review. *Chest* 2009;135(6):1648–1650. doi: 10.1378/chest.08-2922. Review. PubMed PMID: 19497900.

Peña E, Dennie C, Veinot J, et al. Pulmonary hypertension: how the radiologist can help. *Radiographics* 2012;32(1):9–32. doi: 10.1148/rg.321105232. PubMed PMID: 22236891.

16 Answer C. Simple malformations are ones that originate from 1 single segmental artery. Complex malformations are from multiple segmental feeding arteries. There is no intermediate malformation that has been described.

Reference: White RI Jr, Mitchell SE, Barth KH, et al. Angioarchitecture of pulmonary arteriovenous malformations: an important consideration before embolotherapy. *AJR Am J Roentgenol* 1983;140(4):681–686. PubMed PMID: 6601370.

17 Answer A. Pulmonary AVMs are a type of right to left shunt between the unoxygenated blood from the pulmonary artery into the oxygenated blood of the pulmonary veins.

Reference: Martinez-Jimenez S, Heyneman LE, McAdams HP, et al. Nonsurgical extracardiac vascular shunts in the thorax: clinical and imaging characteristics. *Radiographics* 2010;30(5):e41. doi: 10.1148/rg.e41. Epub 2010 Jul 9. PubMed PMID: 20622190.

18 Answer A. Greater than 50% of patients with pulmonary AVM have HHT, while 5% to 15% of HHT patients have pulmonary AVM.

Reference: Martinez-Jimenez S, Heyneman LE, McAdams HP, et al. Nonsurgical extracardiac vascular shunts in the thorax: clinical and imaging characteristics. *Radiographics* 2010;30(5):e41. doi: 10.1148/rg.e41. Epub 2010 Jul 9. PubMed PMID: 20622190.

19 Answer C. The traditional cutoff for treatment of pulmonary AVMs is a 3-mm feeding vessel. However, it is now accepted that treatment of smaller than 3-mm feeding arteries should also be considered given that the smaller AVMs may still cause paradoxical embolization.

Reference: Trerotola SO, Pyeritz RE. PAVM embolization: an update. *AJR Am J Roentgenol* 2010;195(4):837–845. doi: 10.2214/AJR.10.5230. Review. PubMed PMID: 20858807.

20 Answer B. The most common variant of pulmonary venous anatomy is common left trunk.

Reference: Porres DV, Morenza OP, Pallisa E, et al. Learning from the pulmonary veins. *Radiographics* 2013;33(4):999-1022. doi: 10.1148/rg.334125043. Review. PubMed PMID: 23842969.

21 Answer D. Axial image shows complete obstruction of the SVC. Note the prominent collaterals in the mediastinum and vertebral regions. Endovascular stenting has now emerged as a first-line treatment for patients with SVC obstruction.

Reference: Sheth S, Ebert MD, Fishman EK. Superior vena cava obstruction evaluation with MDCT. *AJR Am J Roentgenol* 2010;194(4):W336-W346. doi: 10.2214/AJR.09.2894. Review. PubMed PMID: 20308479.

22 Answer C. Coronal reformat shows narrowing of the left superior pulmonary vein and abnormal left upper lobe airspace opacities. This is consistent with pulmonary vein stenosis post left atrial ablation with pulmonary venous infarct.

Reference: Porres DV, Morenza OP, Pallisa E, et al. Learning from the pulmonary veins. *Radiographics* 2013;33(4):999-1022. doi: 10.1148/rg.334125043. Review. PubMed PMID: 23842969.

23 Answer D. Oblique images show abnormal left pulmonary artery with wall thickening and enhancement. This is suggestive of vasculitis. Takayasu arteritis and giant cell arteritis are large vessel vasculitis that can involve the main pulmonary artery branches. Although the imaging features may be similar, clinical history may be helpful to differentiate. Takayasu arteritis typically occurs in younger patients (< 40 years old), while giant cell arteritis typically occurs in patients greater than 50 years of age.

Reference: Castañer E, Alguersuari A, Gallardo X, et al. When to suspect pulmonary vasculitis: radiologic and clinical clues. *Radiographics* 2010;30(1):33-53. doi: 10.1148/rg.301095103. PubMed PMID: 20083584.

24 Answer B. In adult patients with Marfan syndrome, prophylactic surgery is recommended when the diameter exceeds 5.0 cm. However, earlier surgery may be indicated if there is rapid rate of growth (>1 cm/year).

References: Agarwal PP, Chughtai A, Matzinger FR, et al. Multidetector CT of thoracic aortic aneurysms. *Radiographics* 2009;29(2):537-552. doi: 10.1148/rg.292075080. Review. PubMed PMID: 19325064.

Ha HI, Seo JB, Lee SH, et al. Imaging of Marfan syndrome: multisystemic manifestations. *Radiographics* 2007;27(4):989-1004. Review. PubMed PMID: 17620463.

25 Answer D. MIP axial image shows a nodule with apparent vessel connection. This may be a small simple pulmonary AVM or an artifact due to MIP technique. For the diagnosis of pulmonary AVM, there must be visualization of both a feeding branch and also the draining vein. This one image is not diagnostic so the source images should be consulted to see if this is a nodule versus AVM. The thin axial images show this to be a nodule rather than an AVM.

Reference: Martinez-Jimenez S, Heyneman LE, McAdams HP, et al. Nonsurgical extracardiac vascular shunts in the thorax: clinical and imaging characteristics. *Radiographics* 2010;30(5):e41. doi: 10.1148/rg.e41. Epub 2010 Jul 9. PubMed PMID: 20622190.

26 Answer B. Axial and oblique sagittal views of the aorta show flaps at the arch. This is consistent with an elephant trunk type repair with the arch graft projecting into the aortic lumen in anticipation of future aortic procedure. This patient subsequently received a thoracic endograft connecting to the arch graft to exclude the arch aneurysm. While residual dissection flaps can be present, the appearance of the flaps in continuity with the ascending graft is diagnostic of a normal postoperative appearance of an elephant trunk procedure. This is not a limited intimal tear. There are no findings here to suggest graft infection.

Reference: Sundaram B, Quint LE, Patel HJ, et al. CT findings following thoracic aortic surgery. *Radiographics* 2007;27(6):1583-1594. Review. PubMed PMID: 18025504.

27 Answer C. The false lumen is often the larger diameter lumen and shows the beak sign. In cases where there is the appearance of the lumen being wrapped by another lumen, the true lumen is the one wrapped by the false lumen. Inner wall calcification is not helpful. However, in acute dissection, the outer wall calcification is indicative of the true lumen. This would not be as helpful in chronic dissection since the false lumen can calcify. Cobweb sign indicates false lumen; it is a specific sign but is not always seen.

Reference: LePage MA, Quint LE, Sonnad SS, et al. Aortic dissection: CT features that distinguish true lumen from false lumen. *AJR Am J Roentgenol* 2001;177(1):207-211. PubMed PMID: 11418129.

28 Answer A. Stanford type A dissections are more common (60% to 70% of dissections). There is no such thing as Stanford type C dissection.

Reference: McMahon MA, Squirrell CA. Multidetector CT of aortic dissection: a pictorial review. *Radiographics* 2010;30(2):445-460. doi: 10.1148/rg.302095104. Review. PubMed PMID: 20228328.

11 Devices and Postoperative Appearance

QUESTIONS

1a A 35-year-old male has a history of syncope. There is no family history of sudden death. The patient is scheduled for a cardiac MRI, and the technologist asks you to review a screening chest radiograph.

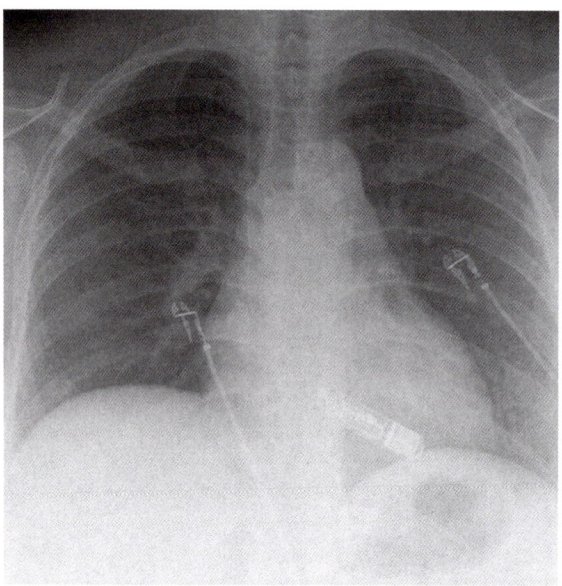

What is the finding on the radiograph?
A. Repeat CXR without device in patient's pocket
B. Previous pacemaker with leads removed
C. Loop recorder
D. External ICD

1b After reviewing the previous screening chest radiograph, how would you proceed with the scheduled cardiac MRI?
A. The x-ray does not have any abnormalities to be concerned with.
B. Discuss the issue with the patient and proceed with the cardiac MRI.
C. Discuss the issue with the patient and postpone until you can discuss with the primary provider.
D. Discuss the issue with the patient and cancel the study because it is contraindicated.

2a A chest radiograph was performed for a patient in the cardiac intensive care unit to check intra-aortic balloon pump placement (below).

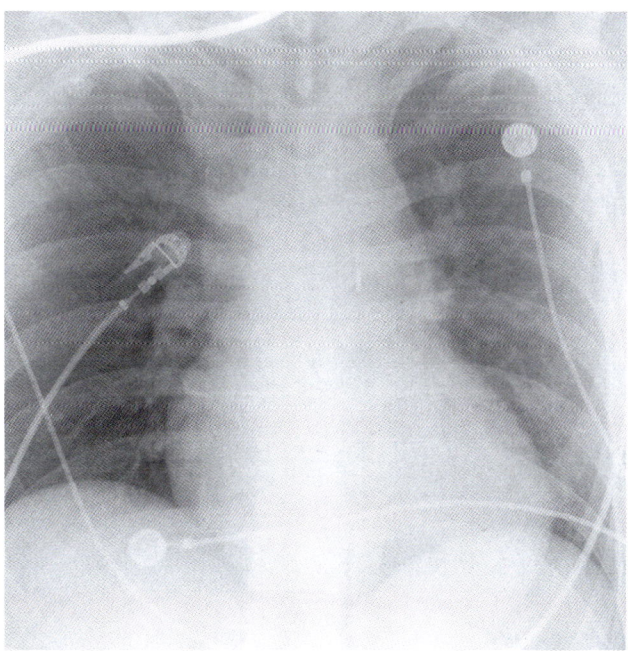

Which of the following are appropriate indications for IABP placement?
A. Aortic dissection
B. Acute tricuspid incompetence
C. Aortic insufficiency
D. Acute mitral incompetence

2b On a follow-up chest radiograph, the tip of the IABP lies just beyond the left subclavian artery. What would you recommend?
A. IABP is adequately positioned and may remain in place.
B. The IABP lies too distal and should be advanced.
C. The IABP lies too proximal and should be retracted.
D. The IABP should be removed.

3 Which of the following devices would present a contraindication to perform cardiac MR?
A. Prosthetic heart valve
B. IVC filter
C. Coronary stent
D. Implantable cardiac defibrillator

4 Which best characterizes the findings of the chest radiograph?

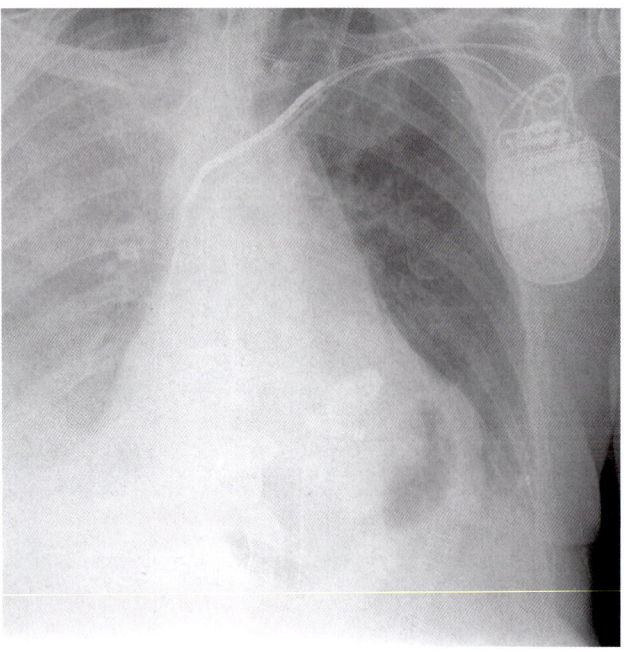

A. Pneumopericardium
B. Artificial heart
C. Mitral and tricuspid valve repair
D. Ventricular assist device

5 Patient is status post ventricular assist device implantation 8 months ago and now presents with the following CT and PET imaging:

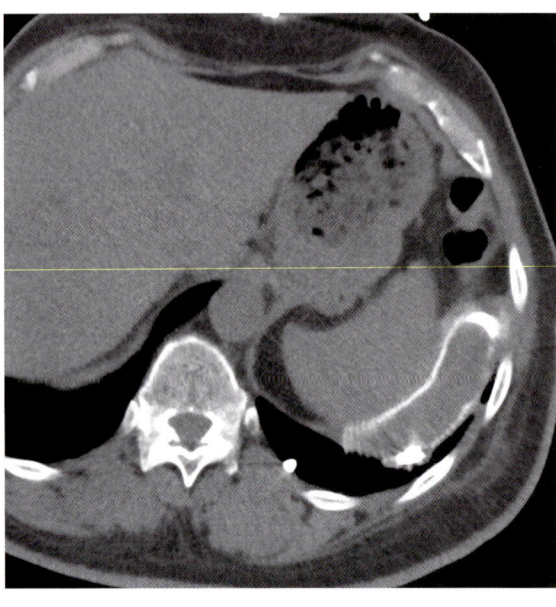
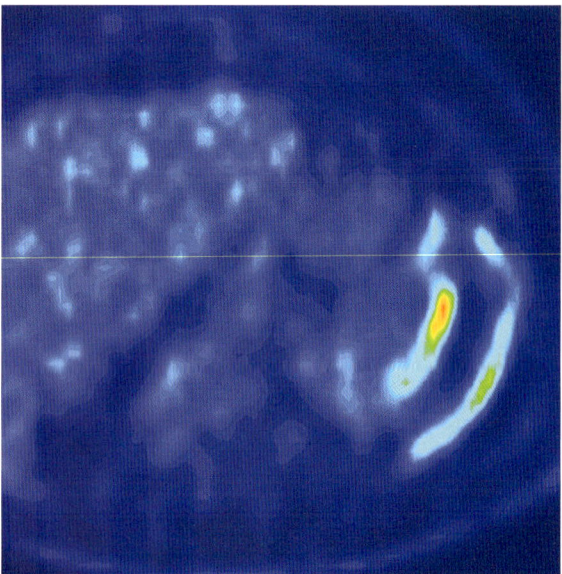

Which of the following is the most likely diagnosis?

A. LVAD infection
B. Cannula fracture
C. LVAD thrombosis
D. Normal activity

6   Patient with ventricular assist device and worsening heart failure presents with the following CT:

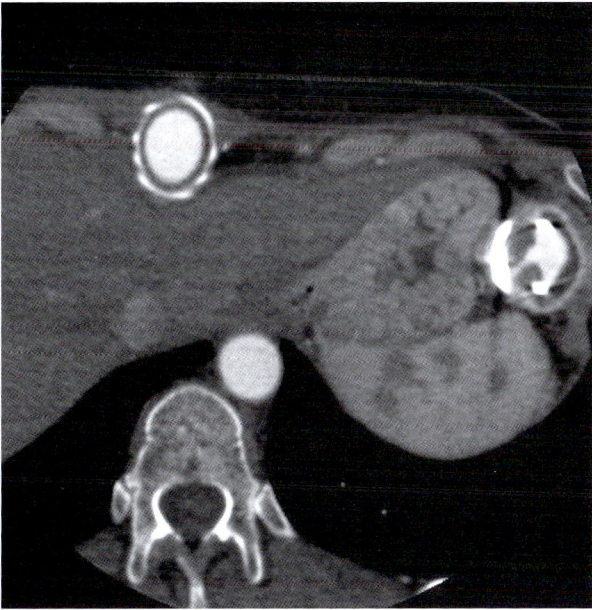

Which of the following is the best diagnosis?

A. LVAD infection
B. Cannula fracture
C. LVAD thrombosis
D. Myocardial infarction

7   A 43-year-old male has a history of ventricular tachycardia and is status post ICD placement 4 months ago now complains of chest pain.

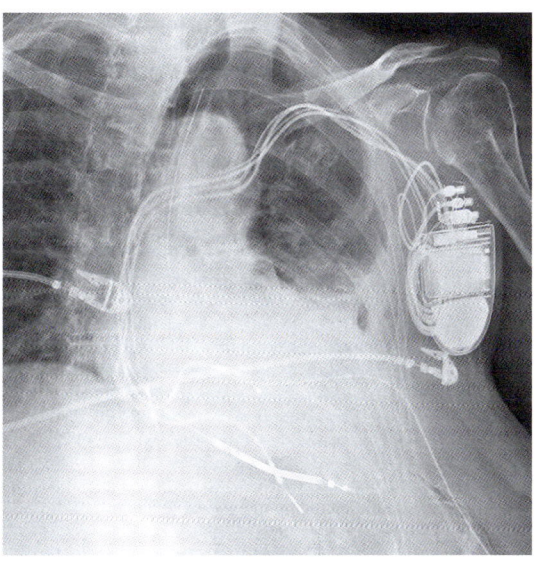 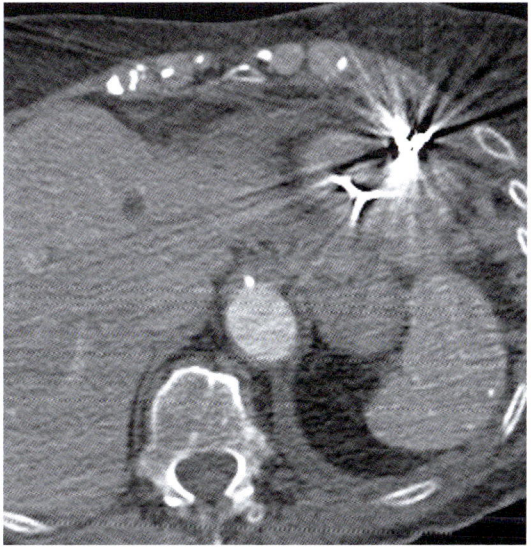

Which of the following is the most likely diagnosis?

A. Myocardial infarction
B. Lead perforation
C. Lead fracture
D. Pneumothorax

8 A radiopaque device is observed overlying the cardiac silhouette on a routine chest radiograph (below). Which of the following is the best diagnosis?

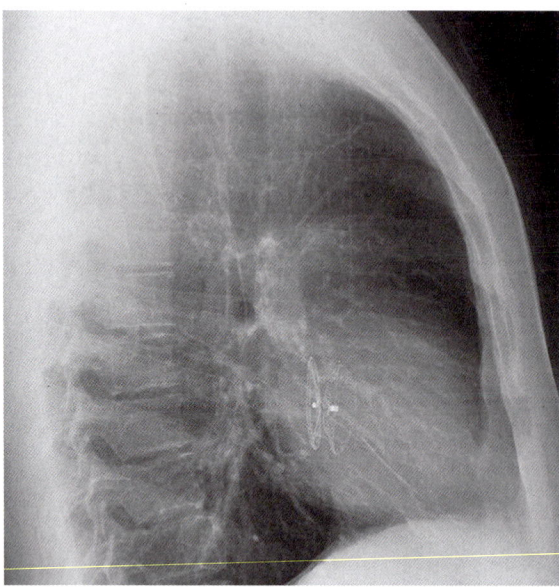

A. Atrial septal occluder
B. Displaced mitral valve
C. Atrial pacing device
D. Left atrial appendage closure

9 Characterize the chest radiograph finding.

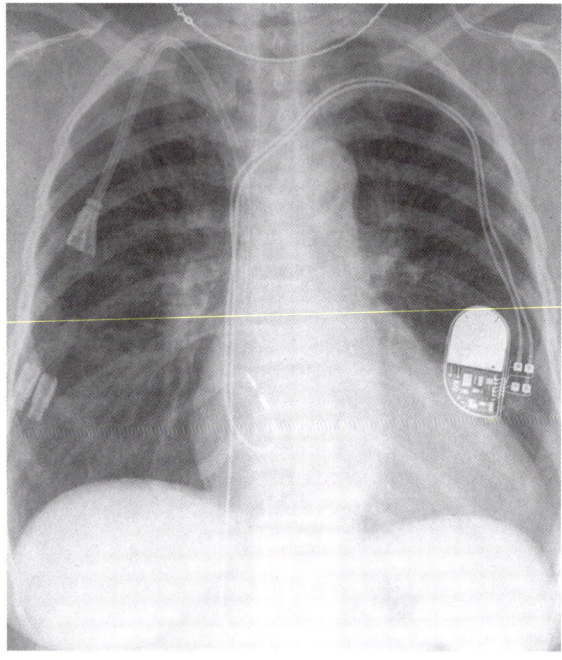

A. Misplaced right atrial lead
B. Misplaced right ventricular lead
C. Biventricular lead
D. Intentional lead placement

10 A 46-year-old female underwent recent revision of her ICD for abnormal lead positioning and failure to capture. She presents for a chest radiograph 2 months after her revision for follow-up.

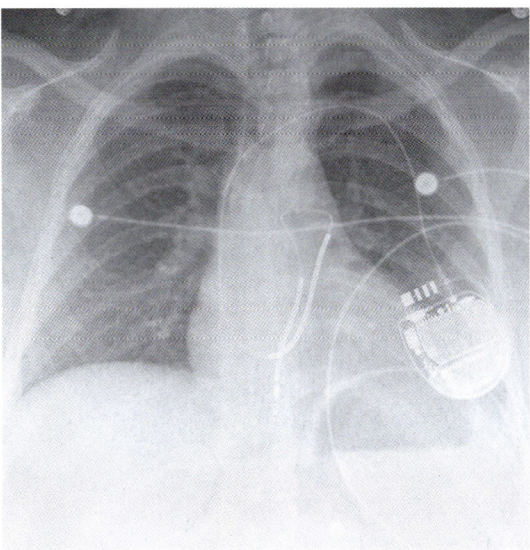

Which of the following best describes the diagnosis?

A. Persistent left SVC
B. Twiddler syndrome
C. Atrial septal defect
D. Arterial placement

11 A patient is scheduled for a brain MRI. Patient admits to a previous ICD but the device was removed over a year ago. A screening chest radiograph was performed prior to the MRI. The MRI technologist is inquiring whether the study is cleared to proceed.

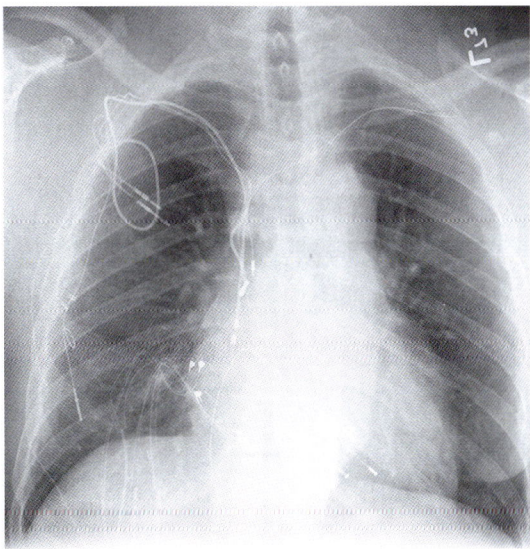

What is your recommendation based on the radiograph?

A. The x-ray is unremarkable and without abnormality.
B. Discuss the issue with the patient and proceed with the cardiac MRI.
C. Discuss the issue with the patient and postpone until you can discuss with the primary attending.
D. Discuss the issue with the patient and cancel the study because it is contraindicated.

12 Patient status post left ventricular assist device placement observed to have widening cardiac silhouette on ICU chest radiographs. A CT is performed for further evaluation.

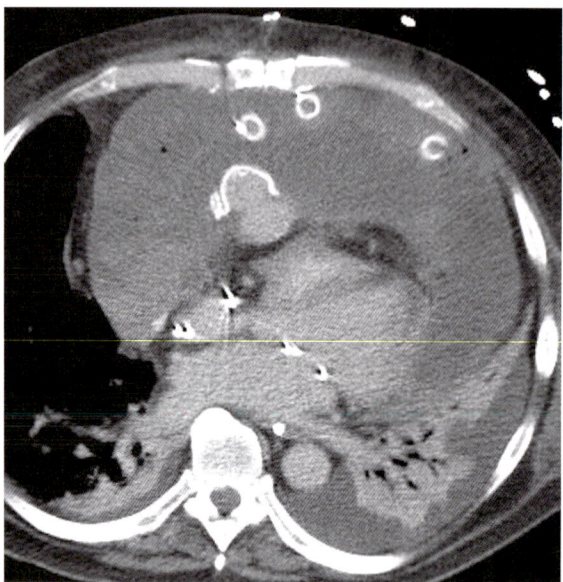

Which of the following is the most likely diagnosis?

A. Unremarkable postsurgical appearance
B. Aortic dissection
C. LV decompensation and acute heart failure
D. Mediastinal hemorrhage

13 You are asked to read these postpacemaker chest radiographs. What is the best next step?

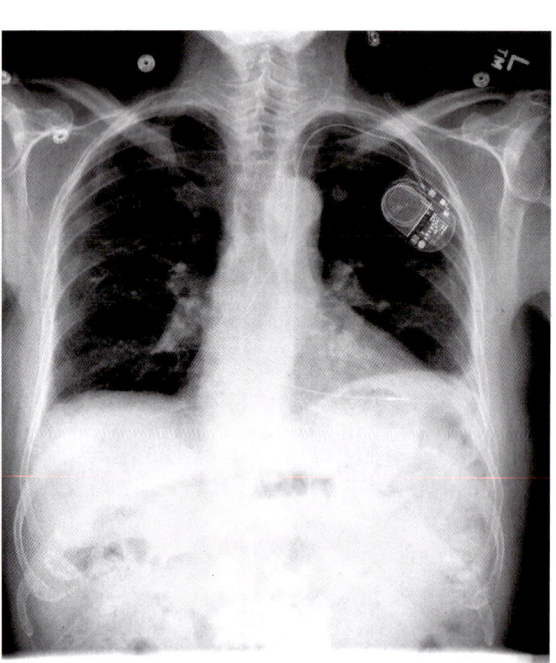
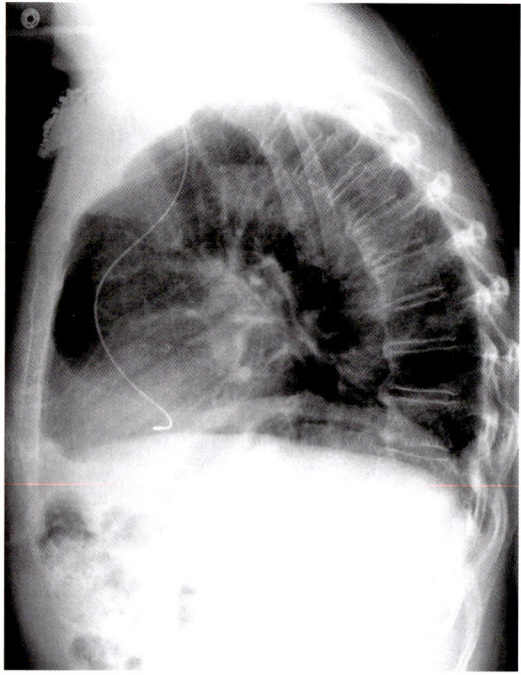

A. Nothing, pacemaker is in a left-sided SVC.
B. Ask for a CT of the chest.
C. Recommend a chest tube.
D. Recommend surgery.

14 The below patient underwent surgery to repair a Type A aortic dissection. The arrow indicates which of the following?

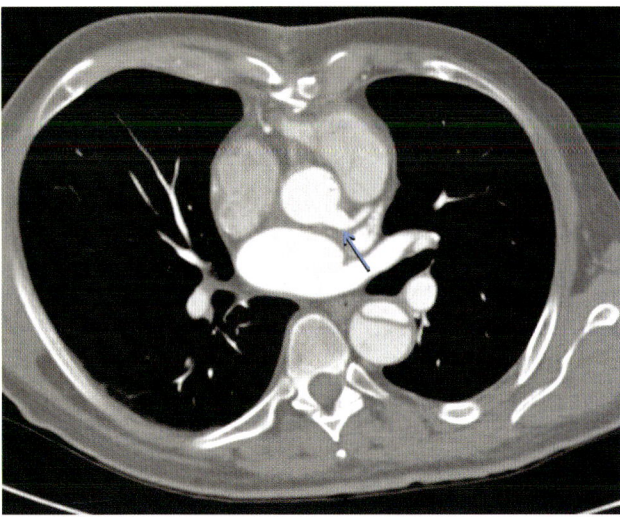

A. Aneurysm of the left main coronary artery
B. Dissection in the left main coronary artery
C. Thrombus in the left main coronary artery
D. Reimplanted left main coronary artery

15 The below images show which of the following?

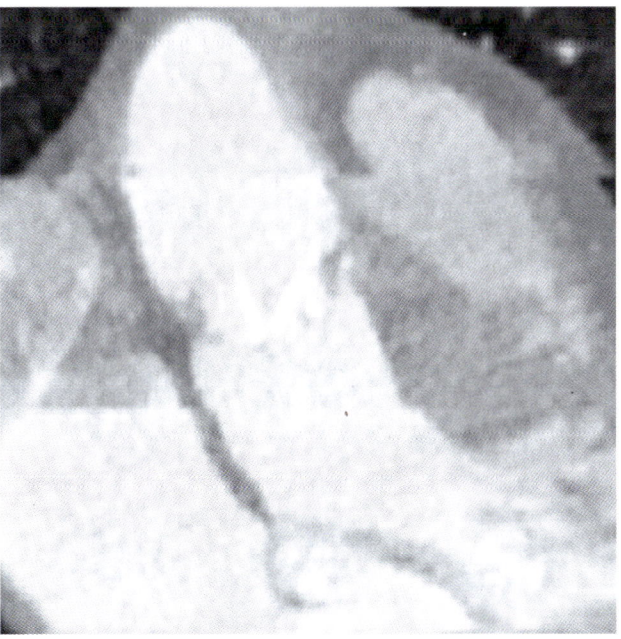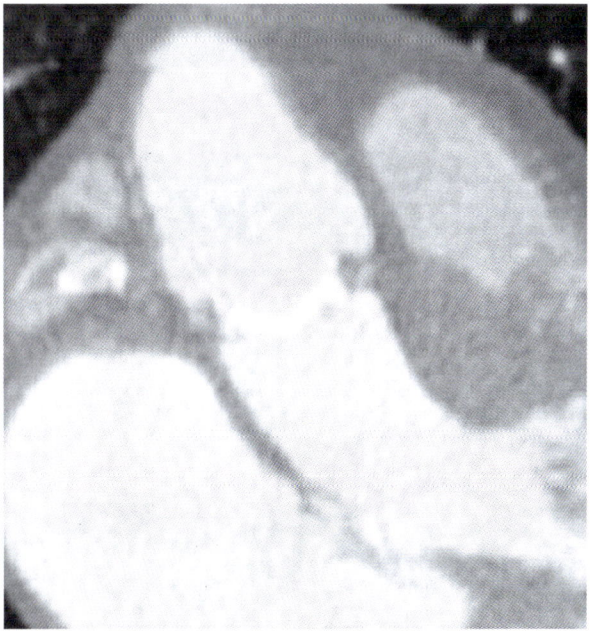

A. Aortic root dissection
B. Paravalvular leak
C. Post surgical ventriculoseptal leaflet
D. Stuck leaflet

16 The below image shows two different patients who have had what type of treatment?

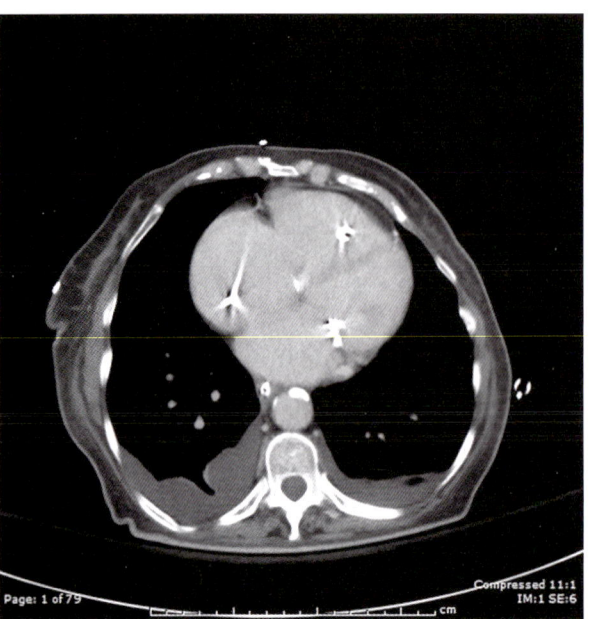
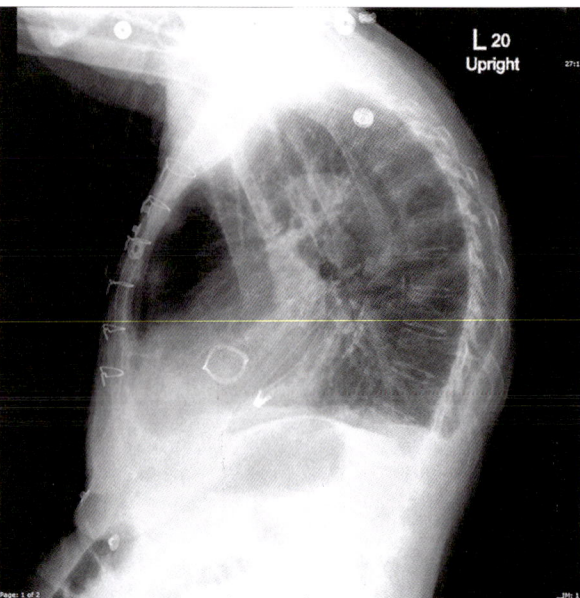

A. Mitral annuloplasty ring
B. Mitral clip
C. Mitral valve in valve
D. Mitral valve replacement

17 A patient with a history of ventricular fibrillation presents with the following chest radiograph:

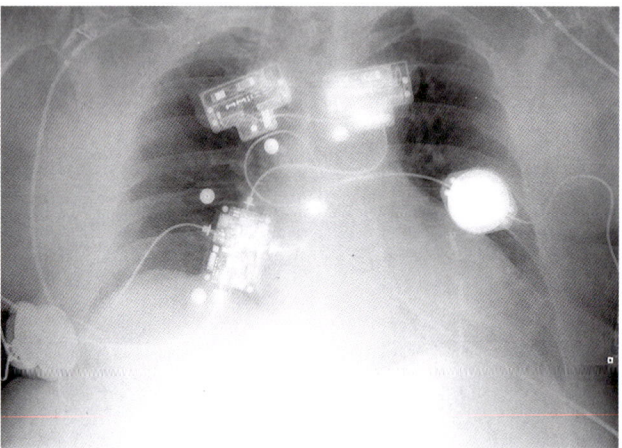

Which best characterizes the imaging findings?

A. Wearable cardioverter-defibrillator
B. Automated external defibrillator
C. Implantable cardiac device
D. Holter monitor

ANSWERS AND EXPLANATIONS

1a Answer C. The chest radiograph demonstrates a radiopaque device overlying the heart, compatible with an implantable loop recorder, and is typically contained in the anterior soft tissues of the chest.

Implantable loop recorders (ILR) are useful in detecting undiagnosed recurrent arrhythmic episodes particularly in unexplained syncope with a significantly higher diagnostic rate than other conventional tests.

ILR not only allows for prolonged monitoring without external electrodes (up to 3 years) but they also have the ability to autoactivate when an arrhythmia is present, allowing episodes to be captured independent of manual patient activation of the device. Once an episode is recorded, the memory is archived by the patient or a relative by applying a nonmagnetic handheld activator. Given prolonged electrocardiographic monitoring, loop recorders can provide more accurate correlations between a patient's symptoms and documented abnormalities in heart rhythm.

Reference: Subbiah RN, Gula LJ, Klein GJ, et al. Ambulatory monitoring (Holter, event recorders, external, and implantable loop recorders and wireless technology). In: *Electrical diseases of the heart*. 2008: 344–352.

1b Answer B. Studies investigating the effect of scanning implantable loop recorders (ILR) in an MRI environment demonstrate no significant translational movement or dislodgement of ILRs in relation to exposure to long-bore and short-bore 1.5 T MRI systems. Thus, MRI scanning of ILR patients can be performed without harm to the patient or device. However, artifacts that could be mistaken for a tachyarrhythmia are seen frequently and should not be interpreted as pathology.

References: Shellock FG, Tkach JA, Ruggieri PM, et al. Cardiac pacemakers, ICDs, and loop recorder: evaluation of translational attraction using conventional ("long-bore") and "short-bore" 1.5 and 3.0 tesla MRI systems: safety. *J Cardiovasc Magn Reson* 2003;5(2):387–397.

Wong JA, Yee R, Gula LJ, et al. Feasibility of magnetic resonance imaging in patients with an implantable loop recorder. *Pacing Clin Electrophysiol* 2008;31(3):333–337.

2a Answer D. The chest radiograph demonstrates an intra-aortic balloon pump with its tip terminating in the descending thoracic aorta, adequately placed.

Intra-aortic balloon pumps (IABP), initially introduced in the 1960s, remain the most widely used form of mechanical circulatory support for patients with critical cardiac disease. As the IABP balloon expands, the volume displacement of blood, which occurs both proximally and distally in the ascending and proximal descending aorta, is termed "counterpulsation." Effectively, balloon inflation in diastole and then rapid deflation in systole results in a decrease in systolic blood pressure and an increase in diastolic pressure. The result is afterload reduction in systole and augmentation of aortic root and coronary artery pressure in diastole, when coronary perfusion pressure is maximal.

The available clinical evidence supports intra-aortic balloon pump placement in cases of cardiogenic shock or refractory angina. Other indications such as mechanical complications of myocardial infarction (i.e., acute mitral regurgitation and ventricular septal defect), intractable arrhythmia, and refractory heart failure are less common, yet generally accepted indications for IABP support.

IABP placement is contraindicated in patients with aortic insufficiency because it worsens the magnitude of regurgitation. IABP insertion should not be attempted in case of suspected or known aortic dissection because inadvertent balloon placement in the false lumen may result in extension of the dissection or even aortic rupture. Similarly, aortic rupture can occur if IABP is inserted in patients with sizable abdominal aortic aneurysms. Patients with end-stage cardiac disease should not be considered for IABP unless as a bridge to ventricular assist device or cardiac transplantation.

References: Tsagalou EP, Drakos SG, Tsolakis E, et al. Intraaortic balloon pump in the management of acute heart failure syndromes. In: Mebazaa A, Gheorghiade M, Zannad FM (eds.). *Acute heart failure*. London: Springer London, 2008:671–683.

White JM, Ruygrok PN. Intra-aortic balloon counterpulsation in contemporary practice—where are we? *Heart Lung Circulation* 2015;24(4):335–341.

2b Answer C. IABP placement is important for successful diastolic augmentation of coronary perfusion. The IABP catheter is inserted percutaneously into the femoral artery through an introducer sheath with a modified Seldinger technique. Once vascular access is obtained, the balloon catheter is inserted and advanced, usually under fluoroscopic guidance, into the proximal descending thoracic aorta, with its radiopaque tip 2 to 3 cm distal to the origin of the left subclavian artery (at the level of the carina).

If the tip is too proximally placed, the balloon may obstruct the great vessels of the aortic arch. If the tip is too distally placed, then the IABP may not be effective enough in increasing coronary blood flow and may also obstruct the splanchnic vessels.

References: Krishna M, Zacharowski K. Principles of intra-aortic balloon pump counterpulsation. *Continuing Educ Anaesthesia Crit Care Pain* 2009;9(1):24–28.

White JM, Ruygrok PN. Intra-aortic balloon counterpulsation in contemporary practice—where are we? *Heart Lung Circulation* 2015;24(4):335–341.

3 Answer D. Patients have to be carefully screened to exclude ferromagnetic implants or ferromagnetic foreign bodies due to effects of the magnetic field. Implantable devices are generally categorized as "MRI safe," meaning they are safe under any, even future, MRI conditions; "MRI conditional," meaning that the implant is safe under certain conditions, which have to be specified in detail for any given device; and "MRI unsafe" which includes any item that is known to pose hazards in all MRI environments.

Passive implants may interact mainly with the main magnetic field (force and torque effects) and RF field, which may induce heating. Most of currently implanted stents, heart valves, sternal wires, cardiac closure, occluder devices, filters, embolization coils, and screws are MRI conditional. Most tested implanted coils, filters, stents, and grafts are unlikely to move or become dislodged as a result of exposure to MRI systems operating at 3 tesla (T) or less. It is unnecessary to wait an extended period of time after surgery to perform an MRI procedure in a patient with a "passive" metallic implant that is made from a nonferromagnetic material. However, new coils, stents, filters, and vascular grafts are developed on an ongoing basis, and attention to the manufacturer's product information or reference manuals is always recommended.

The majority of coronary stents, aortic endografts, and IVC filters are made from nonferromagnetic or weakly ferromagnetic materials. It is generally believed that additional anchoring of these implants into vessel walls occur over 6 to 8 weeks, primarily due to tissue ingrowth. All passive implants, which are nonferromagnetic, may undergo MRI procedures at 3 T or less at any time after implantation. Any implant, which is weakly ferromagnetic, should be scanned preferably 6 weeks after implantation and should be weighed on a case-by-case basis.

The Zenith AAA endovascular graft stent demonstrates high magnetic forces and has been labeled as "MRI unsafe."

Active implants may react on the different electromagnetic fields of an MRI unit, and safety evaluations are much more complicated. Implantable cardioverter-defibrillators (ICDs) are among these devices. ICDs contain metal with variable ferromagnetic qualities, as well as complex electrical systems, and additionally consist of one or several leads implanted into the myocardium. There is potential for movement of the device, programming changes, asynchronous pacing, activation of tachyarrhythmia therapies, inhibition of pacing output, and induced lead currents that could lead to heating and cardiac stimulation.

Current recommendations consider the presence of a pacemaker or ICD a strong relative contraindication to routine MRI examination. Alternative diagnostic tests should be primarily considered, and MR imaging should only be considered when there is a strong clinical indication and in which the potential benefit to the patient clearly outweighs the risks to the patient.

Reference: Levine GN, Gomes AS, Arai AE, et al. Safety of magnetic resonance imaging in patients with cardiovascular devices: an American Heart Association Scientific Statement From the Committee on Diagnostic and Interventional Cardiac Catheterization, Council on Clinical Cardiology, and the Council on Cardiovascular Radiology and Intervention: endorsed by the American College of Cardiology Foundation, the North American Society for Cardiac Imaging, and the Society for Cardiovascular Magnetic Resonance. *Circulation* 2007;116(24):2878-2891.

4   Answer B.   The radiograph demonstrates sternotomy from cardiac surgery and well-circumscribed areas of lucency in the region of the ventricles, which correlate with the ventricular bellows of a total artificial heart. Prosthetic valves are also observed, which are anastomosed to the native atria.

The total artificial heart (TAH) is a biventricular mechanical assist device that is implanted following definitive explantation of the patients failing ventricles. The duration of implantation varies depending on a particular patient's medical condition and the eventual availability of a human heart for orthotopic transplantation. Contraindications for implantation included chronic cardiac cachexia, advanced physiologic age, chronic failure of end organs incompatible with recovery, anticipated to be impossible to recover to transplant candidate status, and judged to have inadequate mediastinal size for the TAH.

Chest radiography is routinely used immediately after TAH implantation, during hospitalization, and until the time of orthotopic transplant to assess the device and monitor for complications. Similar to the case presented here, four mechanical valves are positioned in nonanatomic locations. Air-filled right and left ventricular spaces may mimic the appearance of intracavitary air, pneumomediastinum, pneumopericardium, and abscess.

The TAH is associated with a low but significant risk of thrombosis. As soon as hemostasis allows it, patients need to be placed on a stringent anticoagulation regimen. Postoperative hemothorax or hemomediastinum also occurs in a high percentage of TAH recipients. The need for anticoagulation also increases risk for extrathoracic hemorrhage, including subarachnoid or spontaneous retroperitoneal hemorrhage.

References: Copeland JG, Copeland H, Gustafson M, et al. Experience with more than 100 total artificial heart implants. *J Thorac Cardiovas Surg* 2012;143(3):727-734.

Parker MS, Fahrner LJ, Deuell BP, et al. Total artificial heart implantation: clinical indications, expected postoperative imaging findings, and recognition of complications. *AJR Am J Roentgenol* 2014;202(3):W191-W201.

5   Answer A.   Noncontrast CT demonstrates mild fluid surrounding the outflow cannula that subsequently shows increased metabolic activity on PET imaging. The findings are very suggestive of infection.

The development of left ventricular assist devices (LVADs), first as a bridge to transplant and then as destination therapy, has significantly improved survival and quality of life of patients with end-stage heart failure.

LVAD infections remain among the most frequently encountered adverse events and often lead to significant morbidity and mortality. LVAD-specific infections may be of the hardware itself or the body surfaces that contain them and include infections of the pump, cannula, anastomoses, pocket infections, and the percutaneous driveline or tunnel. Percutaneous driveline infections are the most commonly occurring infections in LVAD patients and may reflect the presence of a deeper infection of the pocket space or pump and/or cannula.

LVAD-related infections include infectious endocarditis, mediastinitis, and sternal wound infection. Evaluation with CT may reveal large valve vegetations and cannula insertion infections. CT may also play a role in characterizing sternal wound infections, particularly to define the extent of deep-seated infection or collection.

References: Hannan MM, Husain S, Mattner F, et al. Working formulation for the standardization of definitions of infections in patients using ventricular assist devices. *J Heart Lung Transpl* 2011;30(4):375-384.

Lima B, Mack M, Gonzalez-Stawinski GV. Ventricular assist devices: the future is now. *Trends Cardiovasc Med* 2015;25(4):360-369.

6 **Answer C.** Axial image from a cardiac CT demonstrates the inflow (left) and outflow (right) cannulas of a ventricular assist device inferior to the base of the heart. Thrombus is observed obstructing the outflow cannula.

The development of left ventricular assist devices (LVADs), first as a bridge to transplant and then as destination therapy, has significantly improved survival and quality of life of patients with end-stage heart failure.

LVAD thrombosis occurs in 2% to 13% of adult patients with a continuous-flow LVAD. This thrombus may form as an acute event or insidiously over a prolonged period of time. Thrombus in the left ventricle, inflow cannula, pump housing, outflow cannula, outflow graft, or aortic root may produce devastating events that include thromboembolic stroke, peripheral thromboembolism, LVAD malfunction with reduced systemic flows, LVAD failure with life-threatening hemodynamic impairment, cardiogenic shock, and death.

For this reason, patients are placed on anticoagulation therapy with warfarin and antiplatelet therapy with aspirin.

Two types of thrombi may develop in an LVAD. Red thrombus forms as stagnating blood coagulates under low pressure. In contrast, white thrombus constructed primarily from activated platelets forms in areas of turbulence. The distinction between the types of thrombi is critical as red thrombi are best treated with anticoagulation, whereas white thrombi are better managed with antiplatelet agents.

An echocardiographic "ramp study" is performed for diagnostic confirmation, whereby stepwise increases to maximal pump speeds fail to elicit complementary augmentation in pump flow. While variable success with thrombolytic therapy has been reported, definitive treatment usually entails operative pump exchange.

The sensitivity of echocardiography surpasses CT to diagnose LVAD thrombus, especially if three-dimensional echocardiography is available. Yet, echocardiography may fail to diagnose LVAD thrombosis, and cases have been described in which CT, but not echocardiography, identified LVAD thrombus. In addition, CT is not limited by acoustic windows and shadowing. Consequently, when suspicion for LVAD thrombosis is high, a negative imaging study should prompt further investigation with additional techniques.

The definitive therapy for LVAD thrombosis is explanation of the device and cardiac transplantation. Unfortunately, the immediate availability of a compatible donor heart leaves this option as a last resort.

References: Bartoli CR, Ailawadi G, Kern JA. Diagnosis, nonsurgical management, and prevention of LVAD thrombosis: LVAD thrombosis. *J Cardiac Surg* 2014;29(1):83-94.

Lima B, Mack M, Gonzalez-Stawinski GV. Ventricular assist devices: the future is now. *Trends Cardiovasc Med* 2015;25(4):360-369.

7 Answer B. Portable AP radiograph demonstrates multiple implanted cardiac leads, which tips overly the right ventricle. Further evaluation by CT demonstrates that the tip has migrated beyond the myocardium and terminates outside the heart.

Cardiac perforation after pacemaker or implantable cardioverter–defibrillator (ICD) implantation is an infrequent complication, more frequently seen in the right ventricle but also in the right atrium. Cardiac perforations may present as acute (events occurring within 24 hours after implantation), subacute (occurring 5 days to 1 month after implantation), or delayed manifestations (occurring more than 1 month after implantation).

The most common symptom is pacing or sensing failure. If a lead perforates the myocardium, capture threshold will be increased and sensing threshold will be reduced in general. In some asymptomatic patients with delayed perforation, pacemaker function and electrophysiologic parameters appear normal and thus cannot exclude cardiac perforation. Hemodynamic stability is mainly determined by the development of hemopericardium.

Sharp chest pain during the insertion, evidence of cardiac tamponade with breathlessness, raised jugular venous pressure, falling systemic blood pressure, and cyanosis, is suggestive of hemopericardium that requires emergency pericardiocentesis and possibly cardiac surgical repair. Echocardiography or computed tomography should confirm hemopericardium and may even show the electrode tip in the pericardial space. Signs and symptoms of pericarditis, including a pericardial friction rub, are also suggestive.

References: Oh S. Cardiac perforation associated with a pacemaker or ICD lead. In: Das M (ed.). *Modern pacemakers—present and future*. InTech, 2011.

Ramsdale DR, Rao A. *Complications of pacemaker implantation. Cardiac pacing and device therapy*. London: Springer London, 2012:249-282.

8 Answer A. The radiograph demonstrates the radiopaque septal occlude in parallel to the interatrial septum.

Patent foramen ovale (PFO) is the most frequent congenital defect of the atrial septum found in approximately 20% to 30% of adults. Anatomically, the foramen ovale corresponds to an opening between the embryologic septum primum and septum secundum interatrial membranes. In some individuals, there is failure to fuse of primum and secundum septa, and there is significant variability in the resultant anatomy. In combination with predisposing morphologic and hemodynamic conditions, this remnant interatrial communication promotes thromboembolic events, which have been linked to cryptogenic stroke, systemic hypoxemia, and migraine headaches.

Transcatheter closure of PFO has proven to be a very safe and effective technique with high success and low complication rates. More than a dozen device designs have been used to percutaneous close PFOs.

Complications though infrequent are serious and include cardiac perforation or air embolization during implantation, induced atrial fibrillation, nonspecific malaise attributed to nickel allergy, and puncture site problems.

References: Franke J, Wunderlich N, Bertog SC, et al. Patent foramen ovale closure. In: Lanzer P (ed.). *Catheter-based cardiovascular interventions*. Berlin, Heidelberg: Springer Berlin Heidelberg, 2013:679-685.

Rohrhoff N, Vavalle JP, Halim S, et al. Current status of percutaneous PFO closure. *Curr Cardiol Rep* 2014;16(5).

9 Answer B. The right ventricular lead from a dual-chamber pacemaker is observed coursing below the diaphragm, terminating in the IVC.

Lead dislodgement is a change in an implantable cardioverter-defibrillator (ICD) lead tip position leading to changes in electrical lead parameters. Although this complication is currently less frequent, due to improvement in lead technology, it still remains one of the most frequent complications of ICD implantation.

Lead dislodgement may be radiographically visible, or there may be microdisplacement, where there is no radiographic change in position, but there is significant increase in pacing threshold and/or decline in the electrocardiogram amplitude.

Displacement can be suspected when stimulation detection abnormalities are observed on telemetry or postimplantation ECG, manifested by a sudden raise in stimulation or detection thresholds. Other manifestations include oversensing that can cause prolonged asystole in pacemaker-dependent patients. In case of implantable defibrillators, it can cause inappropriate shocks or lack of shock delivery.

Reference: Pescariu S, Sosdean R. Complications of cardiac implantable electronic devices (CIED). In: Kibos AS, Knight BP, Essebag V (eds.). *Cardiac arrhythmias*. London: Springer London, 2014:639-651.

10 Answer B. The chest radiograph demonstrates coiling and migration of the ICD lead tips, consistent with Twiddler syndrome.

Twiddler syndrome is an uncommon complication of device implantation with a frequency of 0.07% to 7%. It occurs when the device rotates in the pocket and the leads coil around the generator. It is usually a painless phenomenon and may occur spontaneously or by willful manipulation by the patient.

Twiddler syndrome is more common in the elderly, presumably due to the laxity of their subcutaneous tissues. The disorder may induce lead dislodgment or lead fracture and cause life-threatening symptoms in case of pacemaker dependency. Lead displacement can also produce muscle stimulation or phrenic/brachial plexus stimulation.

Treatment consists in pocket revision and suturing the device to the pectoral muscle or placing the generator subpectorally. Sometimes, replacement of the leads or entire pacemaker system will be necessary.

References: Bhatia V, Kachru R, Parida AK, et al. Twiddler's syndrome. *Int J Cardiol* 2007;116(3):e82. PMID: 17097169.

Ramsdale DR, Rao A. *Complications of pacemaker implantation. Cardiac pacing and device therapy*. London: Springer London, 2012:249-282.

11 Answer D. Multiple abandoned leads are observed on the chest radiograph, disconnected from previous implanted generators.

Abandoned leads do not normally pose a clinically significant additional risk of complication in patients with ICDs. Therefore, a strategy of abandoning nonfunctioning leads is reasonable, and lead extractions should be reserved for cases with system infection or high lead burden.

However, in the setting of MRI, abandoned and pacemaker-attached leads show resonant heating behavior, and maximum heating occurs at different lead lengths due to the differences in termination conditions. For clinical lead lengths (40 to 60 cm), abandoned leads actually exhibit greater lead tip heating compared with pacemaker-attached leads. Therefore, patients with abandoned leads are potentially at a greater risk for RF-induced thermal damage due to MRI exposure.

Reference: Langman DA, Goldberg IB, Finn JP, et al. Pacemaker lead tip heating in abandoned and pacemaker-attached leads at 1.5 tesla MRI. *J Magn Reson Imaging* 2011;33(2):426-431.

12 Answer D. Contrast CT of the chest demonstrates a large and heterogeneous collection in the anterior mediastinum with mass effect on the surrounding mediastinal structures. A portion of the inflow cannula from the LVAD is observed. Multiple mediastinal drains are also in place.

Left ventricular assist devices (LVADs) have become a valuable therapeutic option in the management of advanced systolic heart failure.

Approximately 20% to 30% of patients who get ventricular assist devices will have excessive bleeding subsequently leading to reoperation. Mechanisms responsible for these adverse events include acquired von Willebrand disease, GI tract angiodysplasia formation, impaired platelet aggregation, and overuse of anticoagulation therapy.

Data from the Interagency Registry for Mechanically Assisted Circulatory Support (INTERMACS) have shown the most frequent locations of first bleeding episode after implantation to be mediastinal (45%), thoracic pleural space (12%), lower GI tract (10%), chest wall (8%), and upper GI tract (8%), with no difference in the overall bleeding rates between axial- and pulsatile-flow devices.

References: Jessup M, Goldstein D, Ascheim D, et al. Risk for bleeding after MCSD implant: an analysis of 2358 patients in INTERMACS. *J Heart Lung Transpl* 2011;30(4):S9.

Suarez J, Patel CB, Felker GM, et al. Mechanisms of bleeding and approach to patients with axial-flow left ventricular assist devices. *Circulation* 2011;4(6):779-784.

13 Answer B. Single-lead pacemaker has an abnormal course. It appears to course directly down the aortic arch and the ascending aorta. Of all the choices offered, a CT of the chest is most helpful to further define the course. CT later shows the pacemaker coursing through the left subclavian artery and through the aortic root to end up in the LV apex. A left-sided SVC would be more posterior in course as it goes through the coronary sinus. There is no pneumothorax to warrant a chest tube. Definitive diagnosis of lead malposition should be done before recommending surgery.

References: Bauersfeld UK, Thakur RK, Ghani M, et al. Malposition of transvenous pacing lead in the left ventricle: radiographic findings. *AJR Am J Roentgenol* 1994;162(2):290-292. PubMed PMID: 8310911.

Mazzetti H, Dussaut A, Tentori C, et al. Transarterial permanent pacing of the left ventricle. *Pacing Clin Electrophysiol* 1990;13(5):588-592. PubMed PMID: 1693195.

14 Answer D. The image shows a dissection in the descending thoracic aorta. The left main coronary artery has been reimplanted. The implanted coronary artery has a bulbous origin secondary to a coronary button procedure. In the button procedure a segment of the native aorta is used to attach the aortic graft in the root, creating a slightly enlarged origin.

Reference: Platis IE, Kopf GS, Dwar MS, et al. Composite graft with coronary button reimplantation: procedure of choice for aortic root replacement. *Int J Angiol* 1998;7(1):41-45.

15 Answer D. The image shows a patient who has undergone aortic valve repair with a St. Jude type valve. The valve leaflets are closed during ventricular diastole, however, during systole, only one of the leaflets open, the other is stuck/frozen. The leaflet may be frozen secondary to tissue material at the valve attachment.

Reference: Chen JJ, Mannin MA, Frazier AA, et al. CT angiography of the cardiac valves: normal, diseased, and postoperative appearances. *Radiographics* 2009;29(5):1393-1412.

16 Answer B. The patient has undergone percutaneous treatment for mitral valve regurgitation with one the newest form of treatment, a mitral clip. Patients who have severe mitral regurgitation due to degenerative mitral valve disease may be candidates for the procedure. The clip is placed via a percutaneous approach and the valve is deployed creating a functional bicuspid mitral valve with two openings allowing for blood to transit through the mitral valve.

Reference: Yuksel UC, Kapadia SR, Tuzcu EM. Percutaneous mitral repair: patient selection, results, and future directions. *Curr Cardiol Rep* 2011;13(2):100-106. doi: 10.1007/211886-010-0158-x.

17 Answer A. The chest radiograph demonstrates multiple electrodes that overlie the chest and monitor cardiac activity. These are actually on the back of the patient, and together, they comprise a wearable cardioverter-defibrillator.

The wearable cardioverter-defibrillator (WCD) is an external device for patients who are at significant risk for sudden cardiac arrest, but are not immediate candidates for ICD implantation. It is comprised of two main components: (1) an electrode belt and garment that surrounds the patient's chest and (2) a monitor that the patient wears around the waist or from a shoulder strap. The battery, defibrillator, and response buttons are attached to the belt of the system.

The device monitors the patient's heart continuously, and if the patient goes into a life-threatening arrhythmia, the WCD delivers a shock treatment to restore the patient's heart to normal rhythm. Besides defibrillation, the device acts as a loop recorder that continuously records and transmits via modem both tachyarrhythmias and bradyarrhythmias.

Reference: Adler A, Halkin A, Viskin S. Wearable cardioverter-defibrillators. *Circulation* 2013;127(7):854-860.

INDEX

A

Acute coronary syndrome, negative remodeling, 56, 63
Acute myocardial infarction
　with cardiogenic shock, 58, 64
　myocardial infarction, 58, 64
Amyloidosis, 73, 88
Anatomic structure
　anterolateral papillary muscle, 23, 31
　membranous septum, 21, 30-31
　middle cardiac vein, 20, 29
　obtuse marginal, 21, 30
　pericardium, 20, 29
Annulus and sinotubular junction, 16, 27
Anterior wall, delayed enhancement sequence, 54, 62
Anterolateral papillary muscle, anatomic structure, 23, 31
Aortic dissection, 184, 195, 201, 209-210
Aortic insufficiency, 36, 41, 45, 49, 163, 177
Aortic regurgitation, 185, 196
Aortic root, 15, 27
Aortic wall, 185, 196
Arch abnormality, 192, 198
Arrhythmias, 165, 169, 178, 179
Arrhythmogenic right ventricular dysplasia (ARVD), 67, 77, 81, 92
Arteriovenous malformation, 189, 197
Artifact, incorrect velocity map, 36, 45
ARVD. *See* Arrhythmogenic right ventricular dysplasia (ARVD)
ASD. *See* Atrial septal defects (ASD)
Atherosclerosis, 181, 194
Atherosclerotic plaque, 52, 61
Atrial fibrillation, 40, 47
Atrial septal defects (ASD)
　sinus venosus ASD, 154, 173
　types of, 155, 174
Atrial systole, 34, 43
Atrioventricular groove, 19, 29

B

Beta-blockers, 2, 7, 51, 61
Body mass index (BMI), 5, 11, 52, 62
Bolus geometry, 4, 9
Brachiocephalic vein, 15, 27
Bypass grafting, 53, 62

C

Calcium score, 52, 61
Cardiac arrhythmia, 40, 47
Cardiac CTA (CCTA)
　abnormal nuclear medicine stress test, 37, 38, 45-46
　body mass index (BMI), 5, 11
　cardiac cycle, 5, 11
　flow-limiting stenosis, 38, 46
　intravenous beta blockers, 36, 45
　metoprolol, 34, 43
　obstructed pulmonary vein, 41, 49
　open mitral valve, 32, 42
　reduce radiation dose, 32, 42
　reducing kVp, 32, 42
　renal insufficiency, 6, 11
　sublingual nitroglycerin (SL-NTG), 38, 46, 50, 61
Cardiac masses
　anticoagulation, 97, 114
　atrial fibrillation, 99, 115
　atrial wall mass, 103, 116
　cardiac angiosarcoma, 106, 117
　cardiac fibroma, 105, 117
　cardiac MRI, 113, 119
　Carney complex, multiple myxomas, 104, 116
　central line placement, 110, 119
　chest pain
　　catheter angiography, 100, 115
　　right heart border, 101, 115
　contrast-enhanced CTA, 112, 119
　echinococcus infection, 111, 119
　fossa ovalis, sparing of, 103, 116
　interatrial septum, 106, 117
　left atrial appendage, 98, 114
　left atrium, 107, 117
　left ventricle abnormality, 104, 117
　left ventricular cavity, 97, 114
　left ventricular thrombus, 99, 114
　lymphoma, 110, 118
　metastasis, 99, 115
　metastatic lung cancer, 100, 115
　noncoronary and left coronary cusp, 108, 117
　pericardium, 109, 118
　renal angiomyolipomas, 109, 118
　rhabdomyoma, 104, 117
　right atrial mass, 102, 116
　right coronary artery, 112, 119
　right pericardial cyst, 101, 116
　short tau inversion recovery (STIR), 104, 116
　thrombus, 98, 108, 114, 117
　transient ischemic attack, 109, 117
　transthoracic echocardiogram, 99, 114
Cardiac MRI (CMRI)
　angular phase shift, 34, 44
　aortic insufficiency, 41, 49
　categories, 6, 11
　cavity size, 40, 48
　ejection fraction, 40, 47
　magnitude image and phase velocity map, 36, 45
　mitral valve and aortic valve, 3, 9
　morphologic changes in heart, 41, 49
　myocardial mass, 40, 47-48
　myocardial scar formation, 3, 9
　pressure gradient, 35, 44
　Qp/Qs, 37, 45-46
　scan parameters, 6, 11
　sequence, 3, 8
　temporal resolution, 3, 9
　zone 2, 5, 10
Cardiac support devices, 58, 64
Cardiac valve
　brachiocephalic vein, 15, 27
　mitral valve, 12, 24
　pulmonic, 13, 25
　thebesian, 13, 25
Cardiomyopathy
　AICD, 71, 85-86
　amyloidosis, 73, 80, 88, 95
　arrhythmogenic right ventricular dysplasia (ARVD), 67, 81
　conduction abnormalities, 75, 90
　constrictive pericarditis (CP), 68, 82-83
　Danon disease, 78, 94-95
　dilated cardiomyopathies (DCM), 74, 88-89
　early (E-wave) and late (A-wave) transmitral velocities, 78, 94
　FDG-PET images, 78, 95
　granulocytic sarcoma, 75, 91
　heart transplantation, 80, 95-96
　hemochromatosis, 70, 84
　hypertrophic cardiomyopathy (HCM), 68, 82
　left ventricular noncompaction, 69, 83
　loeffler endocarditis, 72, 86-87
　megacolon, 77, 93
　MR sequence, 75, 92
　myocardial T2*, 75, 92
　myocarditis, 69, 74, 83-84, 89
　nonischemic dilated cardiomyopathy, 73, 87
　pericardial effusions and myocarditis, 77, 93
　peripartum/postpartum cardiomyopathy (PPCM), 77, 94
　and peripheral eosinophilia, 72, 86-87
　premature ventricular complexes (PVCs), 76, 92
　restrictive cardiomyopathy, 72, 87
　RV wall, 79, 95
　severe aortic stenosis, 71, 85
　Staphylococcus infection, 67, 81-82
　stress-induced cardiomyopathy, 70, 85-86
　T2* relaxation, 75, 92
　ventricular compliance and diastolic volume, 75, 91
　ventricular noncompaction, 74, 90

CCTA. *See* Cardiac CTA (CCTA)
Chronic Chagas heart disease, 77, 93
Circumflex coronary artery, 37, 45-46
CMRI. *See* Cardiac MRI (CMRI)
Codominant anatomy, 12, 24
Conduction abnormalities, 75, 90
Congenital heart disease
   abnormal vertical linear opacity, 156, 174
   anomalous pulmonary venous, 156, 174
   aortic insufficiency, 163, 177
   arrhythmias, 165, 169, 178, 179
   arterial switch, 160, 176
   atrial fibrillation, 158, 175
   atrial septal defects (ASD), 153, 155, 173, 174
   bronchi to pulmonary arteries, 167, 178
   commissures, 165, 178
   complication of, 154, 173
   double aortic arch with dominant left arch, 170, 180
   erosion of device, 154, 173
   Kawasaki disease, 172, 180
   lack of adequate rims, 154, 173
   left atrium, shortness of breath, 158, 175
   levotransposition of the great arteries (L-TGA), 161, 176
   membranous, 155, 174
   membranous ventricular septal defect with Eisenmenger syndrome, 157, 174-175
   multiple aortopulmonary collateral arteries (MAPCAs), 171, 180
   muscular ventricular septal defects (VSD), 155, 174
   Mustard/Senning procedure, 162, 176-177
   parachute mitral valve, 163, 177
   polysplenia, 160, 176
   prepulmonic course, 164, 177
   primum atrial septal defect, 166, 178
   pulmonary artery stent, 159, 176
   pulmonary atresia with ventricular septal defect (PA-VSD), 171, 180
   pulmonary vein, 158, 175
   retroaortic left circumflex artery, 161, 176
   right ventricle, rupture of, 170, 180
   Ross procedure, 164, 177
   sail-like anterior leaflet, 166, 178
   Shone complex/syndrome, 163, 177
   shunt, 159, 175
      type of, 164, 178
   sinus venosus atrial septal defect (ASD), 154, 173
   situs ambiguous, 164, 177
   Snowman sign, 167, 168, 179
   stress test, 168, 179
   tricuspid valvular abnormality, 166, 178
   truncus arteriosus, 163, 177
   unroofed coronary sinus, 155, 173, 174
Constrictive pericarditis (CP), 68, 82-83
Contrast flow rate, 4, 9
Coronary arteries, 3, 9, 16, 21, 27, 30, 37, 38, 45-46, 46
   atherosclerotic plaque, 52, 61
   bypass grafts, 51, 61
   right, 16, 27, 30, 38, 46
Coronary CTA, atypical chest pain, 59, 65
Coronary sinus, 13, 25
Coronary venogram, 37, 45

Crista terminalis, 13, 25
CT. *See also* Cardiac CTA (CCTA)
   filtered-back projection (FBP), 1, 7
   scanner, 2, 8

D
Danon disease, 78, 94-95
Devices and postoperative appearance
   aortic dissection, 201, 209-210
   artificial heart, 202, 211
   atrial septal occluder, 204, 213
   brain MRI, 205, 214
   cardiac MRI, 200, 209
   implantable cardioverter-defibrillators (ICDs), 201, 203, 210-211, 213
   intra-aortic balloon pumps (IABP), 201, 209-210
   left ventricular assist devices (LVADs)
      infection, 202, 211-212
      mediastinal hemorrhage, 206, 214-215
      thrombosis, 203, 212
   loop recorder, 200, 209
   mediastinal hemorrhage, 206, 214-215
   mitral clip, 208, 215
   postpacemaker chest radiographs, 206, 215
   reimplanted left main coronary artery, 207, 215
   right ventricular lead, 204, 213-214
   stuck leaflet, 207, 215
   total artificial heart (TAH), 211
   Twiddler syndrome, 205, 214
   wearable cardioverter-defibrillator (WCD), 209, 215-216
Diastolic dysfunction, left ventricular filling rate, 40, 48
Dilated cardiomyopathies (DCM), 48
   idiopathic, 74, 88-89
Dominance, codominant anatomy, 12, 24
Dose length product (DLP), 2, 7
Double-inversion recovery sequence, 1, 7
Dual antiplatelet therapy, 57, 64
Dyssynchronous RV wall motion, 67, 81

E
Effective dose, 2, 7
Effective tube current-time product, 1, 7
Ehlers-Danlos syndrome, 184, 195
Eisenmenger syndrome, 157, 174-175
End ventricular systole, 35, 44
Epicardial fat necrosis, acute chest pain, 145, 152
Etrospective cardiac CTA, 3, 8

F
False lumen, 192, 199
FDG-PET images, cardiomyopathy, 78, 95
Filtered-back projection (FBP), 1, 7
   reconstruction algorithm/kernel, 1, 7
Four-chamber plane, 17, 28

G
Gadolinium
   intravascular injection-extracellular space, 4, 10
   paramagnetic properties, 5, 10
GFR, 6, 11

Graft patency rates, 51, 61
Granulocytic sarcoma, 75, 91

H
Heart rate, 39
Hemochromatosis, 70, 84
Hereditary hemorrhagic telangiectasia (HHT), 189, 197
Hyparterial, pulmonary artery to trachea, 13, 24
Hypertension, 184, 195
Hypertrophic cardiomyopathy (HCM), 68, 82
Hypertrophic obstructive cardiomyopathy (HOCM)
   left atrial pressure, 34, 43
   septal thickening, 34, 43
Hypotension, 39, 46

I
Image acquisition time, 6, 11
Implantable cardioverter-defibrillators (ICDs), 201, 203, 210-211, 213
Infective endocarditis, 67, 81-82
In-stent restenosis (ISR), 57, 64
Interatrial septum, 19, 29
Intra-aortic balloon pumps (IABP), 201, 209-210
Inversion time, 57, 63-64
Iodine flux, 4, 9
Ischemic heart disease
   acute coronary syndrome, 56, 63
   acute infarct, 60, 66
   adenosine stress perfusion, 59, 65
   beta blockers, 51, 61
   body mass index (BMI), 52, 62
   bypass grafting, 53, 62
   chest pain, 55, 63
   chest pain, noncardiac causes of, 54, 63
   dilated cardiomyopathy, 59, 65
   dual antiplatelet therapy, 57, 64
   LAD territory, 60, 66
   microvascular obstruction, 60, 66
   myocardial infarction, 53, 62
   occluded RCA stent, 57, 64
   patent LAD stent, 57, 64
   percutaneous coronary intervention (PCI), 59, 65
   persistent symptoms, with ECG stress test, 54, 62
   right coronary artery
      inferior wall, significant restriction of blood flow, 50, 61
      suboptimal image quality, 59, 65
Isovolumetric contraction, ventricles, 34, 43

K
Kawasaki disease, 172, 180

L
Left atrial appendage, 15, 26
Left circumflex, 12, 30
Left ventricle and parallel to mitral valve, 56, 63
Left ventricular assist devices (LVADs)
   infection, 202, 211-212
   mediastinal hemorrhage, 206, 214-215
   thrombosis, 203, 212
Left ventricular outflow tract, 33, 42-43
Left ventricular systolic ejection fraction, 33, 42

L

Levotransposition of the great arteries (L-TGA), 161, 176
Ligament of Marshall, 22, 30
Loeffler endocarditis, 72, 86–87
Loeys-Dietz syndrome (LDS), 127, 135
Longitudinal magnetization (LM), 5, 10

M

Marfan syndrome, 125, 134, 181, 186, 191, 194, 196, 198
Mediastinal hemorrhage, 206, 214–215
Megacolon, 77, 93
Membranous septum, anatomic structure, 21, 29–30
Metoprolol, 34, 43
Microvascular obstruction, 60, 66
Middle cardiac vein, anatomic structure, 20, 29
Mitral regurgitation, 58, 64
Mitral stenosis
    hemodynamic effects, 124, 133
    pathologic features, 124, 133
Mitral valve prolapse (MVP), 181, 194
    diagnostic criteria, 121, 130
    end diastole (left) and end-systolic images (right), 124, 132
    Marfan syndrome, 125, 134
Mitral valves, 12, 18, 24, 28
    left ventricle and parallel to, 56, 63
MRI. See also Cardiac MRI (CMRI)
    adenosine stress perfusion, 59, 65
MR sequence, spatial modulation of magnetization (SPAMM) tagging, 76, 92
Multiple aortopulmonary collateral arteries (MAPCAs), 171, 180
Mustard/Senning procedure, 162, 176–177
Mycotic aneurysm, 182, 194
Myocardial infarction, 53, 55, 58, 62, 63, 64
Myocardial mass, 40, 47–48
Myocardial nulling, 57, 63–64
Myocardial scar formation, 3, 9
Myocarditis, 69, 74, 83–84, 89

N

Nephrogenic systemic fibrosis (NSF), 4, 9
Nonischemic dilated cardiomyopathy, 73, 87

O

Obtuse marginal, anatomic structure, 21, 30

P

Papillary muscle infarction, 55, 63
Parachute mitral valve, 163, 177
Parallel imaging techniques reduce scan time, 5, 10
Penetrating aortic ulcer (PAU), 196
Percutaneous coronary intervention (PCI), 59, 65
Pericardial disease
    calcifications, 138, 147
    calcific pericarditis, 139, 147
    cardiac MRI
        fat fluid interface, chemical shift artifact, 137, 147
        cardiac tamponade, physiologic findings of, 142, 149
    constrictive pericarditis, 142, 150
    CT, 144, 151
    decreased right ventricular volume, 139, 148
    EKG changes, 142, 150
    epicardial and pericardial fat, separation of, 139, 148
    epicardial fat deposition, cardiovascular disease, 144, 151
    epicardial fat necrosis, 145, 152
    hemopericardium, 143, 150
    lymphangitic extension, 143, 150
    malignant cytology, 144, 151
    malignant pericardial effusion, 140, 148
    metastatic disease, 144, 150
    pericardectomy, 141, 148–149
    pericardial effusion, 137, 147
    pericardial fluid volume, 144, 151
    pericardial lipoma, 138, 147
    pericardial thickness, 145, 151
    pericardial window, 142, 150
    physiologic and morphologic changes, 139, 148
    pneumopericardium, 142, 149
    restrictive cardiomyopathy, 142, 150
    right cardiophrenic angle, mass, 140, 148
    septations, pericardial cyst, 146, 152
    with thickened pericardium and late gadolinium enhancement, 141, 149
    ventricular interdependence, 141, 149
Pericardium, anatomic structure, 20, 29
Peripartum/postpartum cardiomyopathy (PPCM), 77, 94
Phase-contrast images, 2, 8
Phase-encoding steps, 6, 11
Polysplenia, 160, 176
Posteromedial papillary muscle, 16, 27
Pre- and early postgadolinium enhancement, 74, 89–90
Premature ventricular complexes (PVCs), 76, 92
Prepulmonic course, 164, 177
Primum atrial septal defect, 166, 178
Pulmonary artery stent, 159, 176
Pulmonary atresia with ventricular septal defect (PA-VSD), 171, 180
Pulmonary valve, 13, 24
Pulmonary vein, 14, 24, 158, 175
Pulmonary venous anatomy, 189, 198
Pulmonary venous wedge pressure, 41, 48

R

Radiograph, aortic valve, 14, 26
Reduce radiation dose, cardiac CTA (CCTA), 32, 42
Renal insufficiency, 6, 11
Retroaortic left circumflex artery, 161, 176
Right atrial appendage, 17, 28
Right coronary artery, 16, 27, 30, 38, 46
Right superior pulmonary vein (RSPV), 158, 175
Ross procedure, 164, 177

S

Severe aortic stenosis, 71, 85
Shone complex/syndrome, 163, 177
Short tau inversion recovery (STIR), 104, 116
Sildenafil, 39, 50, 61
Sinoatrial node, 5, 17, 40, 47–48
Sinus venosus atrial septal defect, 154, 173
Skin thickening of extremities, nephrogenic systemic fibrosis (NSF), 4, 9
SL-NTG. See Sublingual nitroglycerin (SL-NTG)
Snowman sign, 167, 168, 179
Specific absorption rate (SAR), 4, 10
Stanford classification
    type A, 192, 199
    type B, 184, 195
Staphylococcus infection, 67, 81–82
Stress-induced cardiomyopathy, 70, 85–86
Stress test, 168, 179
Subaortic membrane, 40, 47
Sublingual nitroglycerin (SL-NTG), 38, 46, 50, 61

T

Takayasu arteritis, 191, 198
TAVR. See Transaortic valve replacement (TAVR)
Territories, 37, 38, 45–46
Thebesian valve, 13, 25
Thoracic aorta and great vessels
    annuloaortic ectasia, 184, 195
    aortic dissection, 184, 195
    aortic regurgitation, 185, 196
    aortic wall, 185, 196
    arch abnormality, 192, 198
    arteriovenous malformation, 189, 197
    ascending aorta, noncontrast image, 184, 195
    asymptomatic, 186, 196
    atherosclerosis, 181, 194
    axial images, 192, 198
    complex malformation, 189, 197
    Ehlers-Danlos syndrome, 184, 195
    false lumen, 192, 199
    gated CTA chest, 183, 195
    hereditary hemorrhagic telangiectasia (HHT), 189, 197
    hypertension, 184, 195
    intimal flap, 182, 194
    lumen being wrapped by another lumen, 192, 199
    luminal thrombus, 186, 196
    Marfan syndrome, 181, 186, 191, 194, 196, 198
    mitral valve prolapse, 181, 194
    mycotic aneurysm, 182, 194
    noncontrast images, 183, 195
    pulmonary AVMs, 189, 197
    pulmonary embolism, 187, 197
    pulmonary hypertension, due to left to right shunting, 188, 197
    pulmonary vein stenosis, 190, 198
    pulmonary venous anatomy, 189, 198
    Stanford classification
        type A, 192, 199
        type B, 184, 195
    stent, 188, 190, 197, 198
    Takayasu arteritis, 191, 198
    traumatic pseudoaneurysm *vs.* ductus diverticulum, 182, 194
    Westermark sign, 187, 196

TM. *See* Transverse magnetization (TM)
Total artificial heart (TAH), 211
Transaortic valve replacement (TAVR), 14, 26
Transient interruption, 4, 10
Transverse magnetization (TM), 5, 10
Tricuspid and mitral valves, 12, 24
Tricuspid aortic valve, 35, 44
Tricuspid valvular abnormality, 166, 178
Twiddler syndrome, 205, 214

U
Unroofed coronary sinus, 155, 173, 174

V
Valvular disease
    annular dilation, 121, 130
    annuloaortic ectasia, 126, 127, 135
    aortic peak velocity, 127, 136
    atrioventricular valves, 125, 134
    Bernoulli equation, 120, 129
    bicuspid aortic valve, 125, 134
    bicuspid valve, 124, 132
    carcinoid heart disease, 127, 135-136
    cardiac arrhythmias, 121, 131
    cardiac MR, 124, 133-134
    congenital stenosis, 121, 130
    flail leaflet, 123, 131-132
    infarcted papillary muscle with rupture, 120, 129
    infective endocarditis (IE), complications of, 121, 131
    Loeys-Dietz syndrome (LDS), 127, 135
    mitral stenosis, 124, 133
    mitral valve prolapse (MVP), 121, 124, 125, 130, 132, 134
    papillary fibroelastoma, 122, 131
    paravalvular abscess, 126, 134
    pulmonary valve stenosis, 120, 129
    pulmonary venous waveforms, 122, 131
    rheumatic disease, aortic stenosis, 121, 130
    rheumatic heart disease, 120, 129-130
    rheumatic mitral valve disease, 123, 132
    subvalvular aortic stenosis, 128, 136
    systolic measured area, aortic valve, 120, 129
    transcatheter aortic valve implantation (TAVI), 124, 127, 133, 136
    tricuspid valve leaflets, 127, 135-136
Vascular territory, 37, 38, 46
Ventricles
    atrial systole, 34, 43
    isovolumetric contraction, 34, 43
Ventricular diastole, end-diastolic volume, 35, 44
Ventricular noncompaction, 74, 90
Ventricular preload, 34, 43
Ventricular septal defects (VSD), 155, 174
Voxel value, 3, 9

W
Wall motion abnormalities, 33, 42
Wearable cardioverter-defibrillator (WCD), 209, 215-216
Westermark sign, 187, 196
Wrap around left anterior descending coronary artery, 39, 47